PHYSEO

AF882111

TABLE OF CONTENTS

We would like to extend a special thanks to the following individuals who have spent countless hours and support to make Physeo possible.

Mark Bromberg, MD, PhD
Professor of Neurology
Diagnostic and Clinical Neurology Division Chief
Neuromuscular Medicine Division Interim Chief
University of Utah

Ashleigh Bull
MD Candidate, Class of 2021
University of Utah School of Medicine

Bruce L Horowitz, MD, FASN
Clinical Professor of Medicine
Division of Nephrology & Hypertension
University of Utah School of Medicine

Cara Heuser, MD MS
Assistant Professor, Maternal-Fetal Medicine
Department of Obstetrics and Gynecology
University of Utah Health Sciences Center and
Intermountain Healthcare
Salt Lake City, Utah

David A. Hutcheson, PhD
Research Assistant Professor
Department of Neurobiology and Anatomy
University of Utah School of Medicine

Chizitam F. Ibezim
MD Candidate, Class of 2020
University of Missouri-Kansas City School of Medicine

Pamela S. Ropski
MD Candidate, Class of 2021
University of Utah School of Medicine

Kenneth W. Spitzer, Ph.D.
Professor, Internal Medicine (Cardiovascular Medicine)
Director, Nora Eccles Harrison Cardiovascular Research and
Training Institute
University of Utah School of Medicine
Salt Lake City, UT

Vishnu Sundaresh, MD, FACE
Assistant Professor
Division of Endocrinology, Metabolism, & Diabetes
University of Utah School of Medicine
Salt Lake City, UT

GENERAL PRINCIPLES

Section I - Cell Transport

I. Cell Membranes

A. Composed of phospholipids

B. One hydrophilic phosphate head (water soluble) with two hydrophobic fatty acid tails (lipid soluble)

C. Hydrophobic tails face each other and form a lipid bilayer

D. Lipid soluble (non-polar) substances can cross cell membrane easily (simple diffusion) (Figure 1.1)

1. Steroids
2. Lipids
3. O_2, CO_2, and N_2
4. Numerous drugs and anesthetic gases

E. Water-soluble substances are repelled by the lipid bilayer (Figure 1.2).

1. Charged molecules (H_2O, Na^+, Cl^-, K^+, glucose)
2. Large particles (proteins)

II. Simple Diffusion (Figure 1.1)

A. No carrier/protein transporter

B. No energy required (passive)

C. Follows gradient

1. Driven by transmembrane concentration gradient (substances diffuse down their concentration gradient)

III. Carrier-Mediated Transport

A. Has carrier/protein transporter

B. Conducted via protein

1. Can be saturated → can reach a transport maximum (Tm)
2. Can experience competition

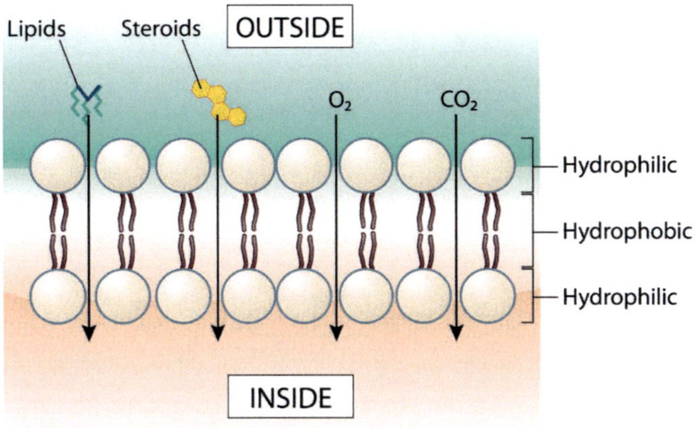

Figure 1.1 - Simple diffusion

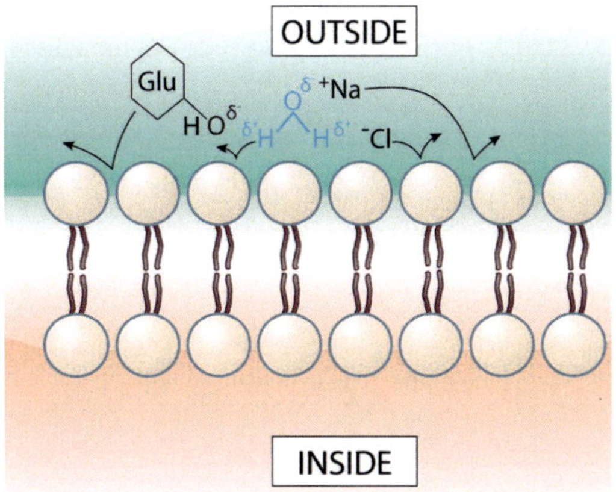

Figure 1.2 - Large and charged substances

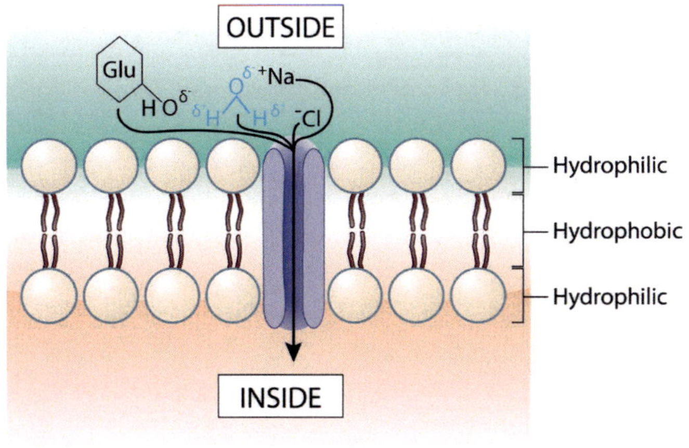

Figure 1.3 - Facilitated Diffusion

C. Types include:
  1. Facilitated diffusion
  2. Primary active transport
  3. Secondary active transport

IV. Facilitated Diffusion (Figure 1.3)

A. Has carrier/protein transporter

B. No energy required (passive)

C. Follows gradient
  1. Driven by transmembrane concentration gradient (substances diffuse down their concentration gradient)

D. Almost any substance that cannot enter via simple diffusion can use facilitated diffusion.

V. Primary Active Transport (Figure 1.4)

A. Has carrier/protein transporter

B. ATP energy required (active)
  1. Examples end with, "ATPase" (Na^+/K^+-ATPase, H^+-ATPase, and Ca^{2+}-ATPase)

C. Moves against gradient
  1. Transported substances move energetically uphill, against their electrochemical gradient.

VI. Secondary Active Transport (Figures 1.5 and 1.6)

A. Has carrier/protein transporter

B. ATP energy required (active)
  1. ATP required indirectly, only to keep intracellular NA^+ low via the Na-K pump

C. Moves against gradient but follows Na^+ gradient created by primary active transport

D. Can be symporters or antiporters
  1. Symporters include: Na^+-glucose cotransporter, Na^+-amino acid cotransporter
  2. Antiporters include: Na^+-Ca^{2+} exchange and Na^+-H^+ exchange

VII. Receptor-Mediated Endocytosis (Figure 1.7)

A. Proteins on ligand bind to proteins on cell surface → cell membrane forms coated vesicle that is then ingested.

B. High yield examples include:
  1. Iron in the serum (transferrin-iron complex stimulate endocytosis)
  2. LDL stimulates LDLR
  3. EGF stimulates EGFR

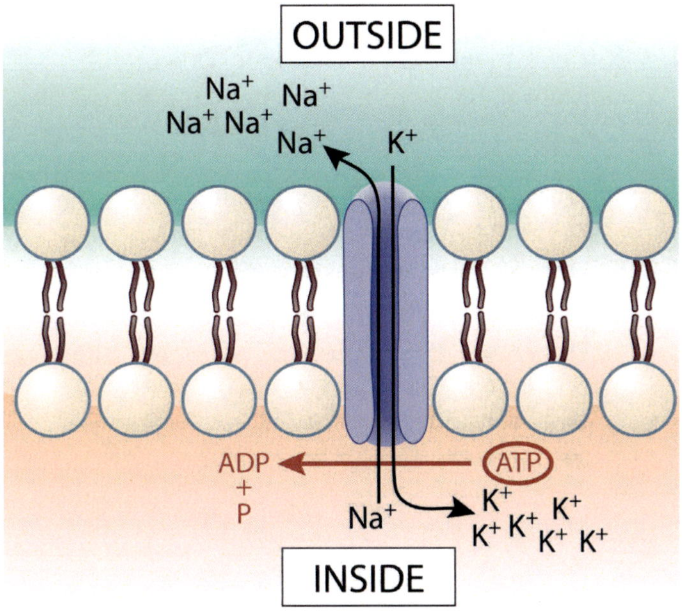

Figure 1.4 - Primary Active Transport

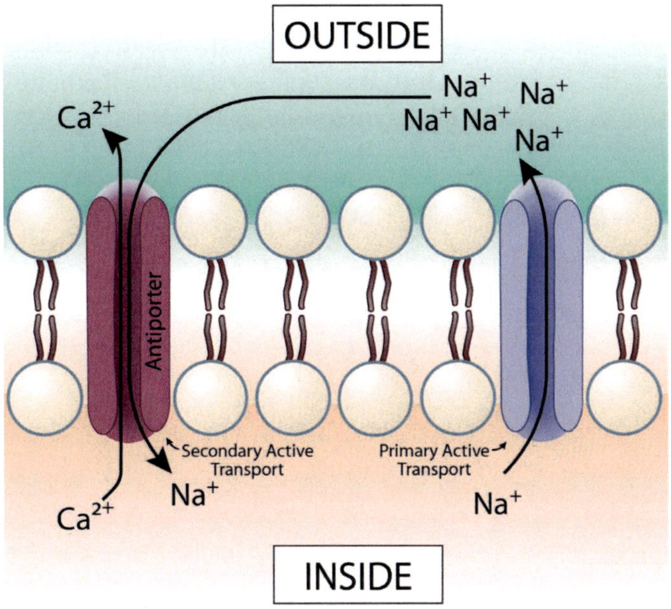

Figure 1.6 - Secondary Active Transport with Calcium

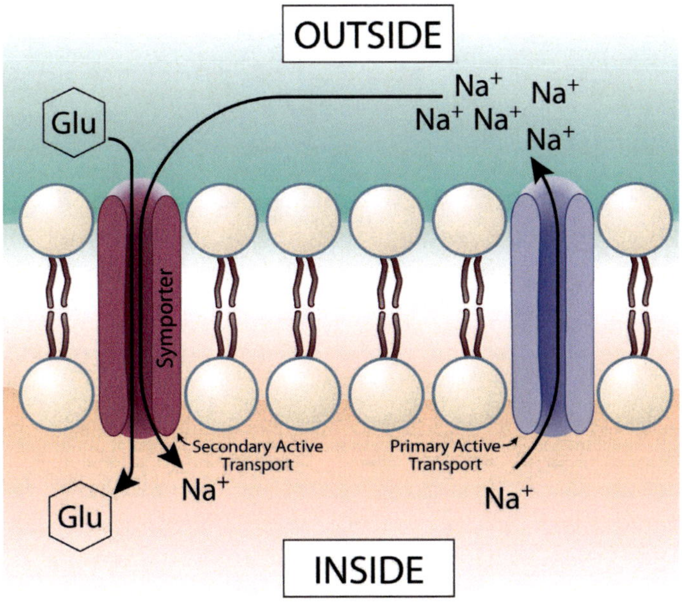

Figure 1.5 - Secondary Active Transport with Glucose

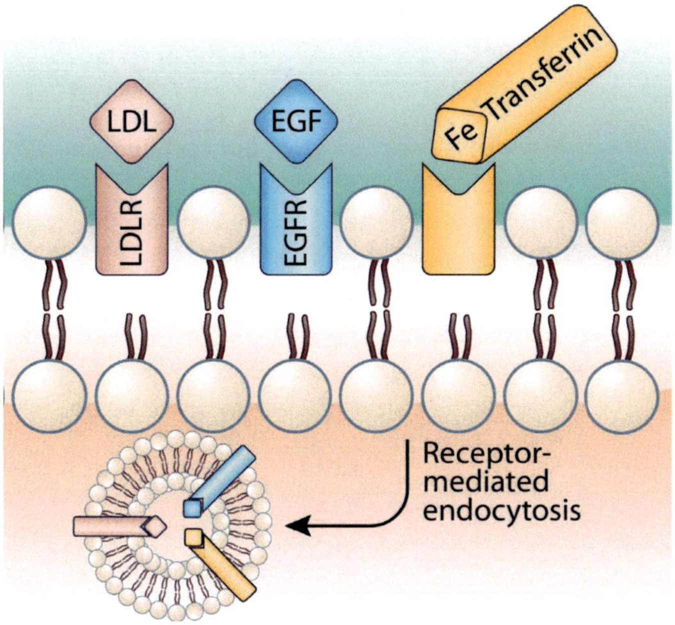

Figure 1.7 - Receptor-mediated Endocytosis

REVIEW QUESTIONS

1. Hemoglobin carries oxygen to the capillaries. How does oxygen leave the capillaries to enter the tissue?

   - **Oxygen can cross the membrane via simple diffusion due to concentration gradient**
   - **Oxygen is high in the capillaries and low in the cell, causing flow of oxygen from the blood into the tissues**
   - **CO_2 is high in the cell (waste product) and diffuses into the capillaries where it can be taken to the lungs and exhaled**

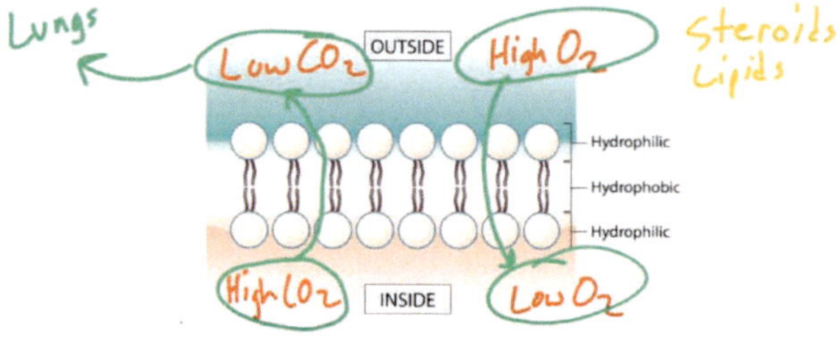

2. In an experimental setting, a cell does not have any protein transporters. The researcher notices that some substances can enter the cell and others cannot. Will glucose be able to enter the cell?

   - **Glucose is not small or lipid soluble**
   - **Glucose requires a protein transporter**

3. A researcher determines that glucose is high in the cell but is still brought into the cell against its concentration gradient. No ATP is used at the transporter glucose uses to enter the cell. What type of transport was used for this glucose?

   - **Glucose is not small or lipid soluble, so simple diffusion is not used**
   - **Facilitated diffusion always moves down a concentration gradient**
   - **Primary active transport requires direct action of ATP**
   - **Secondary active transport can move against a concentration gradient without the direct action of ATP**

4. Measurements are taken for transport of substance A and substance B across distinct and separate cell membranes. Throughout the experiment, both substances are kept low in their respective cells while concentration increases outside the cell. Transfer of substance A increases proportionally as the concentration gradient is increased. However, transfer of substance B does not increase even though its concentration gradient increased. One of the substances is a steroid hormone. Is the steroid likely to be substance A or B?

   - **Protein transporters can be saturated**
   - **The mechanism of transport of substance B was saturated → substance B must require a protein transporter**
   - **Substance A was not saturated → substance A must not require a protein transporter and diffuses freely across the membrane → substance A must be the steroid**

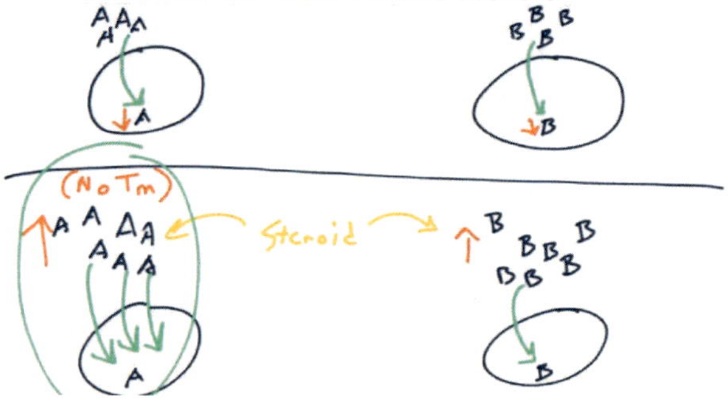

5. The LDLR is dysfunctional in a certain patient. What will happen to the intracellular level of LDL in the adipose tissue of this patient?

   - **Endocytosis of LDL requires LDLR function**
   - **Dysfunctional LDLR means decreased LDL in adipose, keeping it elevated in the serum**

Section II - Signaling Pathways

I. G-protein pathways

Table 1.1 - G-protein pathways

G-protein pathway	Receptor and ligand	Second messenger
G-protein (G_q-alpha subunit)	• H_1 (histamine) • α_1 (Epinephrine, norepinephrine) • V_1 (ADH) • M_1 (acetylcholine) • M_3 (acetylcholine) • GnRH, TRH, Oxytocin, Angiotensin II, Gastrin	↑ IP_3 ↑ DAG
G-protein (G_s-alpha subunit)	• D_1 (dopamine) • H_2 (histamine) • V_2 (ADH) • β_1 (Epinephrine, norepinephrine, Dobutamine, isoproterenol) • β_2 (Epinephrine, Albuterol, isoproterenol) • LH, FSH, CRH, ADH, ACTH, PTH, hCG, MSH, GHRH, Glucagon, Calcitonin	↑ cAMP
G-protein (G_i-alpha subunit)	• M_2 (acetylcholine) • α_2 (Epinephrine, norepinephrine) • D_2 (dopamine)	↓ cAMP

A. G_q-alpha subunit (Figure 1.8)

1. G_q → phospholipase C → cleaves phosphatidylinositol 4,5-bisphosphate (PIP_2) into inositol 1,4,5-trisphosphate (IP_3) and diacylglycerol (DAG)
2. IP_3 binds to the ER → Ca^{2+} release.
3. DAG and Ca^{2+} bind protein kinase C (PKC) which causes a cellular response

B. G_s-alpha subunit (Figure 1.9)

1. G_s → adenylate cyclase → ↑ cAMP → ↑ protein kinase A (PKA)

C. G_i-alpha subunit (Figure 1.9)

1. G_i, adenylate cyclase → ↓ cAMP → ↓ protein kinase A (PKA)

Figure 1.9 - G_s and G_i alpha subunit pathway

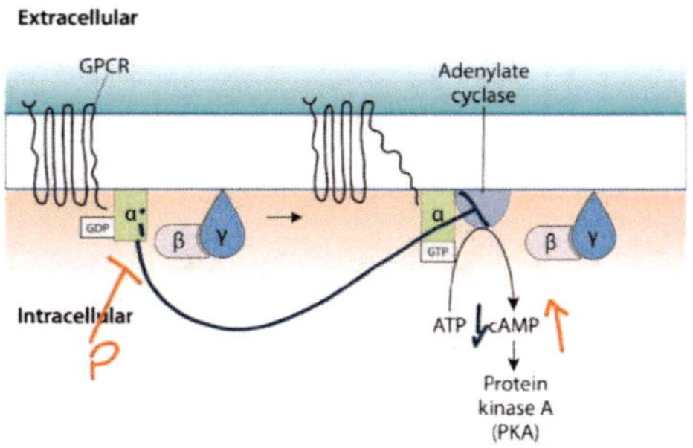

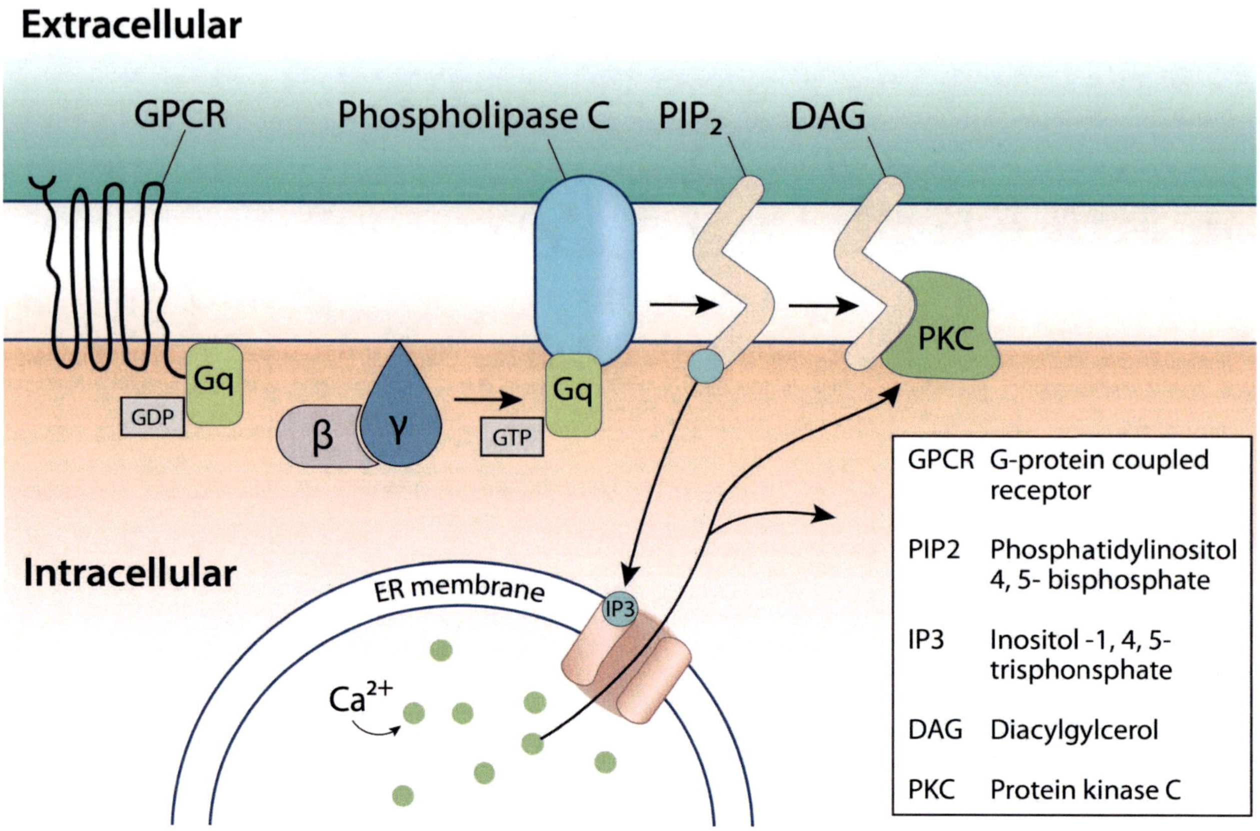

Figure 1.8 - G_q alpha subunit pathway

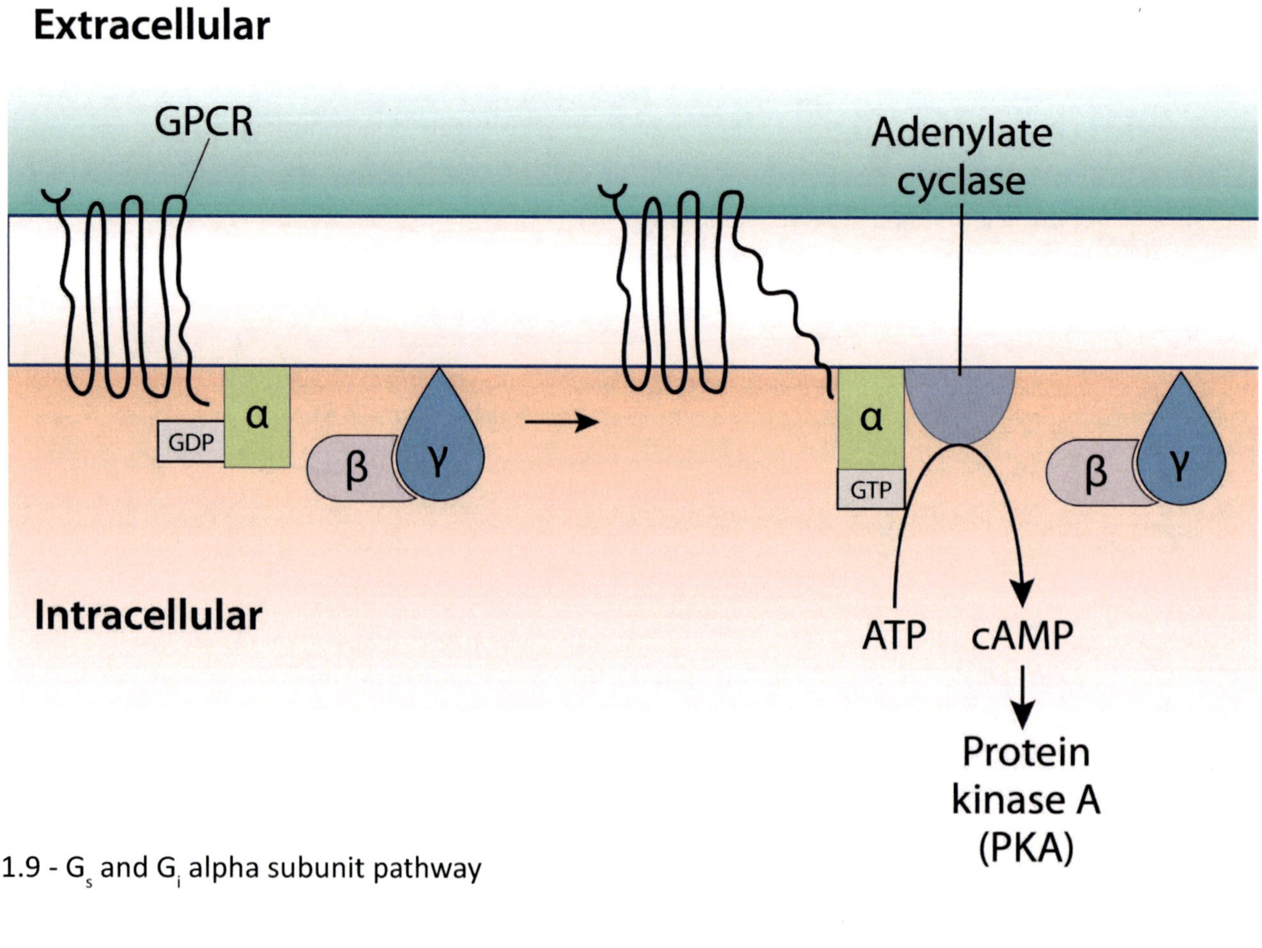

Figure 1.9 - G_s and G_i alpha subunit pathway

II. cGMP receptors (Figure 1.10)

A. Atrial natriuretic peptide (ANP), brain natriuretic peptide (BNP), nitric oxide (NO), and endothelial-derived relaxing factor (EDRF) are ligands that regulate the enzyme guanylate cyclase.

B. Guanylate cyclase → GTP → cGMP → protein kinase G (PKG) → vascular smooth muscle relaxation

III. Steroid hormone receptors

A. Androgens, estrogens, glucocorticoids, mineralocorticoids, progesterone, thyroid hormones, and fat-soluble vitamins are steroid or steroid-like ligands.

B. These ligands bind to an intracellular receptor or a nuclear receptor which ultimately regulate transcription.

IV. Receptor tyrosine kinases (RTK) (Figure 1.11)

A. Insulin, insulin-like growth factor-1 (IGF-1), epidermal growth factor (EGF), platelet-derived growth factor (PDGF), and fibroblast growth factor (FGF) are receptor tyrosine kinase ligands.

B. Receptor tyrosine kinases regulate the RAS/MAP kinase pathway.

Figure 1.11 - Receptor tyrosine kinase (RTK)

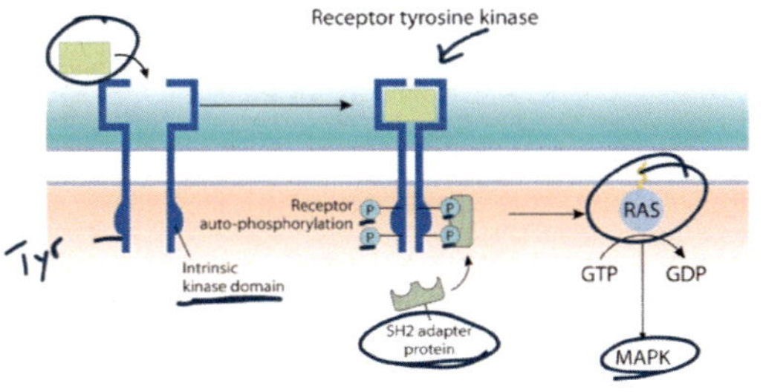

V. Non-receptor tyrosine kinases (Figure 1.12)

A. Immunomodulators (IL-2 and IL-6), prolactin, thrombopoietin, erythropoietin, growth hormone (GH), and granulocyte colony stimulating factor (G-CSF) are non-receptor tyrosine kinase ligands.

B. Non-receptor tyrosine kinases regulate the JAK/STAT pathway.

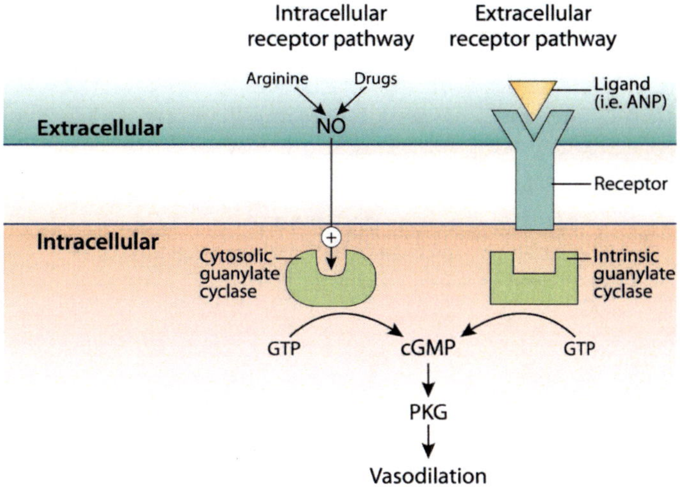

Figure 1.10 - cGMP pathway

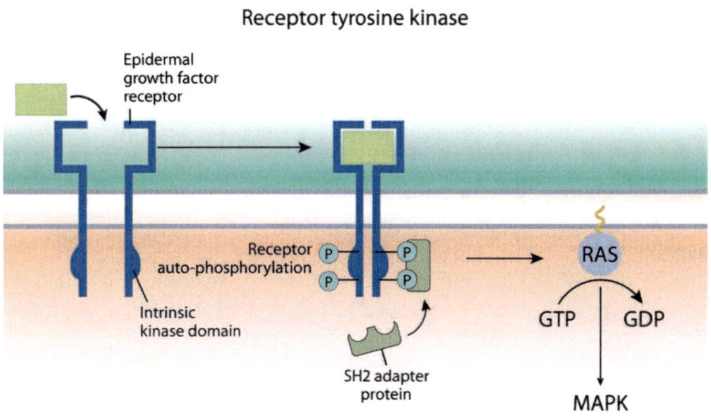

Figure 1.11 - Receptor tyrosine kinase (RTK)

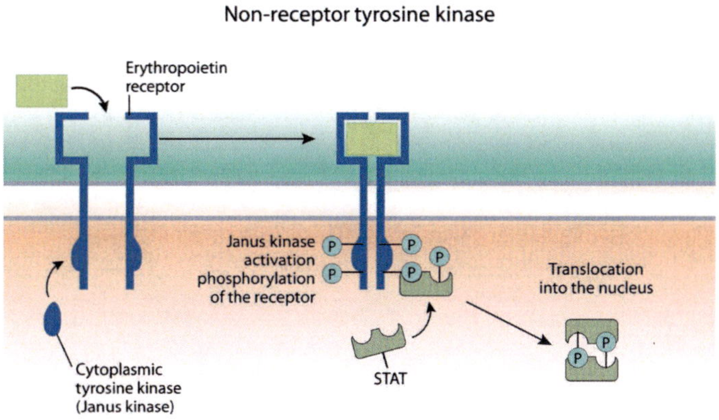

Figure 1.12 - Non-receptor tyrosine kinase

REVIEW QUESTIONS

1. A 2-year-old girl presents with a 5 week history of intense coughing. The physician notices a deep cough on expiration. How will the patient's intracellular signaling most likely be altered as a result of the underlying abnormality?

    - **The Gi alpha subunit pathway normally inhibits cAMP**
    - **Pertussis inhibits the Gi subunit activity → ↑cAMP**

2. A 16-year-old male presents to the ED after abusing his sister's insulin. The physician administers a load of glucose and then injects a drug that normally causes increased gluconeogenesis. This likely drug acts on what second messenger pathway?

    - **Glucagon stimulates Gs subunit activity → ↑cAMP**

3. A 55-year-old male with a 6 month history of stable angina has been prescribed a drug that can relieve acute episodes of chest pain by altering a second messenger pathway. What drug has been prescribed and what is the MOA?

    - **Nitroglycerin converts to nitric oxide (NO) in the body**
    - **NO increases cGMP**
    - **cGMP leads to vasodilation and decreased preload and stress on the heart**

4. A 32-year-old male returned from Africa 2 days ago and presents with complaints of watery diarrhea. Stool examination reveals gram negative organisms that are flagellated and grow in an alkaline environment. What signaling pathway is likely disrupted resulting in the watery diarrhea?

    - **Vibrio cholerae overstimulates Gs subunit pathway**
    - **Gs subunit activity increases cAMP, leading to chloride and water secretion into gut lumen (watery diarrhea)**

5. A 68-year-old female presents with a 2 week history of intense itching and burning after her weekly routine of exercising at the pool and sitting in the hot tub. What intracellular signaling pathway is abnormally activated?

    - **Polycythemia Vera (high Hb)**
    - **A JAK2 mutation leads to increased STAT pathway activity, causing increased Hb**

6. A 19-year-old male is taking anabolic steroids for muscle growth. Where within the cell does this drug likely act?

    - **Steroids act on intracellular receptors to alter gene transcription within the nucleus**

Section III - Sympathetic and Parasympathetic Signaling

I. Autonomic Receptors (Figure 1.13)

A. Sympathetic receptors

Table 1.2 - Sympathetic receptors

Receptor	Actions
α_1	Mydriasis Vasoconstriction (↑ BP, ↑ VR to heart) Gastrin
α_2	↓ NE release (negative feedback) ↓ Aqueous humor production (↓ IOP)
β_1	↑ HR ↑ Contractility ↑ Renin (RAAS) (↑ BP)
β_2	Vasodilation (skeletal muscles) Bronchodilation ↑ Aqueous humor production (↑ IOP)
M_3	Sweating

1. α_1, α_2, β_1, β_2
2. Norepinephrine is the primary sympathetic neurotransmitter.
3. Epinephrine is released from adrenal medulla and can stimulate β2 receptors.

B. Norepinephrine and Epinephrine overview (Figure 1.14)

1. Direct sympathetic agonists will directly stimulate the sympathetic receptors.
2. Indirect sympathetic agonists can increase a sympathetic response by:

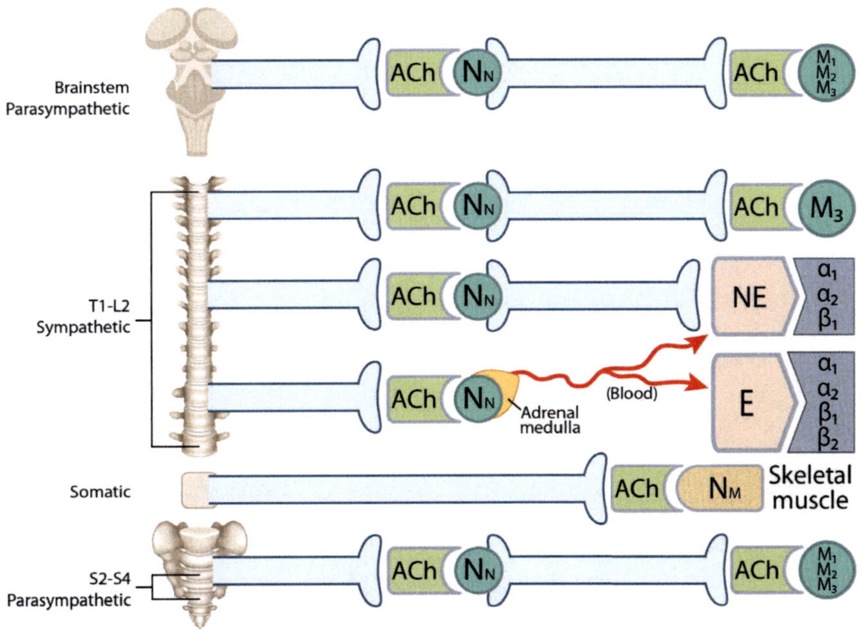

Figure 1.13 - Autonomics Overview

a) Blocking the reuptake of norepinephrine at the presynaptic neuron

b) Stimulating release of norepinephrine from the presynaptic neuron

c) Stimulating release of norepinephrine and epinephrine from the adrenal medulla

3. Sympathetic blockers can block the α_1, α_2, β_1, or β_2 receptors (e.g. α or β blockers)

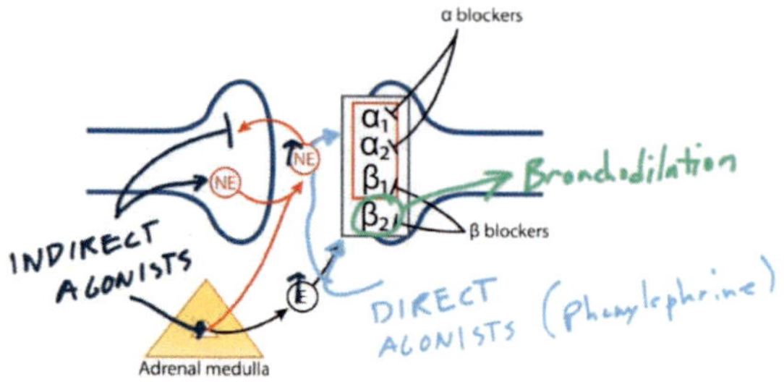

4. M_1, M_2, M_3

5. Acetylcholine is the parasympathetic neurotransmitter.

Table 1.3 - Parasympathetic receptors

Receptor	Actions
M_1	CNS
M_2	↓ HR ↓ Contractility
M_3	Miosis Lens accommodation ↑ Lacrimation Bronchoconstriction ↑ Gastric acid secretion ↑ Salivation ↑ Peristalsis

C. Acetylcholine Overview (Figure 1.15)

1. Acetylcholine (ACh) is released from presynaptic neuron and can stimulate muscarinic receptors or nicotinic receptors in the skeletal muscle (N_M).

2. Can be emulated by ACh agonists (bethanechol, carbachol, methacholine, and pilocarpine)

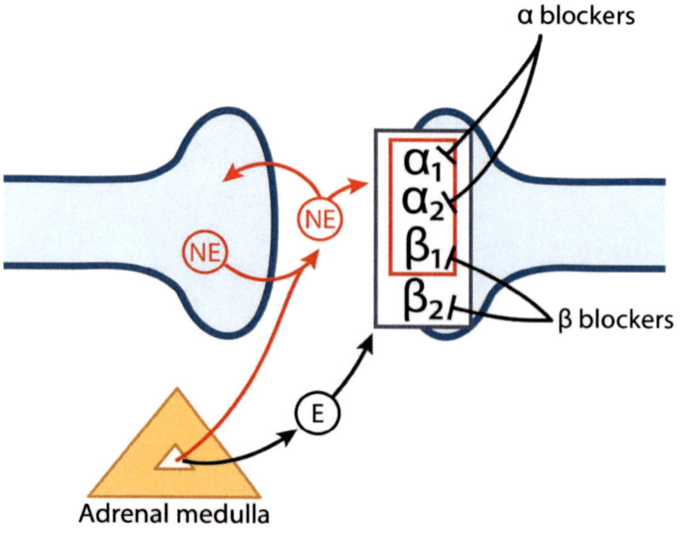

Figure 1.14 - Norepinephrine and Epinephrine Overview

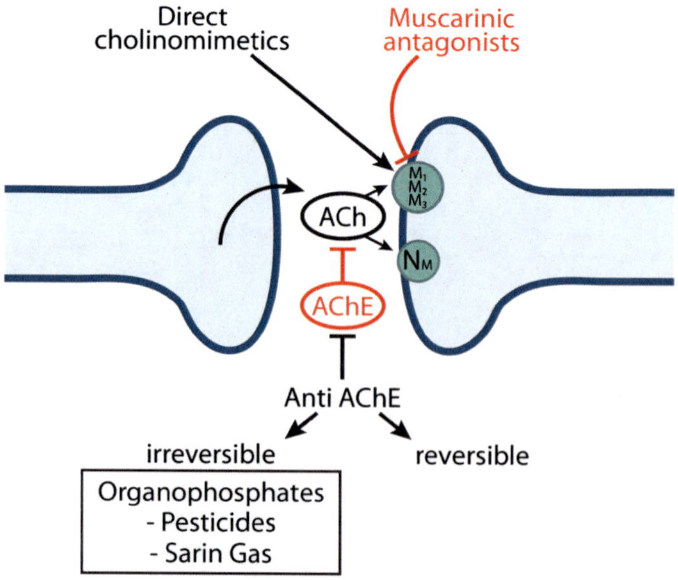

Figure 1.15 - Acetylcholine Overview

3. ACh is broken down by acetylcholinesterase (AChE) → modulates effect of ACh.
   a) Anticholinesterases breakdown AChE → decreased breakdown of ACh → increased ACh → increased muscarinic or nicotinic effect

II. Muscarinic Antagonists

A. Example drugs: Ipratropium, atropine.

B. Function to block M_1, M_2, and M_3 receptors

C. Inhibition of M_1 can lead to disorientation.

D. Inhibition of M_2 can lead to a relative increase in HR and contractility.

E. Inhibition of M_3 can lead to constipation, urinary retention, red and warm skin and blurry vision.

F. Popular mnemonic: Hot as a hare. Dry as a bone. Red as a beat. Blind as a bat. Mad as a hatter.

III. H_1 Receptor Functions

A. Increased mucus production in airways and nasal passages

B. Antihistamines decrease rhinorrhea in colds

C. Bronchoconstriction and vasodilation

D. Histamine released from mast cells during allergic reaction causes difficulty breathing (bronchoconstriction) and edema (vasodilation).

IV. H_2 Receptor Functions

A. Increased HCl secretion from gastric parietal cells

B. H_2 blockers decrease acid production (helpful in GERD).

V. V_1 Receptor Functions

A. Vasoconstriction

B. Vasopressin can be administered to cause vasoconstriction to increase blood pressure or to decrease variceal bleeding.

VI. V_2 Receptor Functions

A. Increased aquaporins in collecting tubule → increased H_2O reabsorption from kidneys

B. ADH (aka vasopressin) can act on both receptors.

REVIEW QUESTIONS

?

1. Would an indirect agonist, that functions only by blocking the reuptake of NE back into the presynaptic neuron, be able to cause the intended bronchodilation in a patient experiencing anaphylaxis

   - **β_2 receptors cause bronchodilation**
   - **NE does not stimulate β_2 receptors**

2. A patient is exposed to a chemical which leads to increased sweating, diarrhea, and a dangerously low heart rate. What single neurotransmitter, in excess, could lead to all of the symptoms demonstrated in this patient?

   - **M_3 receptor stimulation increases sweating and peristalsis**
   - **M_2 receptor stimulation decreases heart rate**
   - **ACh stimulates M_2 and M_3 receptors**

3. The previous patient is treated with atropine to diminish the symptoms of organophosphate poisoning. However, the atropine is continued for longer than necessary and at a much higher dose than necessary. What symptoms could he develop?

   - **Atropine blocks M receptors**
   - **Inhibition of M_1 can lead to disorientation**
   - **Inhibition of M_2 can lead to a relative increase in HR and contractility**
   - **Inhibition of M_3 can lead to constipation, urinary retention, red and warm skin and blurry vision**

4. A 6-year-old boy with a severe peanut allergy is exposed to peanuts. He begins to have difficulty breathing and demonstrates widespread edema. What receptor, if stimulated, can counteract his difficulty breathing?

   - **β_2 receptors cause bronchodilation and can be stimulated by epinephrine, improving breathing**
   - **M_3 receptors cause bronchoconstriction. This should not be stimulated in this patient**
   - **H_1 receptors cause bronchoconstriction and are stimulated during this allergic reaction**

5. Upon administration of epinephrine, the boy experiences a reduction in edema in addition to normalized breathing. Why is that?

   - **H_1 receptors cause vasodilation, leading to edema in this allergic reaction**
   - **α_1 receptors cause vasoconstriction Epinephrine stimulation of α_1 would reduce edema**

6. A patient is hypotensive and the physician would like to cause vasoconstriction to increase blood pressure. However, the physician would like to do this without increasing heart rate or contractility. What drug would be most appropriate out of the following: epinephrine, vasopressin, or a muscarinic antagonist?

   - **Epinephrine acts on α_1, α_2, β_1, and β_2. Stimulating only α_1 would increase blood pressure (α_1) but would also increase heart rate and contractility (β_1)**
   - **Muscarinic antagonists block M_1, M_2, and M_3 (parasympathetic) which would indirectly lead to an overall sympathetic response (α_1, α_2, β_1, and β_2 activity). Blood pressure would increase, but so would heart rate and contractility**
   - **Vasopressin can directly cause vasoconstriction without stimulating other adrenergic receptors (α_1, α_2, β_1, and β_2)**

Section IV - Gradients and Action Potentials

I. Gradients

A. Ion channels are integral membrane proteins that are selective for the passage of anions or cations.

1. Permeability of an ion channel is determined by the probability that the channel is open.
2. Voltage-gated channels are regulated by changes in membrane potential.
3. Ligand-gated channels are regulated by second messengers, hormones, or neurotransmitters.

B. Chemical gradient

1. The difference in ion concentration across a permeable membrane produces a driving force in which ions diffuse from the high concentration compartment to the low concentration compartment.
2. This force is sometimes also referred to as diffusion potential.
3. The chemical gradient, or potential, increases when the concentration gradient is large and decreases when the concentration gradient is small.

C. Electrical gradient

1. The difference in charge across a membrane produces a driving force in which ions are attracted or repelled depending on the size and sign of the gradient.

D. Equilibrium potential

1. The difference in electrical potential across a cell membrane that exactly balances the chemical, or concentration gradient.

E. Resting membrane potential

1. Measured as the potential difference (mV) across the cell membrane
2. The resting membrane potential is determined, in part, by multiple ions attempting to reach their individual equilibrium potentials.
3. The negative resting membrane potential is primarily a result of potassium leak channels.

II. Action potentials

A. Definitions

1. Current
   a) Inward current is the movement of positively charged molecules into the cell.
   b) Outward current is the movement of positively charged molecules out of the cell.
2. Depolarization is when the membrane potential becomes more positive.
3. Hyperpolarization is when the membrane potential becomes more negative.
4. Threshold is the membrane potential at which an action potential must occur.

B. Steps

1. Resting membrane potential
2. Depolarization and upstroke
3. Repolarization
4. Hyperpolarization

REVIEW QUESTIONS

1. $E_{Na} = (-65\ mV/z)\log_{10} [C_i]/[C_e]$; $C_i = 10$ mM; $C_e = 100$ mM; $E_{Na} = ?$

- **The above question represents the Nernst Equation**
- **The answer tells us how strong the electrical gradient must be to prevent additional ions from entering the cell (+65 mV)**

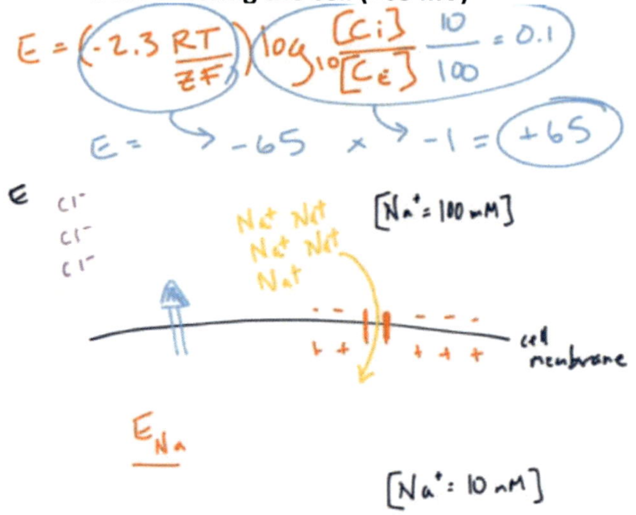

2. How would the administration of diazepam alter the resting membrane potential of neurons?

- **Benzodiazepines such as diazepam potentiate GABA-A → chloride influx**
- **Increased intracellular chloride results in hyperpolarization (the cell must now receive a greater stimulus in order to reach threshold)**

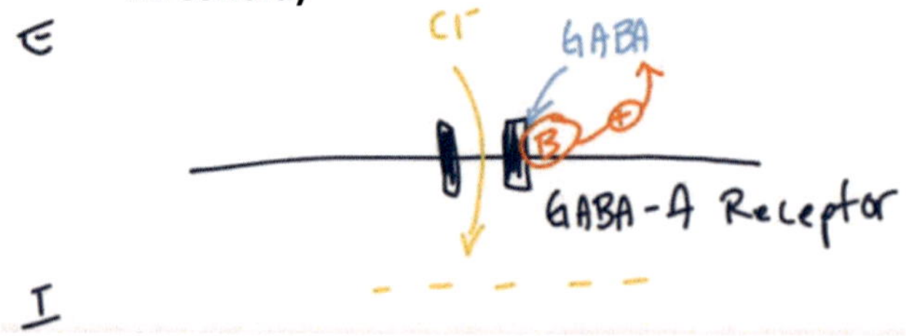

3. How would exposure to ciguatoxin alter the resting membrane potential?

- **Ciguatoxin promotes the influx of sodium into neurons → cellular depolarization**
- **The sodium gate remains open → no additional depolarization can occur → paralysis**

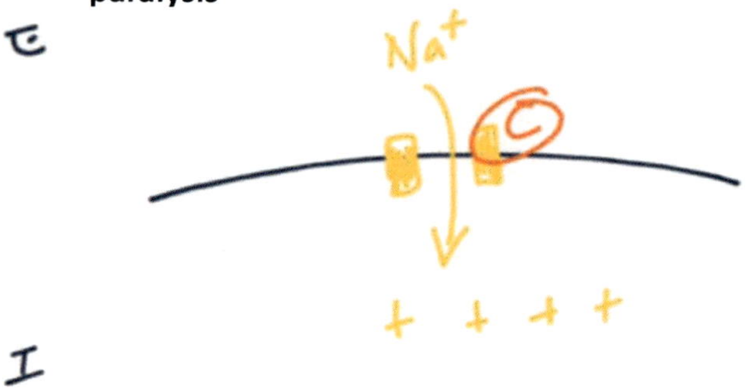

4. The nerve tissue of a mouse is found to have a resting membrane potential of -70 mV. The equilibrium potential (E) for sodium is +60 mV and is +125 mV for calcium. Where will these ions move after opening their associated channels?

- **Sodium and calcium are more concentrated in the extracellular space**
- **Sodium and calcium will move down their concentration gradients into the cell until the cell reaches +60 mv and +125 mv respectively**

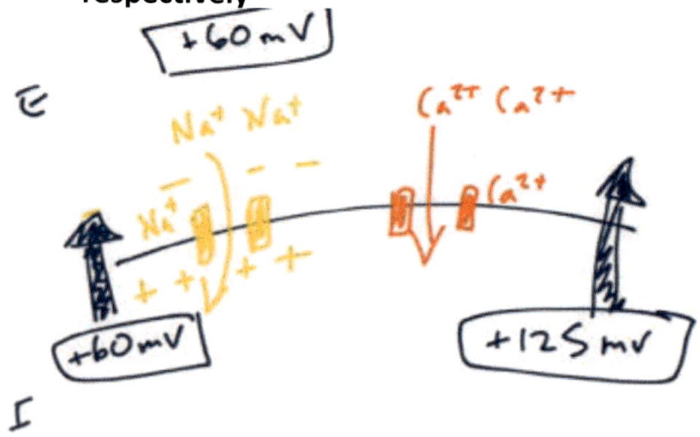

CARDIOLOGY

Section I - Introduction to Cardiology

I. Basic Principles

A. Figures 2.1 and 2.2 provide a basic overview of the anatomy of the heart.

B. Coronary circulation

1. Blood from the coronary sinus drains into the right atrium → right ventricle → pulmonary arteries → pulmonary veins → left atrium → left ventricle → aortic root → coronary arteries → coronary sinus.

2. Coronary Vessels

a) The coronary arteries provide oxygenated blood to the heart.

b) The left coronary artery (LCA) branches into the circumflex artery (LCX) and the left anterior descending artery (LAD).

c) The LCX supplies blood to the lateral and posterior walls of the left ventricle.

d) The PDA branches off of the LCX 10% of the time. These patients are considered to have a left-dominant circulation.

e) The LAD supplies blood to the anterior wall of the left ventricle and the anterior ⅔ of the interventricular septum.

f) The right coronary artery (RCA) branches into the right marginal artery

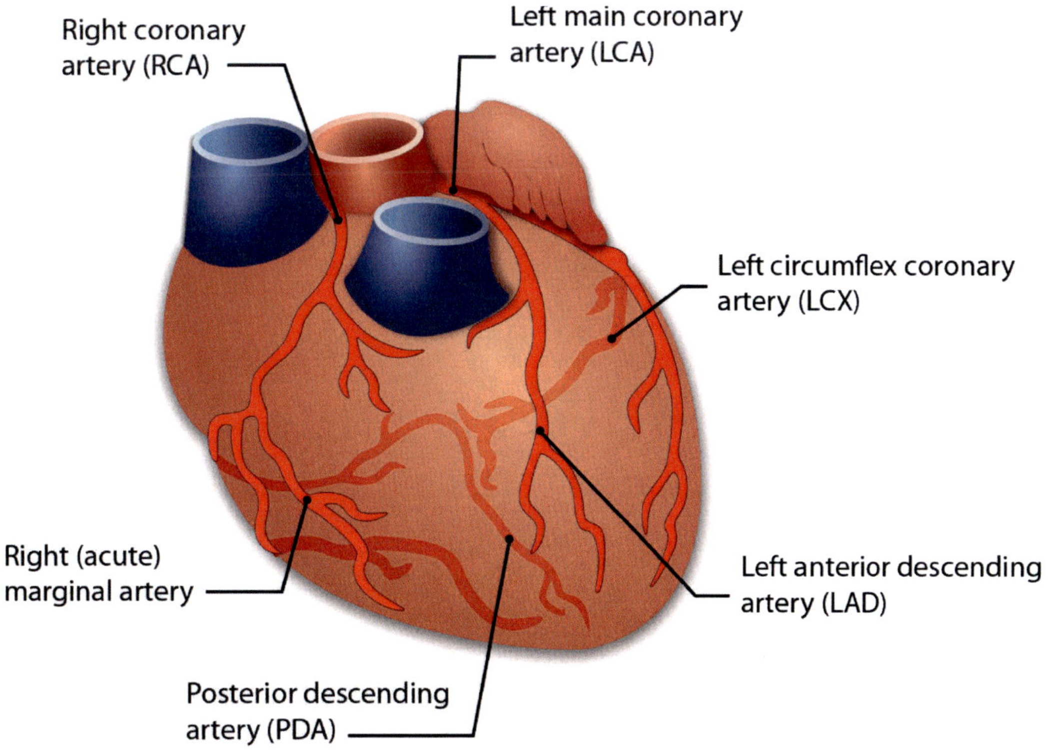

Figure 2.1 - Anterior view of the heart

and the posterior descending artery (PDA) 80% of the time.

(1) The right marginal artery supplies the right ventricle.

(2) Also supplies the papillary muscles of the right ventricle and the posterior wall of the heart.

(3) The RCA gives rise to the PDA in patients with right-dominant circulation.

C. Systemic and pulmonary circulation

1. Blood from the vena cava drains into the right atrium → right ventricle → pulmonary arteries → pulmonary veins → left atrium → left ventricle → aorta → systemic circulation (arteries, arterioles, capillaries, venules, veins) → vena cava.

2. Oxygen exchange between the blood and tissues occurs at the capillaries.

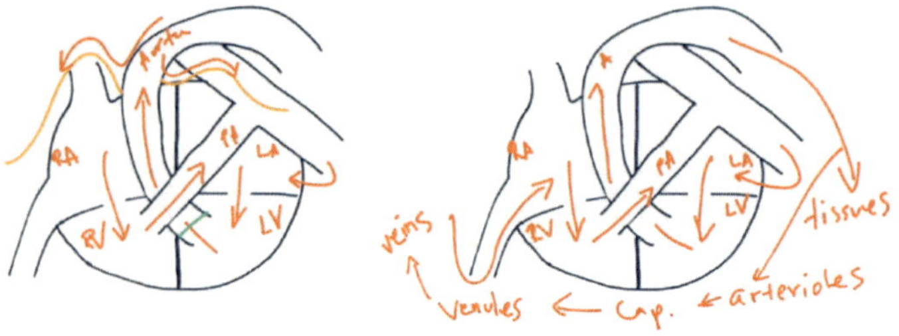

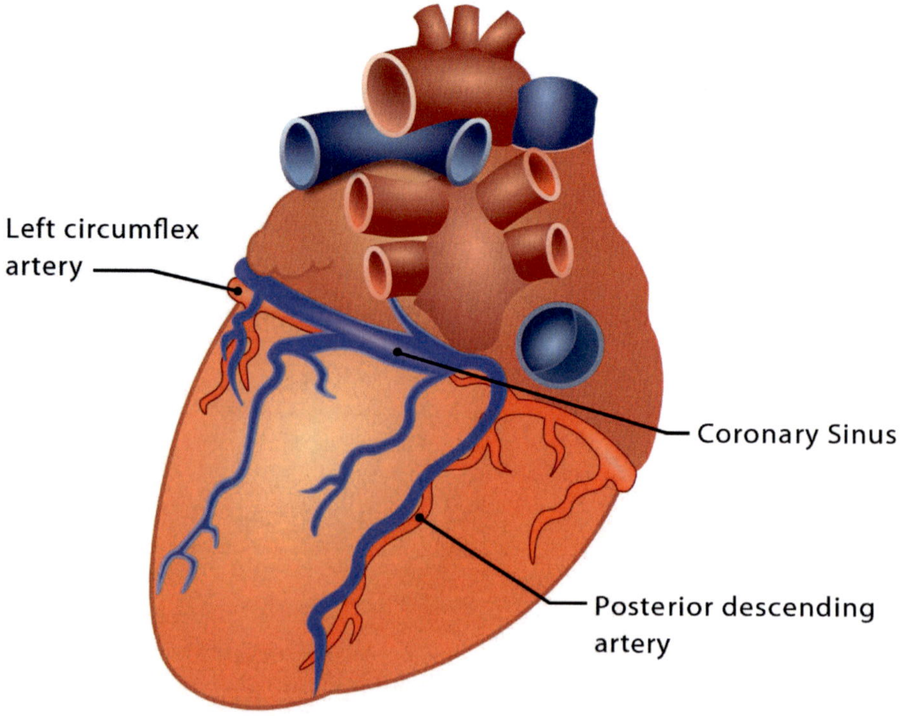

Figure 2.2 - Posterior view of the heart

REVIEW QUESTIONS

1. What part of the systemic circulation contributes the most to total peripheral resistance?

- **The arterioles**

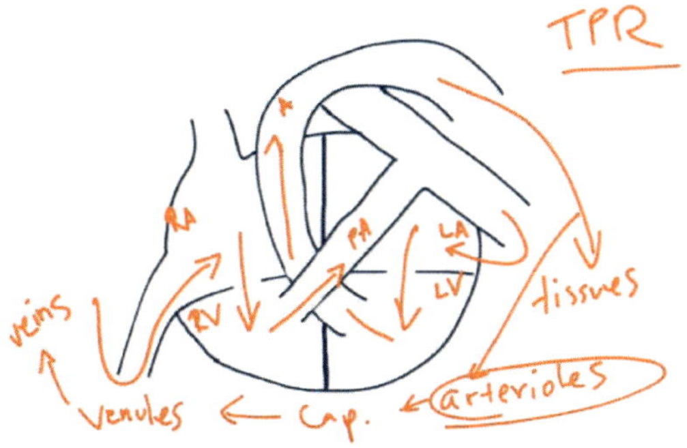

2. How would an arteriovenous (AV) shunt alter the oxygen content in the tissues?

- **In an AV shunt, oxygen bypasses the capillaries and goes directly from the arteries to the veins**
- **Less oxygen enters the tissues → ↑ oxygen in the veins**

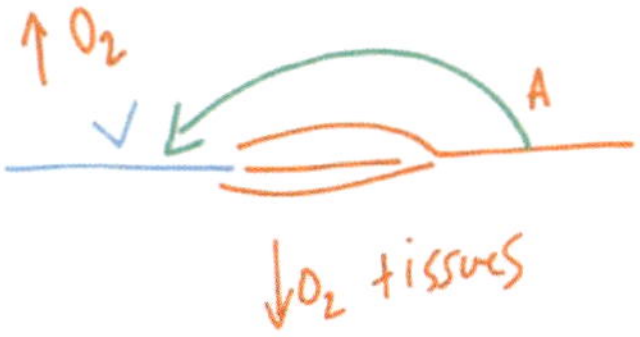

3. How would the right ventricle appear on an echocardiogram in a patient with stenosis of the right coronary artery?

- **The RCA supplies blood to the posterior aspect of the heart**
- **Stenosis of the RCA would result in decreased activity of the posterior aspect of the right ventricle**

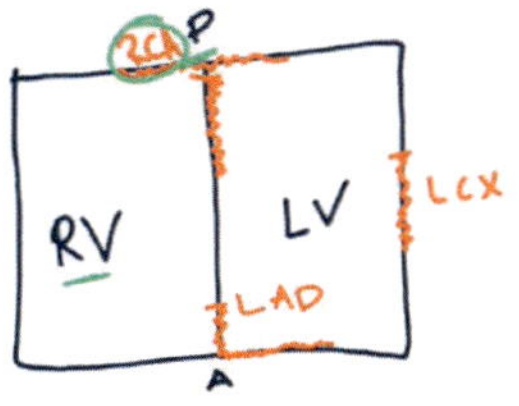

4. Dilation of what part of the heart can cause dysphagia?

- **The esophagus is directly posterior to the left atrium**
- **Dilation of the left atrium can compress the esophagus → dysphagia**

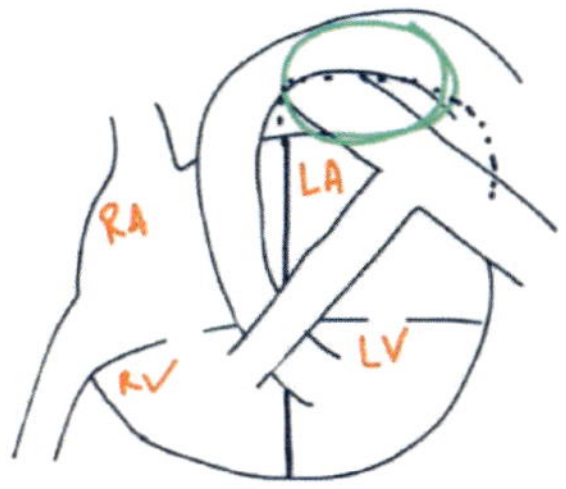

5. What vessel in the body contains the most deoxygenated blood?

- **The heart is more metabolically active than the peripheral tissues**
- **It extracts more oxygen from RBCs than the peripheral tissues**
- **Therefore, the last part of the coronary circulation (the coronary sinus) contains the most deoxygenated blood**

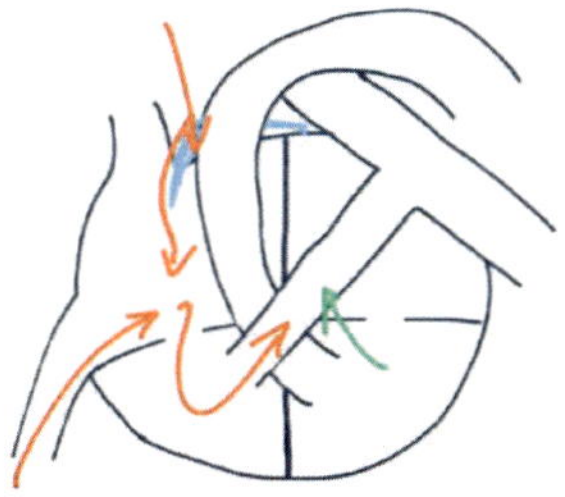

6. How would stenosis of the pulmonary artery alter the pressure in the right ventricle, right atrium, and coronary sinus?

- **Stenosis of the pulm. artery → ↑ volume in the right ventricle and right atrium → ↑ pressure**

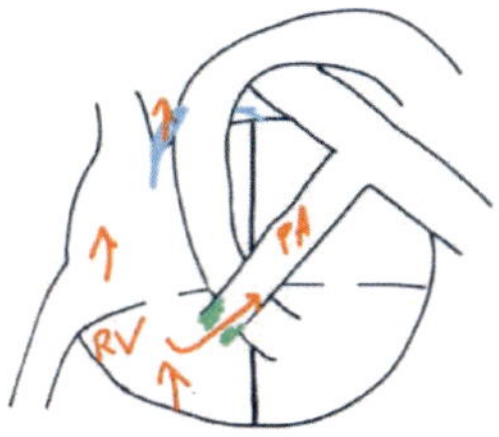

Section II - Cardiology Equations

I. Equations

A. Stroke volume (SV)

$$SV = EDV - ESV$$

Where:
SV = stroke volume (mL/beat)
EDV = end diastolic volume
ESV = end systolic volume

1. Stroke volume represents the volume of blood pumped by the heart every beat.

B. Cardiac output (CO)

$$CO = SV \times HR$$

Where:
CO = cardiac output (mL/min)
SV = stroke volume (mL/beat)
HR = heart rate (beats/min)

$$CO = \text{rate of } O_2 \text{ consumption} / (\text{arterial } O_2 \text{ content} - \text{venous } O_2 \text{ content})$$

Where:
CO = cardiac output (mL/min)
Rate of O_2 consumption (mL O_2/min)
Arterial O_2 content (mL O_2/100 mL blood)
Venous O_2 content (mL O_2/100 mL blood)

1. Known as the Fick equation
2. Cardiac output represents the volume of blood pumped by the heart every minute.

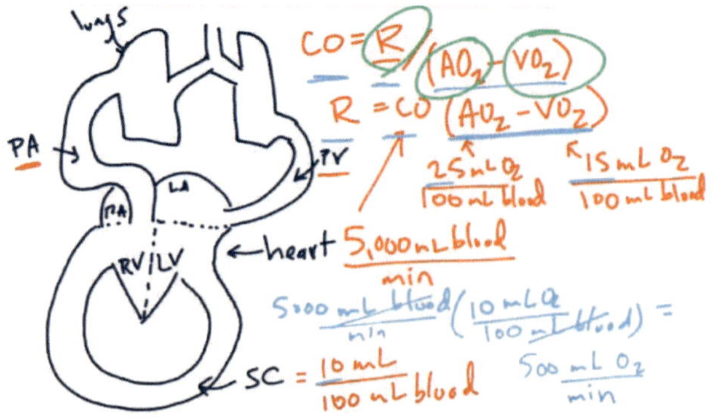

C. Ejection fraction (EF)

$$EF = (EDV - ESV) / EDV$$

Where:
EF = ejection fraction
EDV = end diastolic volume (mL)
ESV = end systolic volume (mL)
SV = stroke volume (mL)

1. EF is the fraction of EDV ejected from the ventricle during each contraction.

D. Stroke Work

Stroke work = aortic pressure × stroke volume

1. The work created by the heart in a single beat

E. Resistance

$$R = 8L\eta / \pi r^4$$

Where:
R = resistance (mmHg × min/mL)
L = length of blood vessel
η = viscosity
r = radius of blood vessel

1. The total resistance in series can be calculated as follows:
   a) $R_{total} = R_1 + R_2 + R_3 +.. R_n$

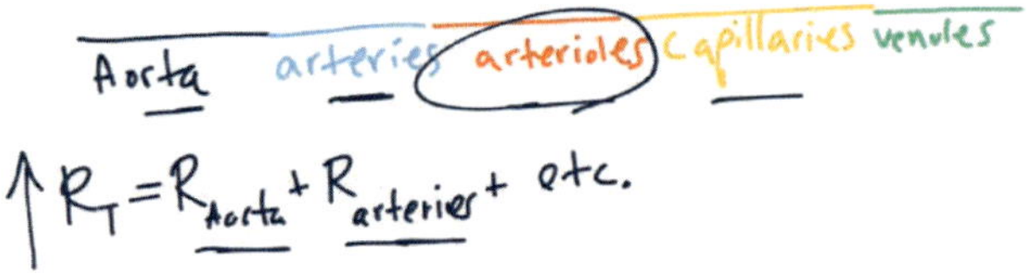

2. The total resistance in parallel can be calculated as follows:
   a) $1/R_{total} = 1/R_1 + 1/R_2 + 1/R_3 + ...1/R_n$

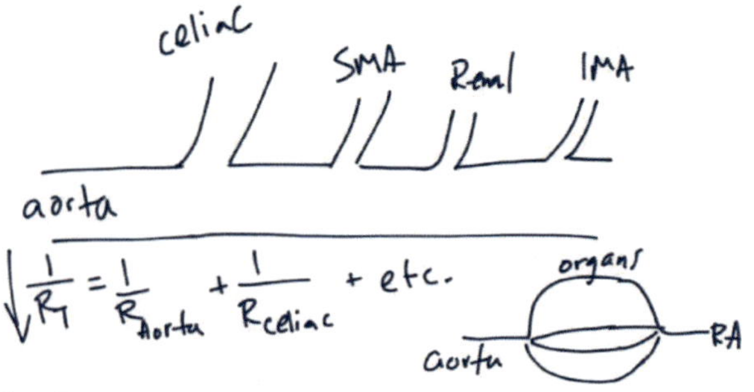

F. Pressure

$$MAP = CO \times TPR$$

Where:
MAP = mean arterial pressure (mmHg)
CO = cardiac output (mL/min)
TPR = total peripheral resistance (mmHg × min/mL)

1. MAP is determined by the cardiac output and TPR, primarily at the arterioles.

Pulse Pressure = systolic blood pressure - diastolic blood pressure

2. Normal is between 30-50 mmHg.
3. Increased, or widened pulse pressures occur when systolic pressure rises and/or diastolic pressures decrease.
   a) Decreased arterial compliance and increased stroke volume will increase pulse pressure.

G. Blood flow

$$Q = \Delta P / R$$

Where:
Q = flow (mL/min)
ΔP = change in pressure (mmHg)
R = resistance (mmHg × min/mL)

1. Blood flow describes the movement of blood over a given period of time.

$$V = Q / A$$

Where:
V = velocity (cm/s)
Q = flow (mL/min)
A = cross-sectional area (cm^2)

2. Velocity is inversely proportional to cross-sectional area.
3. Velocity is proportional to the blood flow.

H. Capillary fluid exchange

$$J_v = K_f \, [(P_c - P_i) - \varsigma(\pi_c - \pi_i)]$$

Where:
J_v = net fluid movement between compartments
K_f = filtration coefficient
P_c = capillary hydrostatic pressure
P_i = interstitial hydrostatic pressure
ς = permeability of the capillary to protein
π_c = capillary oncotic pressure
π_i = interstitial oncotic pressure

1. Positive Jv = filtration, or fluid movement out of the capillary
2. Negative Jv = absorption, or fluid movement into the capillary
3. Increased fluid movement from the capillaries to the interstitium results in increased lymphatic flow.

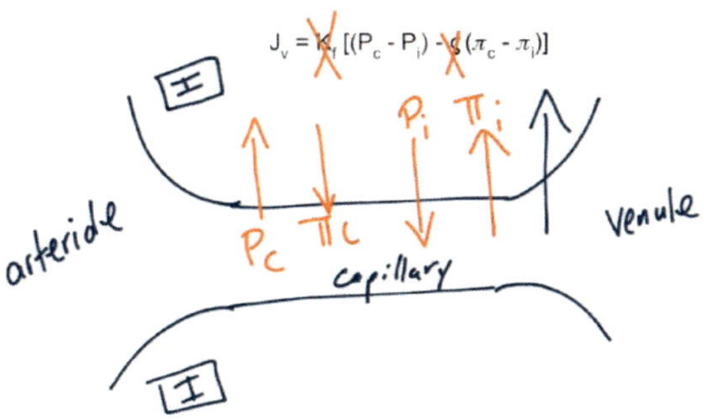

I. Compliance

$$C = V / P$$

Where:
C = compliance (mL/mmHg)
V = volume (mL)
P = pressure (mmHg)

1. Compliance indicates the ability of the tissue to expand as pressure rises.

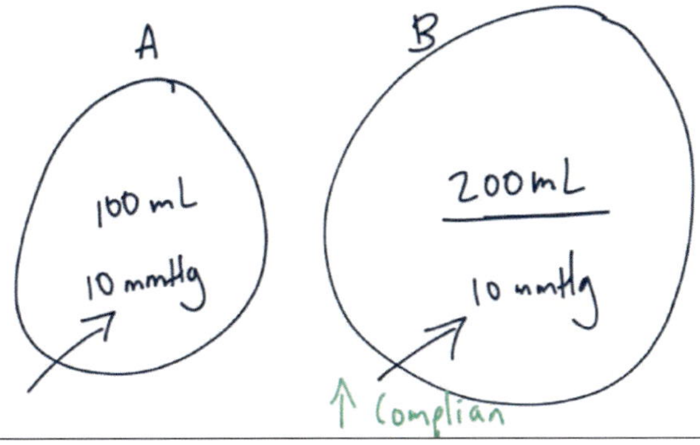

J. Elastance

$$E = P / V$$

Where:
E = elastance (mmHg/mL)
P = pressure (mmHg)
V = volume (mL)

1. Elastance is the ability of the tissue to recoil upon distension.

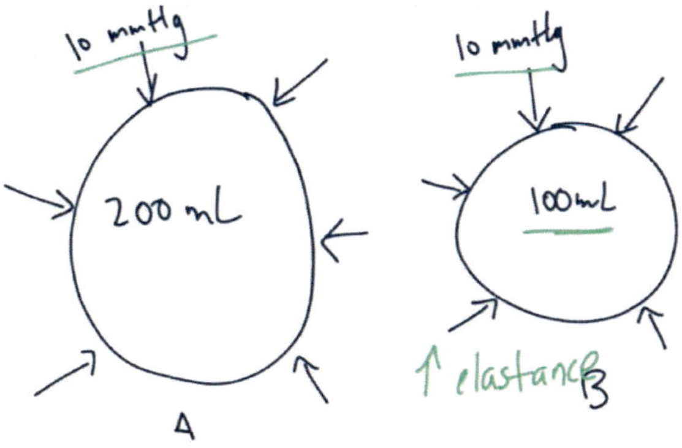

REVIEW QUESTIONS

1. How would the stroke volume be altered in a patient with aortic regurgitation?

- **In AR, blood leaks from the aorta back into the left ventricle during diastole**
- **The volume at the end of diastole (EDV) increases**
- **This results in ↑ stroke volume**

Aortic regurgitation | SV = ? ↑

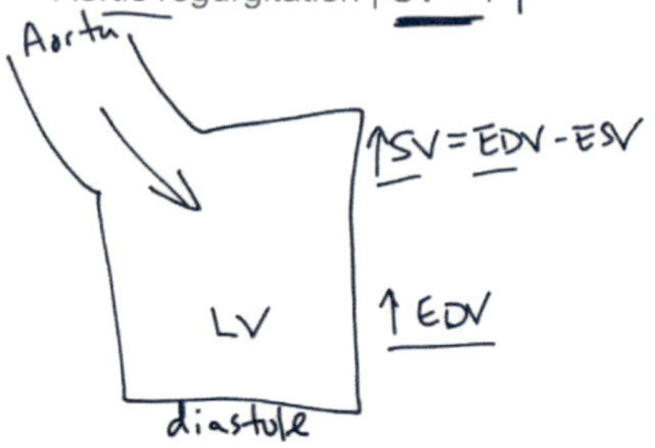

2. How would acute hemorrhagic shock alter stroke volume and cardiac output?

- **Hemorrhagic shock → blood loss → decreased blood returning to heart → decreased EDV**
- **↓ EDV → ↓ SV**
- **Although SV is decreased, HR is increased resulting in a constant CO**

Shock | SV = ? | CO = ?

Blood loss → ↓ EDV

$\downarrow SV = \downarrow EDV - ESV$

$CO = SV \times \uparrow HR$

3. What would be the cardiac output if the end diastolic volume is 110 mL, the end systolic volume is 50 mL, and the RR interval from an EKG is 0.7?

- **The RR interval represents a single heartbeat (seconds/heart beat).**
- **This can be used to calculate heart rate.**
- **With the heart rate, EDV, and ESV, cardiac output can be calculated**
- **CO = 5,148 mL/min**

EDV = 110 | ESV = 50 | RR = 0.7 | CO = ?

$CO = SV \times HR \quad \frac{60\ mL}{beat} \times \frac{85.8\ beats}{min} =$

$RR = 0.7 \frac{s}{beat} \qquad 5,148\ mL\ minute$

$HR = \frac{1}{0.7\ s/beat} = 1.43 \frac{beats}{s} \Big| \frac{60\ s}{min} =$

$SV = EDV - ESV \qquad 85.8\ beats/min$

$110 - 50 = 60\ mL$

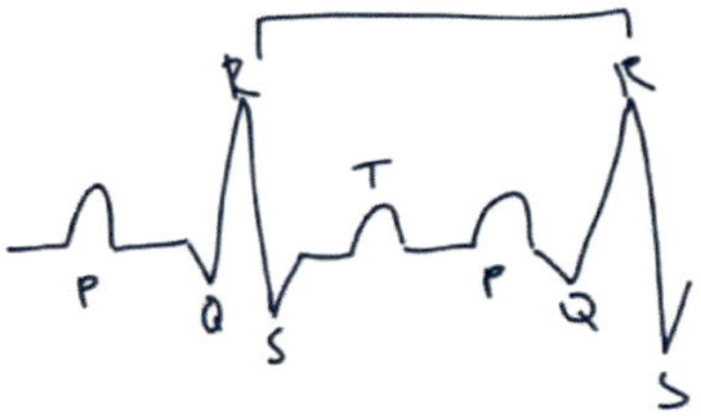

4. If the rate of oxygen consumption is 600 mL of O_2 / min, the arterial oxygen content is 30 mL of O_2 / 100 mL of blood, and the venous oxygen content is 20 mL of O_2 / 100 mL of blood, what is the cardiac output?

- **Equation is CO = R / (AO_2 - VO_2)**
- **Plugging the numbers in → 6,000 mL/min**

$CO = R / (AO_2 - VO_2)$

$CO = \frac{600\ mL\ O_2}{min} \Big/ \left(\frac{10\ mL\ O_2}{100\ mL\ blood}\right) =$

$\boxed{CO = 6,000 \frac{mL}{min}}$

REVIEW QUESTIONS

5. If a patient has an end systolic volume of 70 mL and an end diastolic volume of 130 mL, what is the ejection fraction?

- **Plug numbers in using the equation EF = EDV - ESV / EDV**
- **EF = 130 - 60 / 130 = 0.46**
- **The heart pumped 46% of the blood from the left ventricle into the aorta during a single contraction**

ESV = 70 mL | EDV = 130 mL | EF = ?

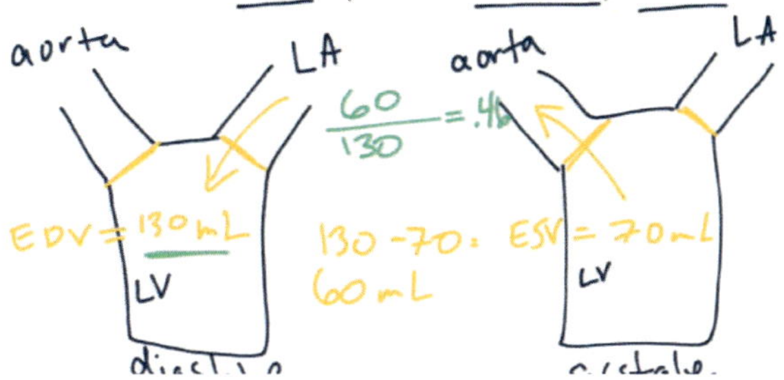

6. Imagine a parallel circuit that involves the aorta and the celiac artery. In this the resistance of the aorta is 10 and the resistance of the celiac artery is 10. What would the total resistance be? How will the resistance change if the superior mesenteric artery is added to the system which also has a resistance of 10?

- **Use the equation 1/Rt = 1/R1 + 1/R2**
- **Total resistance = 5**
- **If a component is added to a parallel circuit (10), then the resistance decreases = 3.33**

$$\frac{1}{R_T} = \frac{1}{R_{aorta}} + \frac{1}{R_{celiac}} \quad (10,\ 10)$$

$$\frac{1}{R_T} = 0.1 + 0.1 = 0.2$$

$$R_T = \frac{1}{0.2} = 5$$

$$\frac{1}{R_T} = \frac{1}{R_{aorta}} + \frac{1}{R_{celiac}} + \frac{1}{R_{SMA}} \quad (10,\ 10,\ 10)$$

$$\frac{1}{R_T} = 0.1 + 0.1 + 0.1 = 0.$$

$$R_T = \frac{1}{0.2} = 5$$

$$\downarrow R_T = \frac{1}{0.3} = 3.33$$

7. How would removing a kidney, or a nephrectomy, alter the total resistance?

- **This describes a parallel circuit**
- **Use the equation 1/Rt = 1/R1 + 1/R2**
- **The resistance would increase**

Nephrectomy | R_{total} = ?

$$\uparrow \frac{1}{R_T} = \frac{1}{R_1} + \cancel{\frac{1}{R_2}} + \text{etc.}$$

8. How would squatting relieve symptoms of hypoxia in a patient with Eisenmenger syndrome?

- **Pressure on the L side of the heart is normally > R side**
- **In a chronic L → R shunt the pressure on the R can become greater than L**
- **This results in reversal of the shunt → hypoxia**
- **Squatting increases the resistance throughout the systemic vasculature → decreased cardiac output → increased volume/pressure on R side of heart → temporary reversal of shunt**

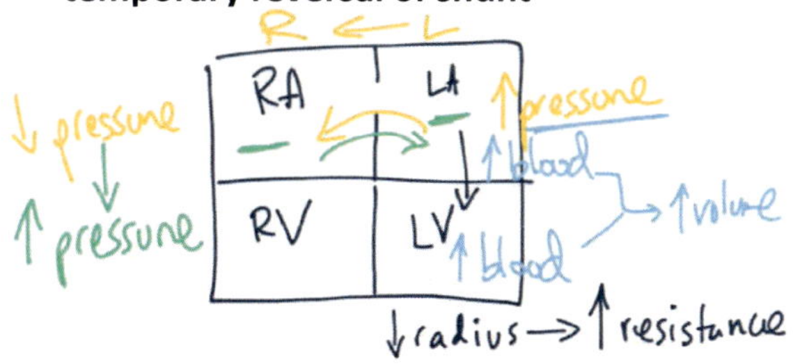

REVIEW QUESTIONS

9. If the radius of the lumen of a blood vessel has been decreased by 75%, by what factor has the blood flow been altered?

- **Flow is proportional to the radius to the fourth power**
- **A 75% decrease in vessel size → the lumen is ¼ its original size**
- **Decreasing the radius by ¼ → decrease in flow by a factor of 256**

Radius of the lumen ↓ by 75% | Q = ?

$$Q = \Delta P / R$$
$$R = \eta L / \pi r^4$$
$$Q = \Delta P \pi r^4 / \eta L$$
$$\downarrow Q = r^4 \rightarrow \left(\frac{r}{4}\right)^4 = 4 \times 4 \times 4 \times 4 = 256$$

10. The pressure at the beginning of a parallel circuit is 120 mmHg and 15 mmHg at the end. There are six segments to the circuit and each segment has a resistance of 9 mmHg/mL/min. What is the flow rate?

$$Q = \Delta P / R \quad (105)$$

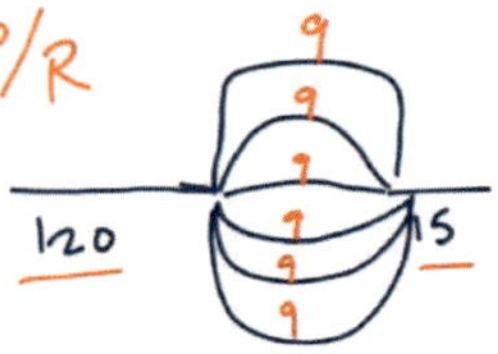

$$\frac{1}{R_T} = \frac{1}{R_1} + \frac{1}{R_2} + \text{etc}$$
$$\frac{1}{R_T} = 6\left(\frac{1}{9}\right) = 0.667$$
$$R_T = \frac{1}{0.667} = 1.50$$
$$Q = \Delta P / R = \frac{105}{1.50} = \boxed{70 \text{ mL/min}}$$

11. Where is the velocity of blood lowest in the circulatory system?

- **V = Q / A**
- **It can be deduced from the above equation that when the cross-sectional area is increased, the velocity will be decreased.**
- **The capillaries have the greatest cross-sectional area so velocity is lowest here. What would happen to the net fluid of movement between the compartments in a patient with liver failure?**

Liver failure | J_v = ? ↑

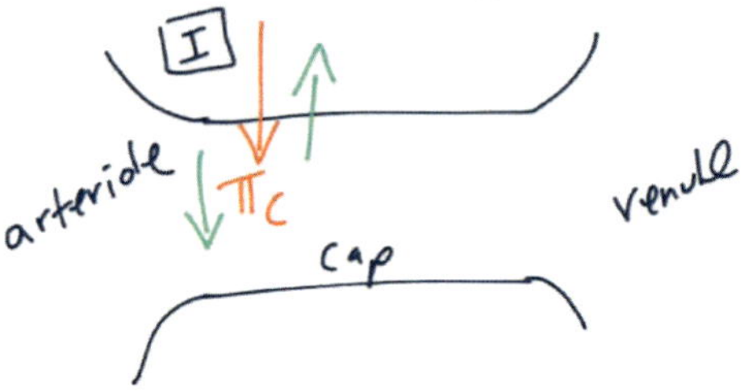

12. What would happen to the net fluid of movement between the compartments in a patient with liver failure?

- **The liver produces proteins and other factors that contribute to the oncotic pressure**
- **In liver failure the oncotic pressure decreases → fluid leaves the capillary into the interstitium → edema**
- **↑ Jv**

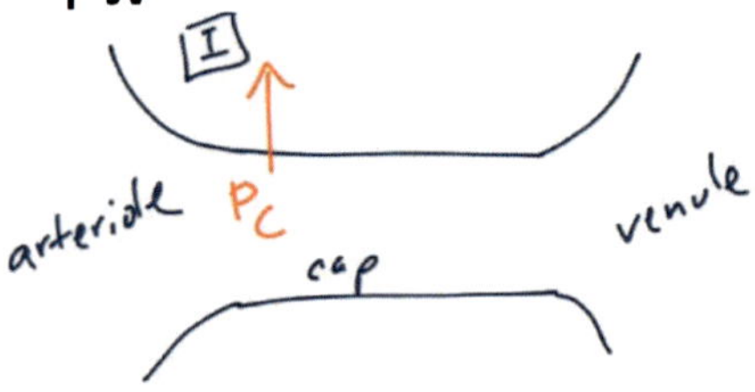

↑ pressure → ↑ RV hypertrophy → ↑ volume

REVIEW QUESTIONS

13. What would happen to the net fluid of movement between the compartments in a patient with pulmonary hypertension?

- **Chronic ↑ pulmonic pressure → heart failure →↑ hydrostatic pressure**
- **↑ Jv**

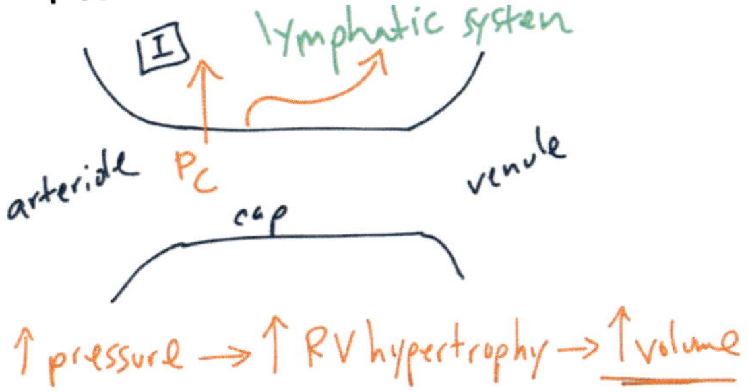

14. At the very early stages of right sided heart failure there is an increase in fluid throughout the vasculature, but patients don't typically have edema. Why would these patients have edema initially?

- **The lymphatic system increases the rate of reabsorption**

15. How would sitting in a warm bath impact the net fluid of movement between the compartments, antidiuretic hormone, and atrial natriuretic peptide?

- **Heat increases permeability of capillaries →↑ Jv →↓ blood volume →↑ ADH**
- **ANP normally rises in response to ↑ blood volume; hence, a ↓ blood volume →↓ ANP**

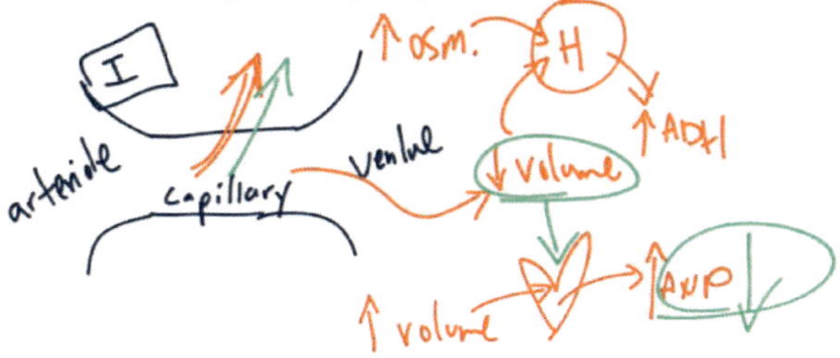

16. How would increased arterial compliance of the aorta alter the pulse pressure?

- **Compliance = volume / pressure**
- **↑ aortic compliance →↑ radius →↓ resistance →↓ systolic pressure**
- **Pulse pressure = systolic pressure - diastolic pressure; hence, a ↓ systolic pressure →↓ pulse pressure**

↑ arterial compliance | pulse pressure = ?

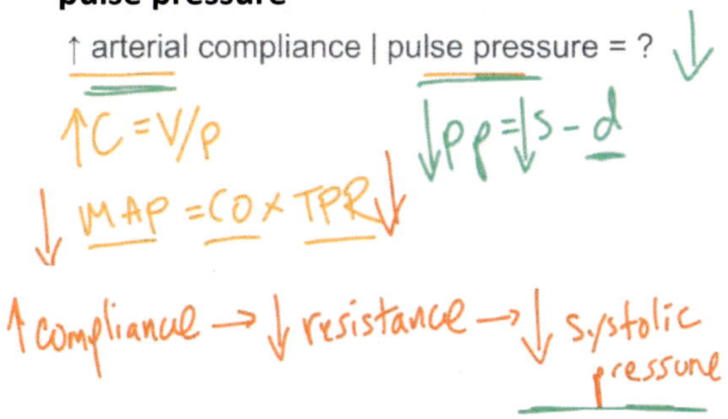

Section III - Electrophysiology

I. Electrophysiology

A. Cardiac Electrical System

1. Figure 2.3 shows the normal anatomy of the cardiac electrical system.
2. The electrical system consists of the sinoatrial (SA) node, the atrioventricular (AV) node, the Bundle of His, the right and left bundle branches, and the Purkinje fibers.
3. The SA node normally sets the pace of the heart with spontaneous depolarization occurring approximately every 60-100 seconds.
4. Other components of the electrical system (AV node, Bundle of His, and Purkinje fibers) spontaneously depolarize less frequently and become eclipsed by the SA node.
5. Fastest to slowest rate of spontaneous depolarization: SA > AV > Bundle of His & Purkinje fibers.

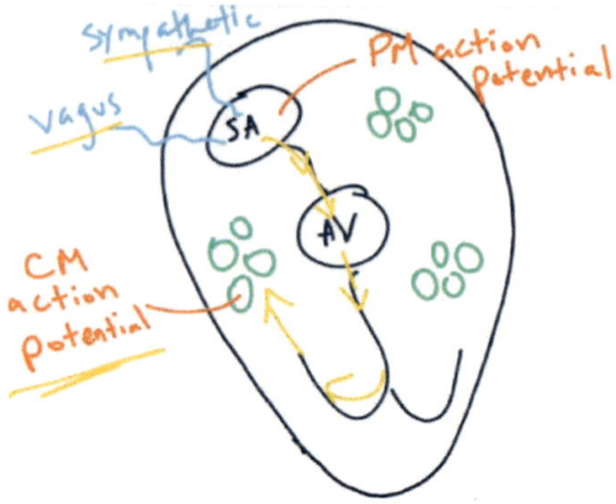

B. Conduction Velocity

1. The time required for an electrical signal to spread throughout cardiac tissue.
2. The conduction speed is fastest to slowest as follows: Purkinje fibers > SA node > AV node.

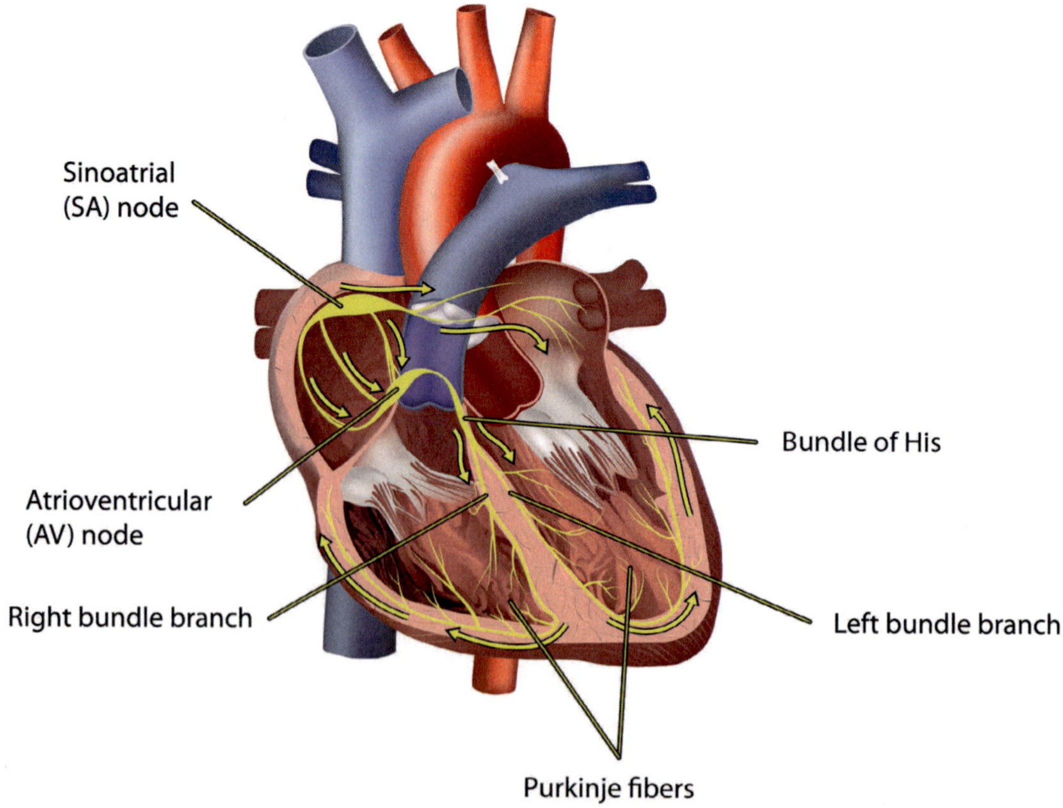

Figure 2.3 - Cardiac electrical system

C. Action Potentials

1. Cardiac myocyte action potentials occur throughout cardiac muscle tissue in response to depolarizing signals generated by cardiac pacemaker cells (Figure 2.4).

   a) Phase 0 (upstroke) is a caused by voltage-gated Na^+ channels opening and subsequent Na^+ influx.

   b) Phase 1 (initial repolarization) is a caused by voltage-gated K^+ channels opening and subsequent K^+ efflux.

   c) In phase 2 (plateau), the K^+ channels remain open and Ca^{2+} channels open resulting in Ca^{2+} influx. The combination of positively charged K^+ leaving the cell and positively charged Ca^{2+} entering the cell results in a delay of repolarization.

   d) In phase 3 (rapid repolarization) the Ca^{2+} channels close and the K^+ channels remain open.

   e) Phase 4 is caused by permeability of the K^+ channels and is responsible for the resting membrane potential.

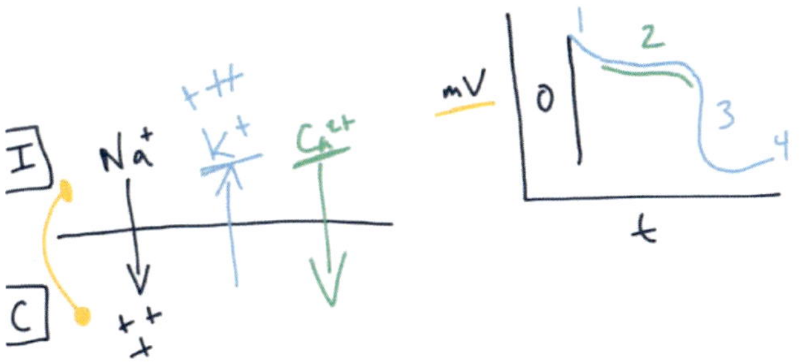

2. Pacemaker action potentials occur in specialized cells of the heart (SA node, AV node, Bundle of His, Purkinje fibers) that are responsible for controlling the speed at which the heart contracts (Figure 2.5).

   a) Phase 0 (upstroke) is a result of L-type voltage-gated Ca^{2+} channels opening and subsequent Ca^{2+} influx (Ca^{2+} moves from the interstitium into the cell) .

   b) Phases 1 and 2 are absent in pacemaker action potentials.

   c) Phase 3 (repolarization) is a result of K^+ channels opening and subsequent K^+ efflux (K^+ moves from the cell to the interstitium).

   d) Phase 4 (spontaneous depolarization) is a result of increased Na^+ influx and decreased and K^+ efflux through I_f (funny channels).

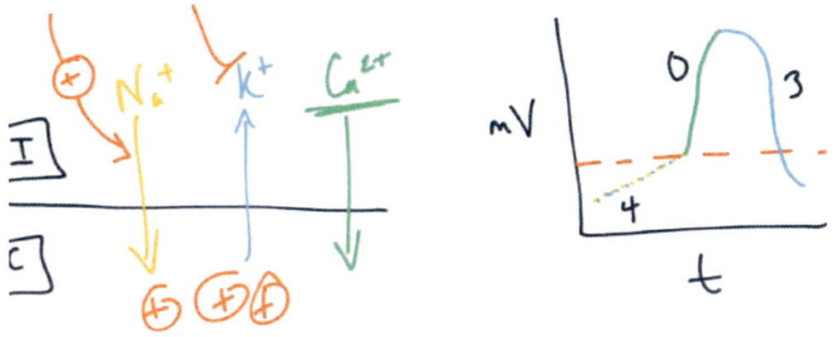

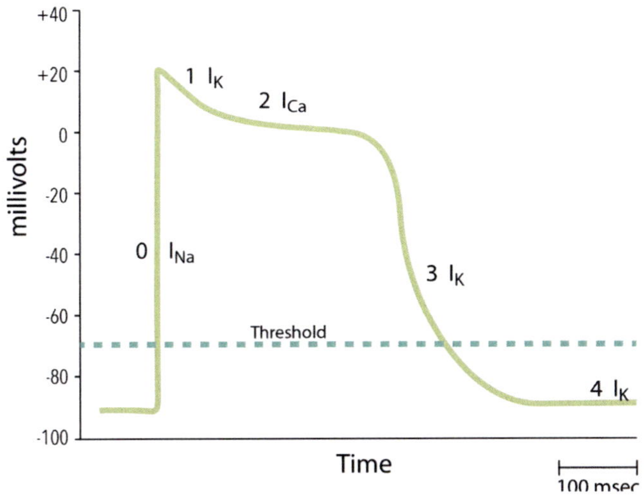

Figure 2.4 - Cardiac myocyte action potential

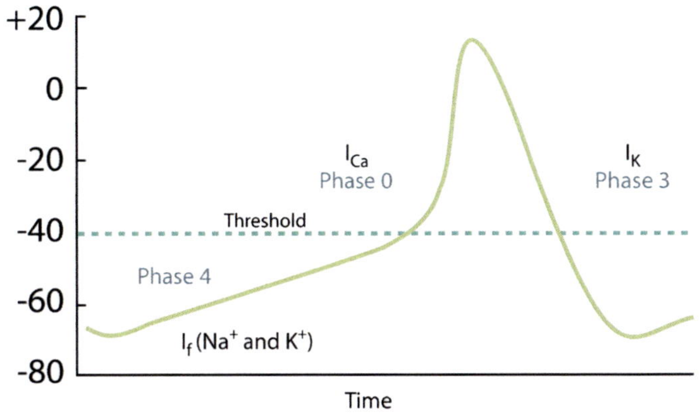

Figure 2.5 - Pacemaker action potential

D. Contraction and relaxation

1. Contraction

a) Voltage-gated Na^+ channels open resulting in depolarization.

b) Ca^{2+} enters the cell through L-type Ca^{2+} channels.

c) Ca^{2+} binds ryanodine receptors on the sarcoplasmic reticulum (SR).

d) Ryanodine receptors interact with Ca^{2+} channels which release Ca^{2+} from the SR.

e) Ca^{2+} release from the SR results in increased cytosolic Ca^{2+} which binds to troponin C.

f) Troponin C moves tropomyosin from actin allowing myosin to bind actin and cause muscle contraction.

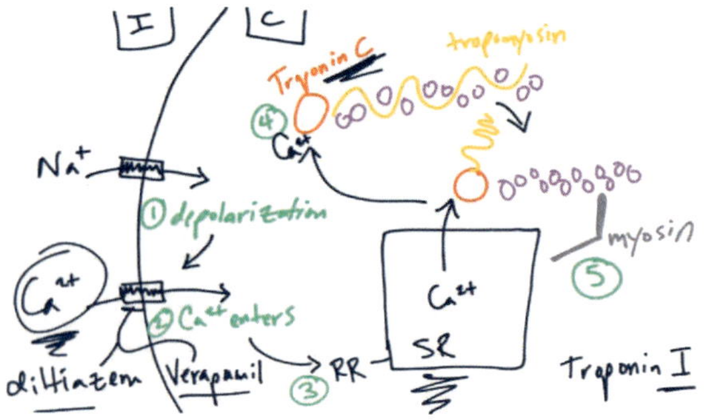

2. Relaxation

a) Cytosolic Ca^{2+} is moved into the SR through Ca^{2+}-ATPase channels (SERCA).

b) The protein phospholamban inhibits SERCA.

c) When phospholamban is phosphorylated via protein kinase A (PKA), phospholamban is unable to block SERCA.

d) Catecholamines up-regulate PKA, resulting in increased SR uptake of Ca^{2+}.

e) Increased storage of Ca^{2+} in the SR allows the following contraction cycle to release more Ca^{2+}, resulting in a stronger contraction.

f) Ca^{2+} is also removed from the cytosol into the extracellular space through Na^+/Ca^{2+} antiporter. Three Na^+ molecules are exchanged for one Ca^{2+} molecule.

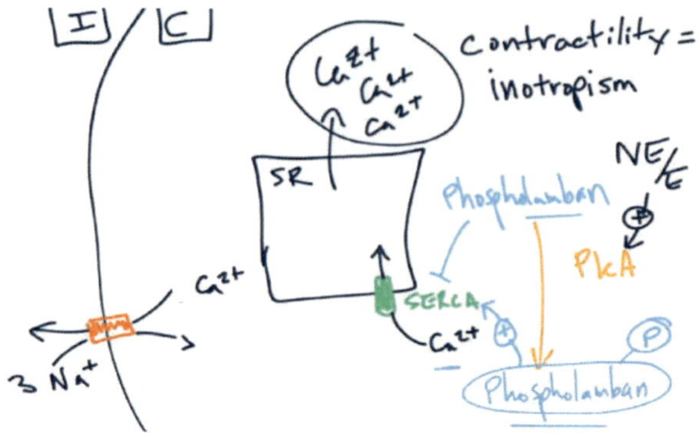

3. Inotropes produce changes in contractility.

a) Regulate the intracellular concentration of Ca^{2+} in cardiac myocytes.

4. Chronotropes produce changes in heart rate.

a) Alter the firing rate of the SA node by regulating the influx of Na^+ in the SA nodal cells.

(1) Dromotropes produce changes in conduction velocity.

(a) Alter the conduction velocity through the AV node by regulating the influx of Ca^{2+} in the AV nodal cells.

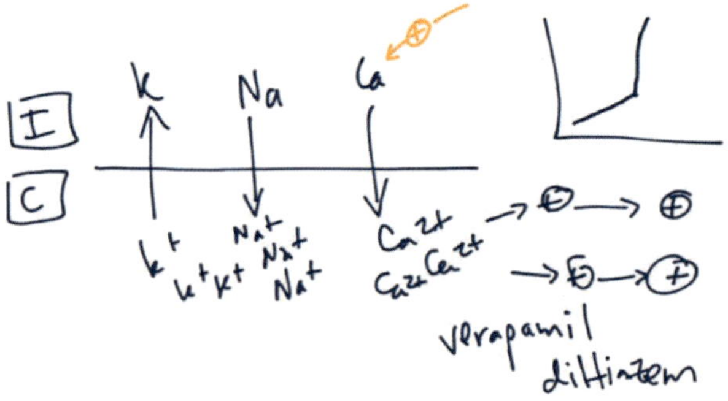

II. EKGs (Figure 2.6)

A. P wave represents depolarization of the atria.

B. The QRS complex marks the depolarization of the ventricles.

1. Repolarization of the atria occurs during the QRS complex but is obscured by depolarization of the ventricles.

C. T wave represents repolarization of the ventricles.

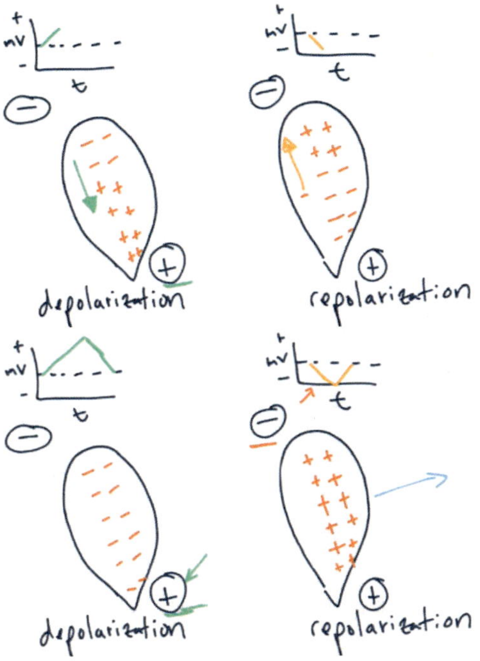

D. Abnormal Electrical Activity

1. First degree heart block

a) Prolongation of the PR interval.

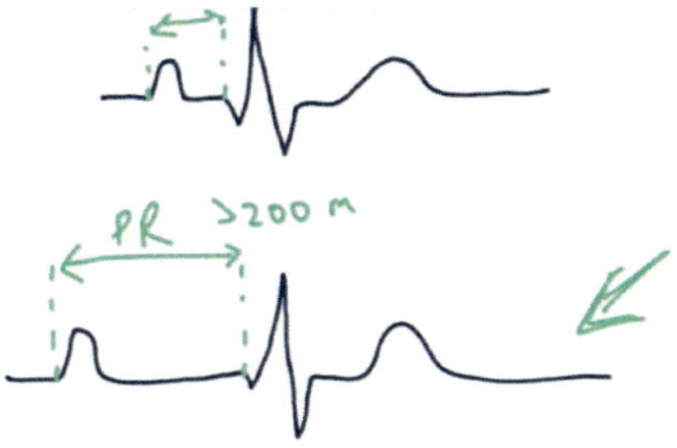

2. Second degree heart block

a) Mobitz type I

(1) Progressive lengthening of the PR interval until the QRS complex is dropped.

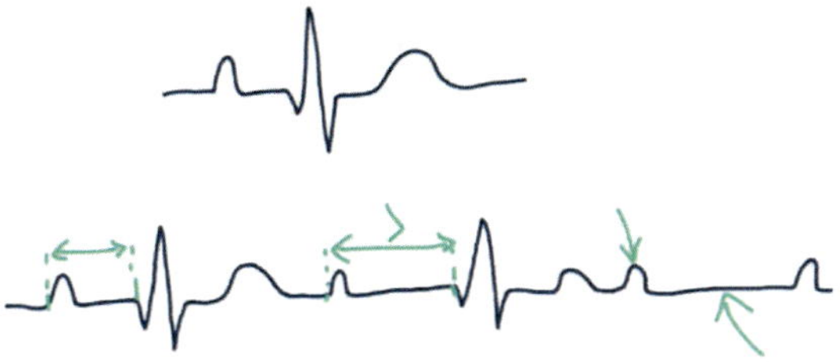

b) Mobitz type II

(1) Normal PR intervals with a sudden drop in the QRS complex.

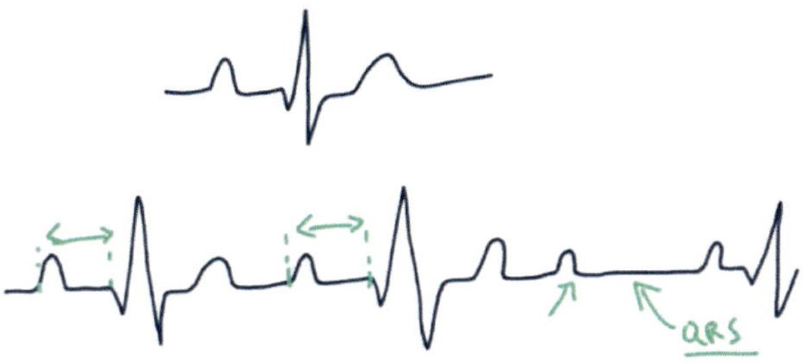

3. Third degree heart block

a) The SA and AV nodes become desynchronized with the SA node pacing the atria and the AV node pacing the ventricles.

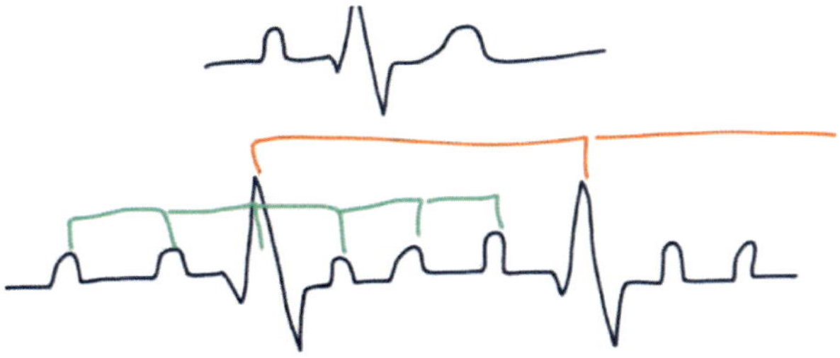

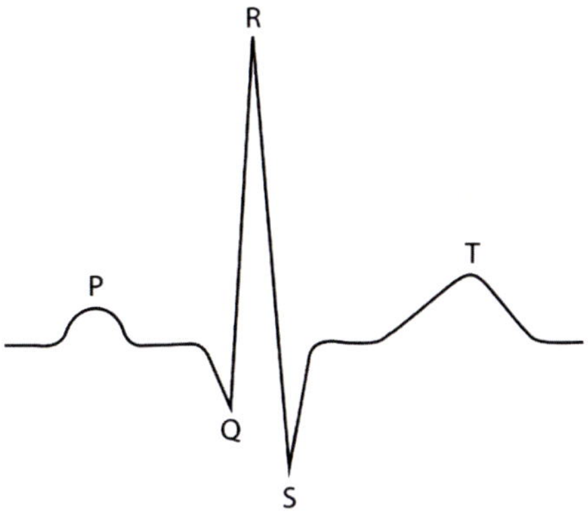

Figure 2.6 - EKG

REVIEW QUESTIONS

1. What drugs prolong phase 3 of the cardiac myocyte action potential?

   - **Potassium channel blockers (Ibutilide, sotalol, amiodarone, and dofetilide)**

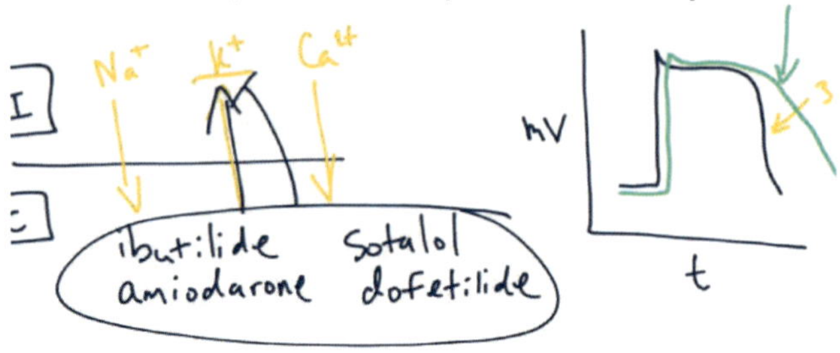

2. Which phase or phases of the pacemaker action potential is altered by adenosine?

   - **Adenosine ↓ influx of calcium and ↑ the efflux of potassium**
   - **This results in a ↓ resting membrane potential →↑ phase 4 and phase 0**

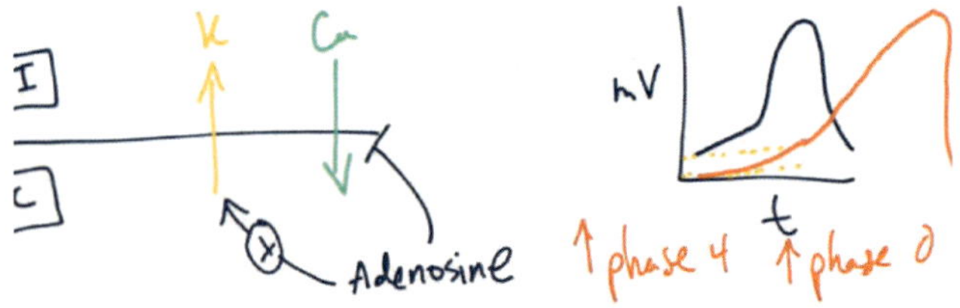

3. What marker is elevated in a patient with a myocardial infarction?

   - **Troponin I**

4. What drugs block the L-type calcium channel?

   - **Non-dihydropyridine calcium channel blockers (Diltiazem & Verapamil)**

5. What component of the EKG is disrupted in a patient with atrial fibrillation?

   - **P-wave deflection on an EKG represents atrial depolarization**
   - **In a-fib, electrical remodeling occurs and abnormal pacemaker-like regions form**
   - **The bombardment of electrical signals disrupts atrial depolarization → absent p-waves**

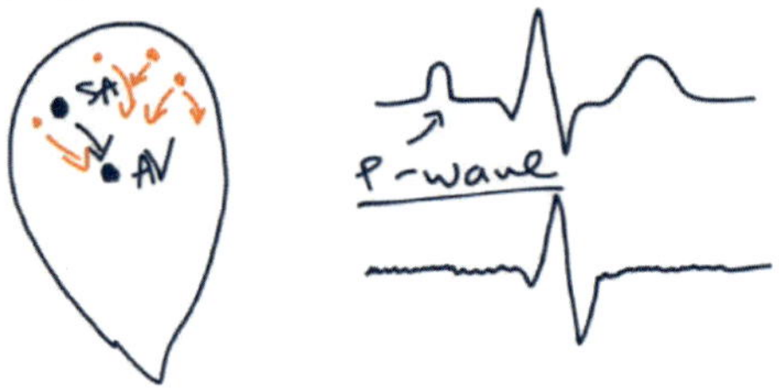

6. How would a supraventricular tachycardia alter stroke volume?

   - **↑ EDV →↑ stroke volume**

7. What does a delta wave on an EKG indicate?

   - **The QRS complex represents ventricular depolarization**
   - **A delta wave indicates early depolarization of the ventricles**

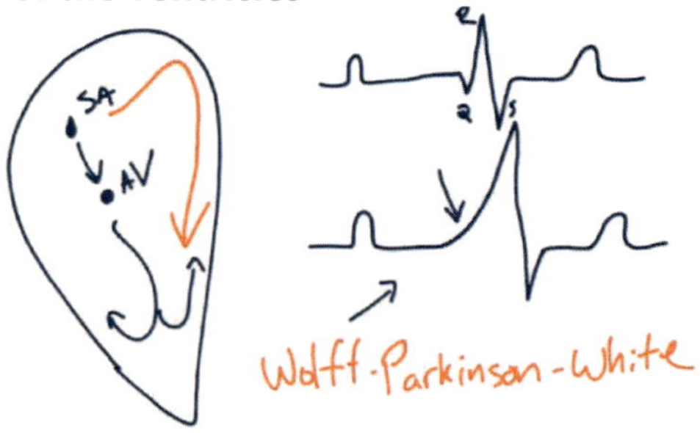

REVIEW QUESTIONS

8. What ion channel is defective in a patient with QT prolongation?

- **The QT interval represents depolarization and repolarization of the ventricles**
- **In QT prolongation, the T wave is particularly long → delayed ventricular repolarization**
- **Phase 3 of the action potential is responsible for repolarization (potassium channels)**

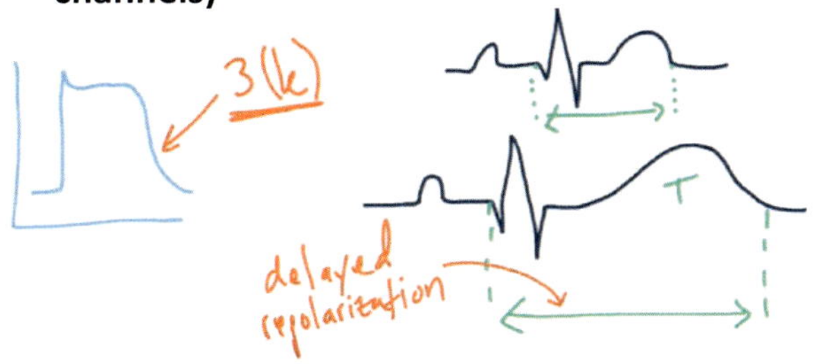

9. How would the end diastolic volume (EDV) change if the QRS complex was not preceded by a P wave?

- **Absent p-waves → atria are not depolarizing →↓ blood volume reaches ventricles →↓ EDV**

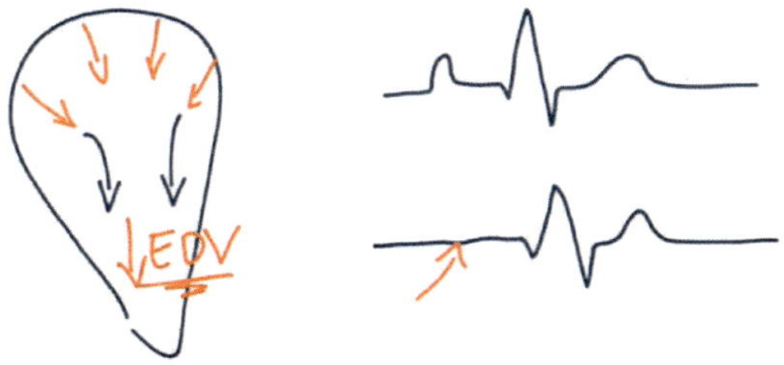

Section IV - Pressure-Volume Loops and Cardiac Cycle

I. Pressure-Volume Loops and Cardiac Cycle

A. Pressure-Volume Loop (Figure 2.7)

1. Isovolumetric contraction
   a) Isovolumetric means the volume is not changing while the pressure increases.
   b) Begins after the mitral valve closes and the left ventricle begins to contract against closed valves.
2. Systolic ejection
   a) Systolic pressure begins the moment the aortic valve opens and blood enters the aorta.
   b) Systolic pressure is the pressure during the period the left ventricle is contracting (mitral valve closing to aortic valve closing).
3. Isovolumetric relaxation
   a) Isovolumetric means the volume is not changing while the pressure decreases.
   b) Begins after the aortic valve closes and the left ventricle begins to relax.
4. Diastolic filling
   a) Begins once the mitral valve opens and blood enters the left ventricle from the left atrium.
   b) Diastolic pressure is the pressure during the period the left ventricle is relaxed (aortic valve closing to mitral closing).

B. Preload

1. Determined by end-diastolic volume (EDV).

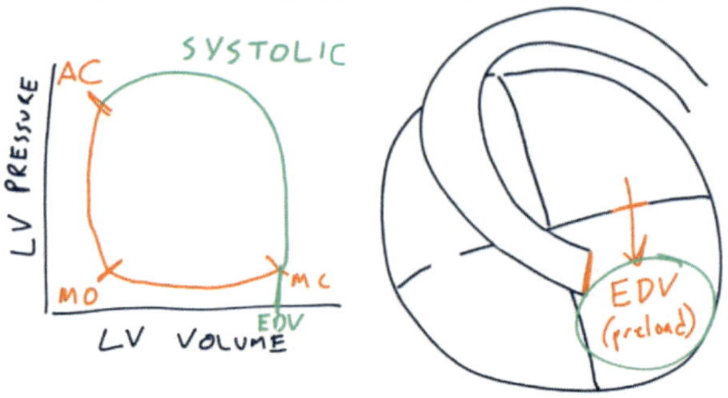

2. EDV is proportional to right atrial pressure (RAP); therefore, increased RAP or EDV indicates increased preload.

C. Afterload

1. Determined by what the ventricle is working against when ejecting blood. For the left ventricle, afterload is determined by aortic pressure. Higher aortic pressure means higher afterload. For the right ventricle, afterload is determined by the pressure in the pulmonary artery.

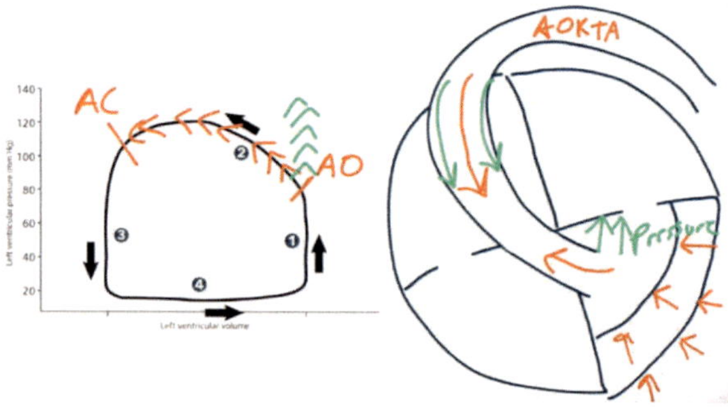

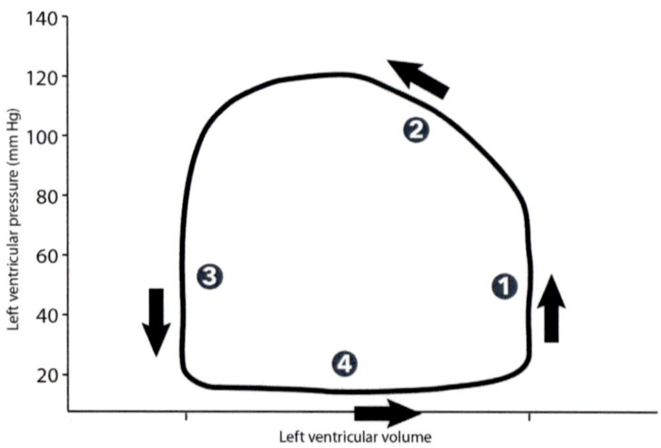

Figure 2.7 - Pressure volume loop

1. Isovolumetric contraction
2. Systolic ejection
3. Isovolumetric relaxation
4. Ventricular filling

D. Stroke Volume

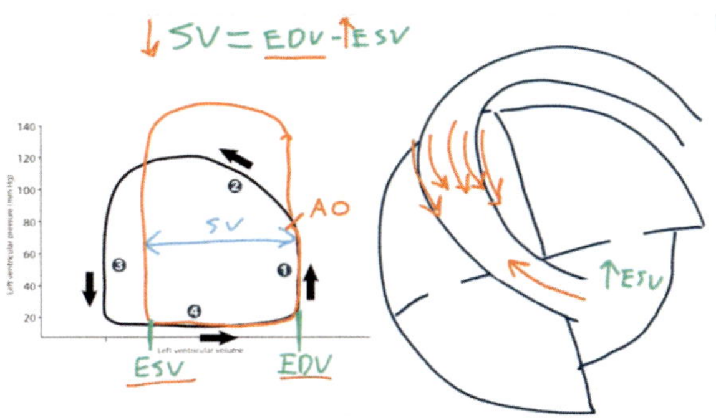

1. The volume of blood leaving the heart (left ventricle) with every contraction
2. Can be increased by increased contractility because the heart is contracting harder and will therefore increase the volume expelled
3. Can be increased by increased preload because there is more volume in the heart to be expelled
   a) Can be increased by decreased afterload because there is less resistance to blood flowing out of the left ventricle

E. Stroke Work

1. Determined by the area that the pressure-volume loop contains. Therefore, certain diseases could demonstrate a bigger sized loop which would indicate an increase in work.
2. See also stroke work in Section II.

F. Contractility

1. A function of how much intracellular Ca^{2+} is present
2. More Ca^{2+} → more troponin C can bind and remove tropomyosin from actin → myosin heads can bind actin → increased force of contraction → more blood ejected from heart → decreased ESV.

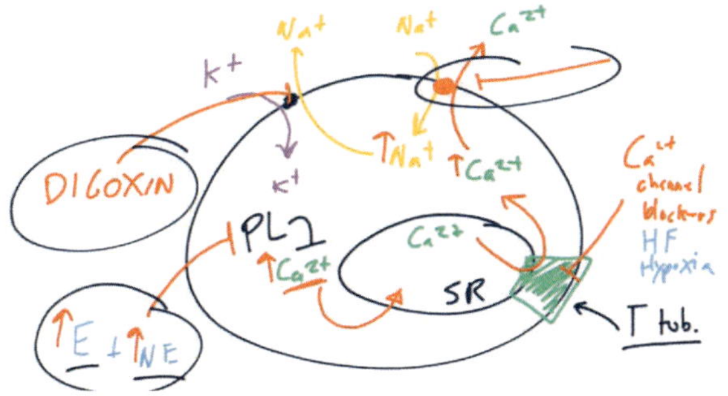

3. Both increased preload and contractility increase stroke volume, but only increased contractility results in decreased ESV. Preload will not decrease ESV. Preload results in the heart contracting with greater force because the sarcomere gets stretched more such that the myosin can bind the actin with greater leverage.
4. Shifting the loop to the right will decrease contractility.
5. Shifting the loop to the left will increase contractility.

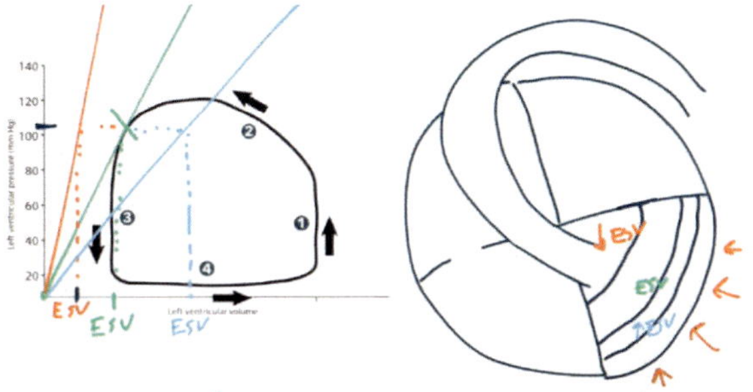

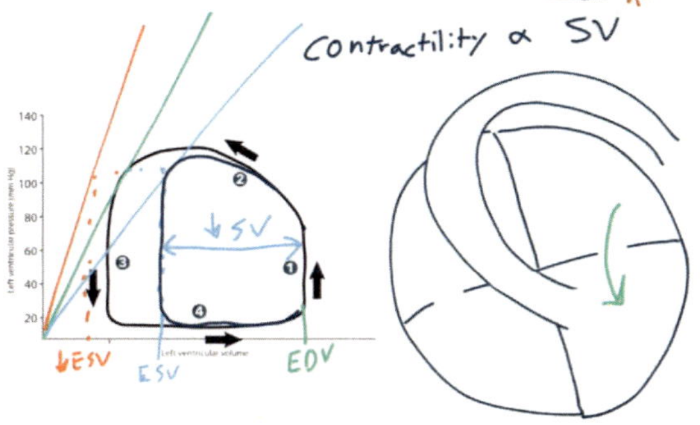

G. Compliance

1. The ability of the heart to expand with increased volume
2. Changes in compliance

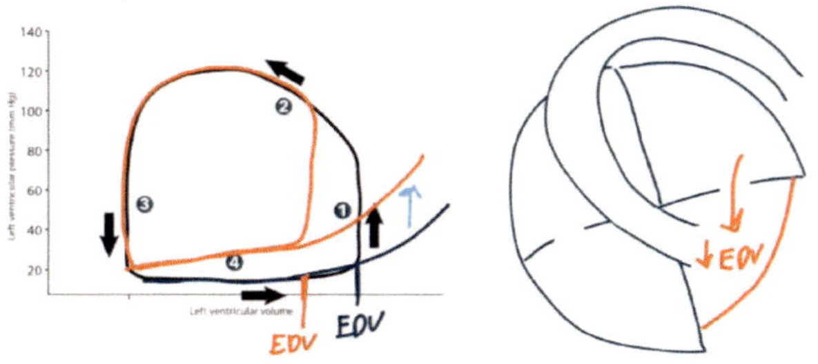

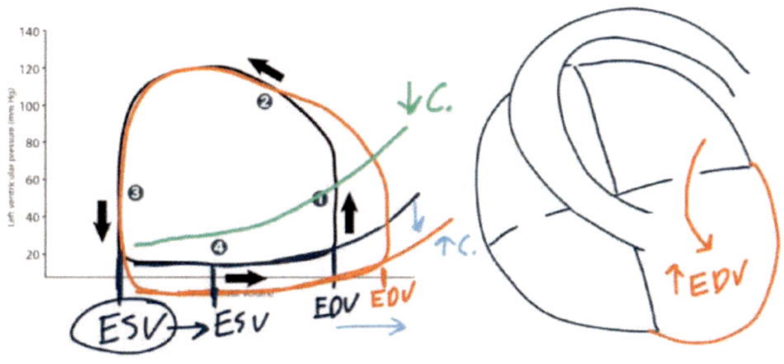

REVIEW QUESTIONS

1. At what point on the pressure volume loop would you likely hear the diastolic rumble in a pt with mitral stenosis?

    - **The sound comes from the turbulence created by the stenotic mitral valve**
    - **This can be heard during diastole between the mitral valve opens normally to when it should close normally**

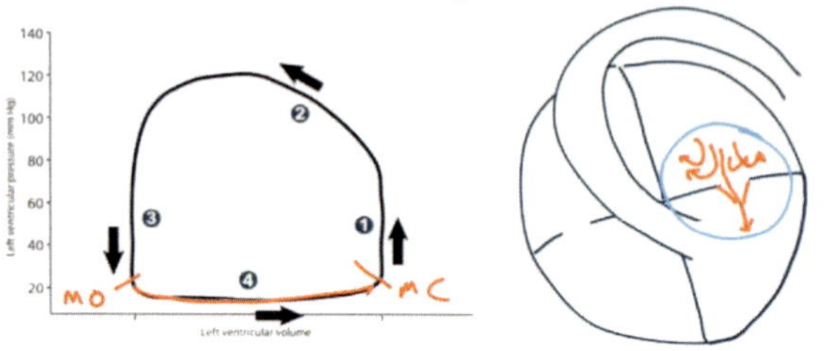

2. How would nitroglycerin alter the PV loop?

    - **Nitroglycerin dilates the veins (via product NO)**
    - **Venous dilation decreases the pressure gradient of blood returning to the heart, decreasing preload (EDV moves left on the graph)**

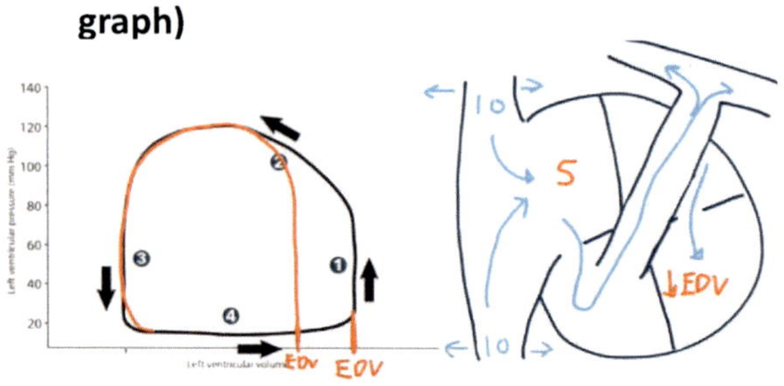

3. How would hydralazine alter the PV loop and why?

    - **Hydralazine primarily dilates the arteries more than veins, decreasing afterload**
    - **Decreased afterload will allow the aortic valve to open earlier and at a lower pressure (aortic valve will open lower along x-axis)**
    - **Decreased afterload will also cause more blood to be ejected during systole (ESV will decrease, left shift on graph)**

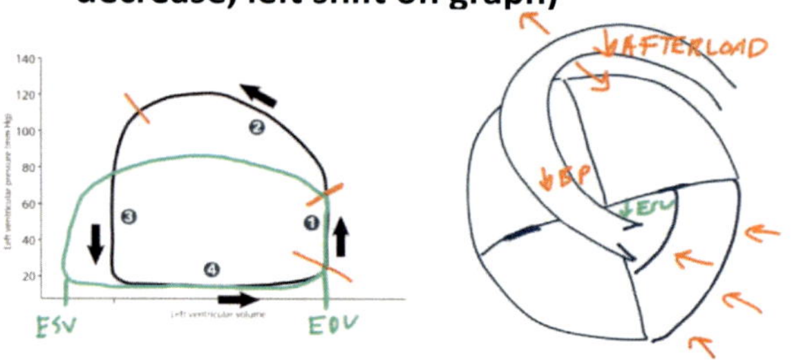

4. What would increased preload do to oxygen levels in the coronary veins?

    - **Increased preload means increased EDV (thus increased SV)**
    - **Increased SV without changing aortic pressure (AP), would cause stroke work to increase**
    - **Increased stroke work causes increased O_2 consumption from the capillaries, resulting in lower venous O**

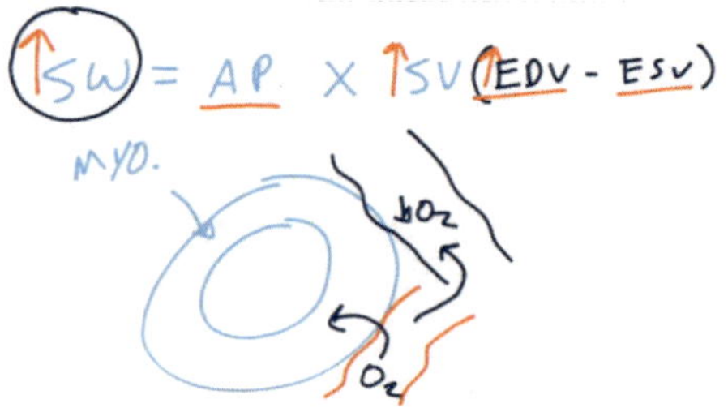

REVIEW QUESTIONS

5. How would dobutamine alter the PV loop?

- **Dobutamine is a β_1 agonist, which increases sympathetic activity on the heart, thereby inhibiting phospholamban, increasing Ca^{2+} return to the sarcoplasmic reticulum (SR)**
- **Increased SR Ca^{2+} increases contractility which will increase blood ejection during systole (decreased ESV)**
- **Increased Ca^{2+} and contractility should also remind you that the line for contractility will have a steeper slope**

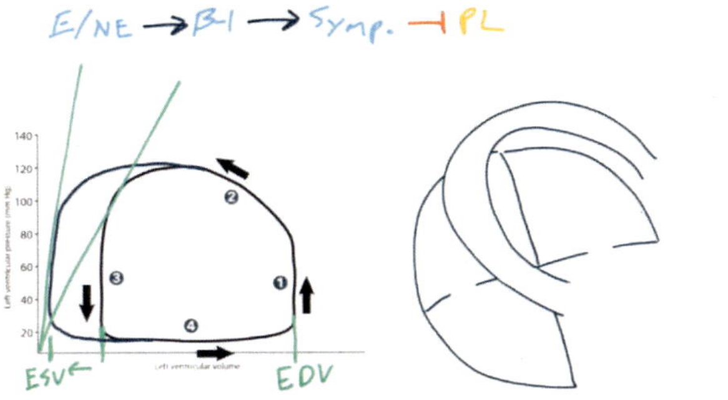

6. How would amyloidosis alter compliance and contractility on the PV loop?

- **Amyloidosis invades wall and decreases compliance, decreasing the ability of the LV to expand during diastole (diastolic heart failure)**
- **Decreased expansion means decreased preload (EDV shifts left on graph)**
- **Decreased compliance means higher pressure is reached faster (i.e. at a lower volume), causing the compliance line to rise**
- **Changes in compliance will not alter ESV or contractility**

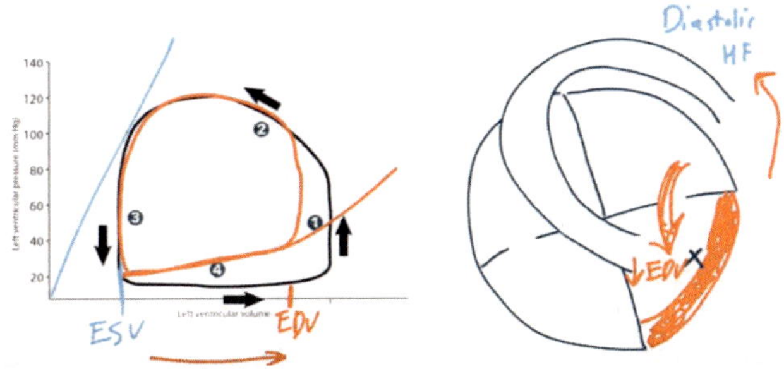

7. What would happen to contractility and compliance in a patient with mild congestive heart failure with severe anxiety?

- **EDV will increase as a result of increased compliance in mild systolic CHF**
  - **Note: In advanced CHF, ESV would increase as a result of inability to eject blood during systole**
- **ESV will decrease as a result increased contractility of increased sympathetic action on the heart (β_1 receptors)**

8. What would chronic hypertension do to the PV loop?

- **Chronic HTN causes increased afterload → decreased ability to eject blood during systole → increased ESV**
- **Increased afterload from HTN will also cause gradual hypertrophy of the LV → decreased LV compliance → PV loop will increase along y axis**
- **Contractility will not change**

9. How would ventricular dilatation alter the PV loop and why?

- **Dilatation will cause increased EDV**
- **With increased stretch on LV wall, stretching of sarcomeres will compensate for the dilatation, resulting in normal contractility (not increased contractility) → ESV will not change**

Section V - Heart Pressures

I. Pressures in the Heart

A. Systole

1. Left atrial pressure < 12 mmHg. This can be measured using a balloon catheter which can be inserted into the pulmonary artery and inflated. Once inflated, it estimates the left atrium, which lies adjacent to the pulmonary artery. This pressure doesn't change significantly during diastole, as can be seen on the pressure tracing of the left atrium.

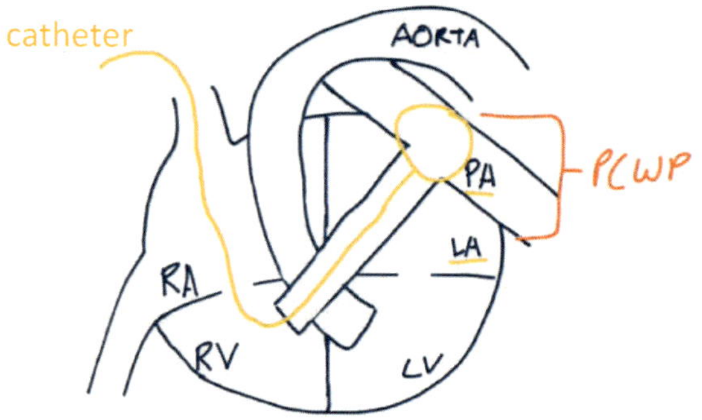

2. Left ventricular pressure is roughly 130 mmHg.
3. Right atrial pressure is roughly 5 mmHg. Like the left atrium, the pressure in the right atrium does not change significantly from systole to diastole.
4. Right ventricular pressure is roughly 25 mmHg.

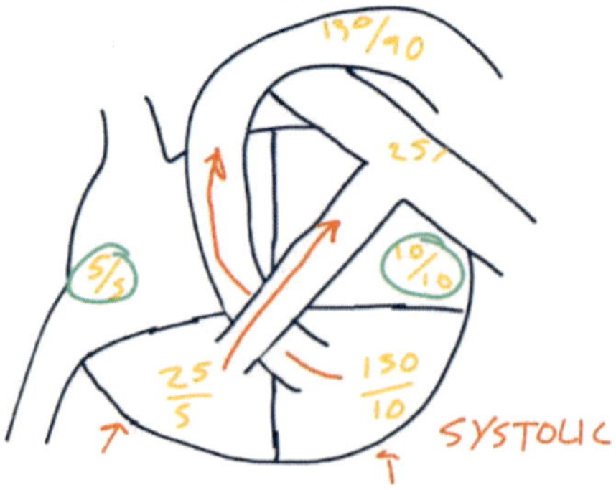

B. Diastole

1. Left ventricular pressure is roughly 10 mmHg.
2. Right ventricular pressure is roughly 5 mmHg.

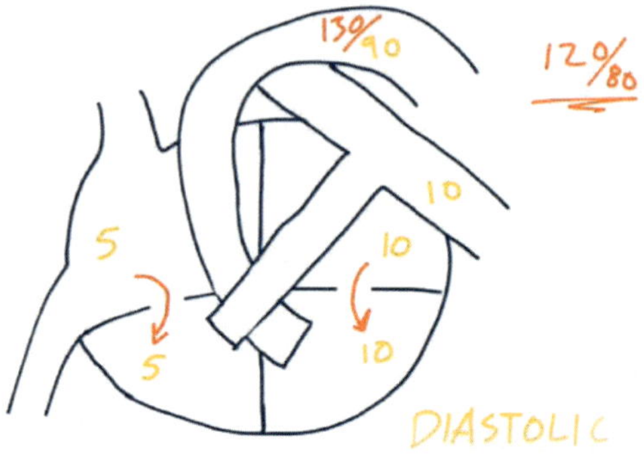

C. Pressures on the right side of the heart are typically lower than the left because the RV pumps blood into a lower resistant circuit (the pulmonary vasculature). The pulmonary vasculature is more compliant than the systemic circuit so the RV can maintain homeostasis with lower pressures (typically 1-30 mmHg with the lower spectrum occurring during diastole and the higher spectrum occurring during systole).

REVIEW QUESTIONS

1. How would heart pressures change in a patient with mitral stenosis?

- **During diastole, pressures in the LA and LV should be roughly the same (~10 mmHg)**
- **Mitral stenosis would increase LA pressure and decrease LV pressure**

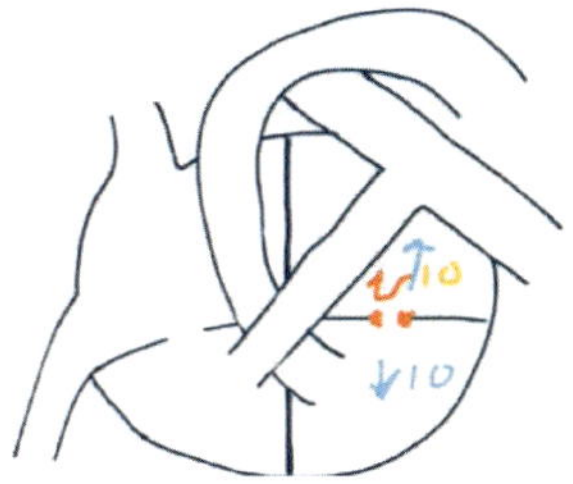

2. If left ventricular pressure increased significantly, what pathology would this implicate?

- **With increased LV pressure, aortic stenosis should be suspected**
- **Notice that aortic pressure would decrease**

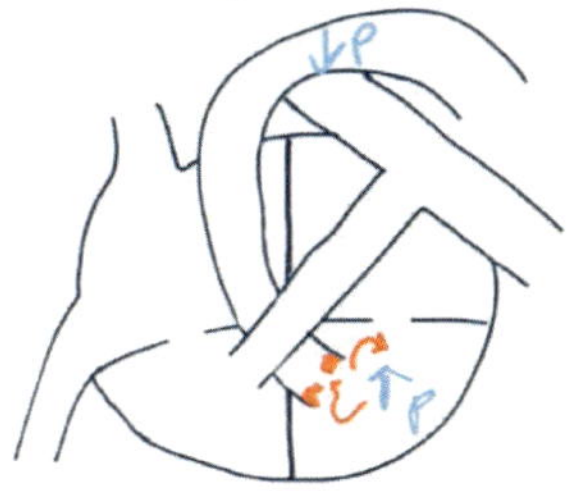

3. What would happen to heart pressures in a patient with a ventricular septal defect (VSD)?

- **Pressures in the left heart are higher than the right heart, so blood would travel from L→R through the VSD**
- **Increased blood in the RV (and subsequently RA), will cause increased pressures in these chambers**
- **Increased RV pressure results in increased pulmonary flow and ultimately increased LA pressure**
- **LV pressure will remain lower than normal**

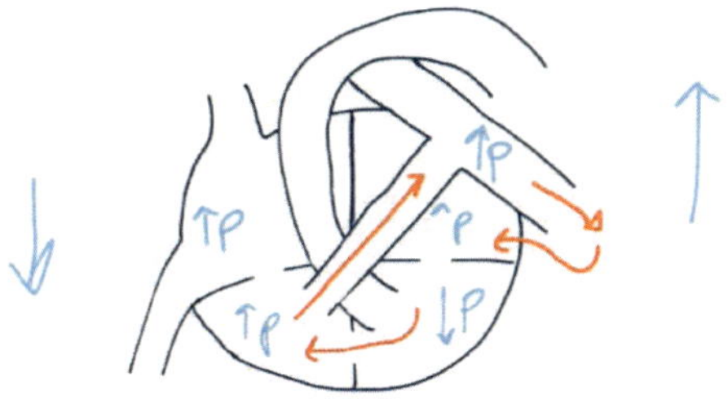

4. What would happen to heart pressure in a patient with an atrial septal defect (ASD)?

- **Pressures in the left heart are higher than the right heart, so blood would travel from L→R through the ASD**
- **Pressures in the RA and RV will increase, thereby increasing pulmonary flow**
- **Even with increased pulmonary blood flow, LA pressure (and subsequently the LV) will be lower than normal**

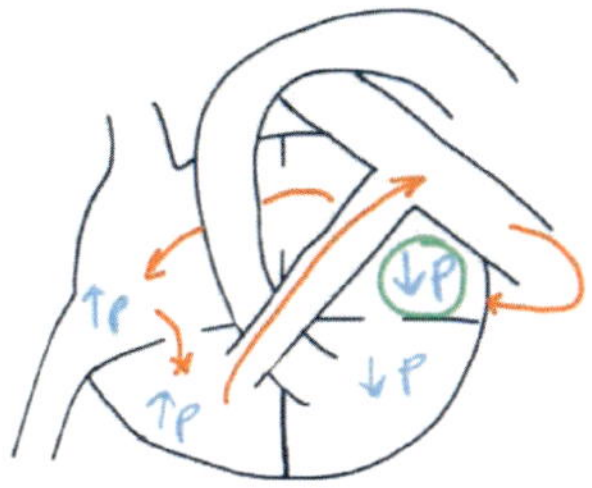

Section VI - Starling Curve and Cardiac/Vascular Function Curves

I. Starling Curve (Figure 2.8)

A. Starling curves graphically measure cardiac output (CO) as a function of preload.

1. CO increases as preload increases up to a point.

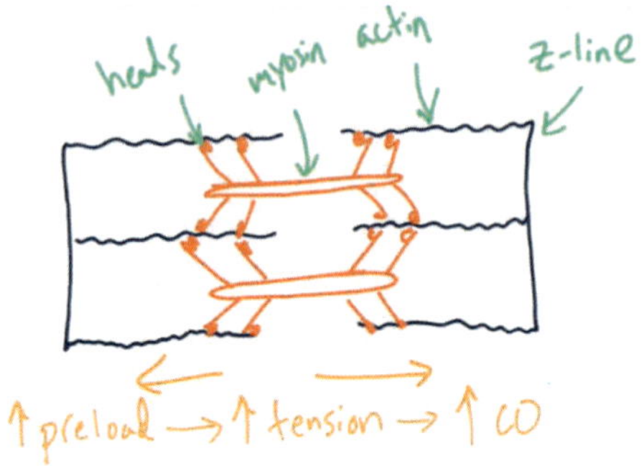

2. Changes in inotropy cause shifts in the Starling curve.

3. Changes in afterload cause shifts in the Starling curve.

B. Cardiac and Vascular Function Curves (Figure 2.9)

1. Measures venous return and cardiac output

2. The line with the positive slope represents cardiac output at increasing levels of end diastolic volume.

a) Inotropy and afterload cause the cardiac output curve to shift.

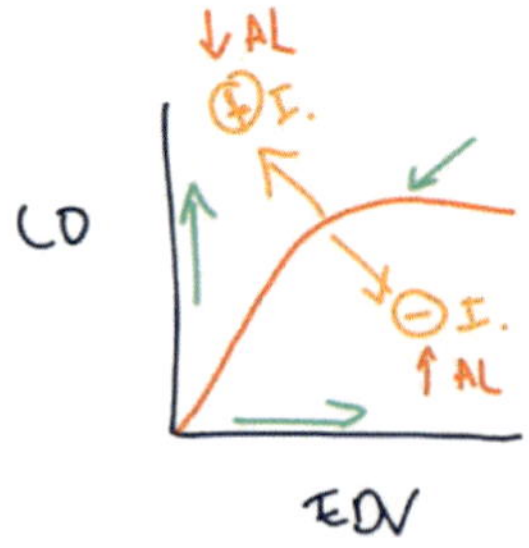

3. The line with the negative slope represents venous return at increasing levels of right atrial pressure (RAP).

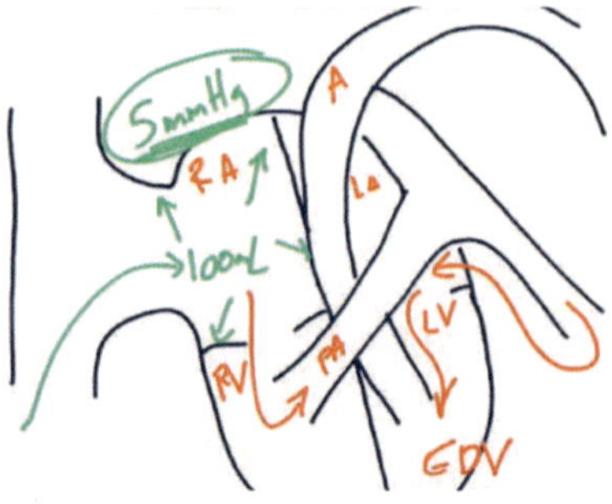

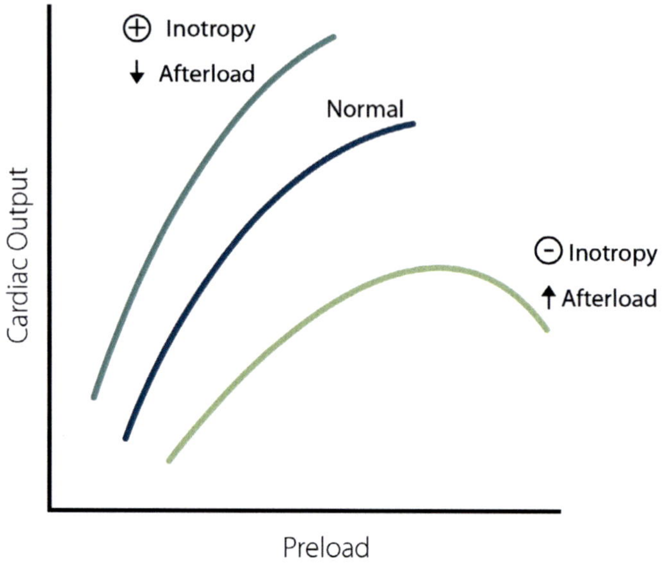

Figure 2.8 - Starling curve

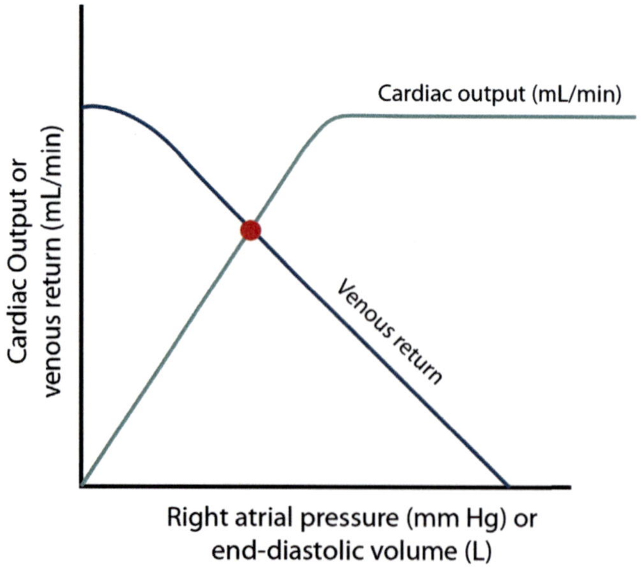

Figure 2.9 - Cardiac and vascular function curve

a) The slope of the venous return curve changes with changes in arterial resistance.

b) The mean systemic filling pressure (MSFP) is seen in figure 2.9 where the venous return curve intersects with the x-axis. MSFP is determined experimentally and can be measured in the right atrium when the cardiac output is zero.

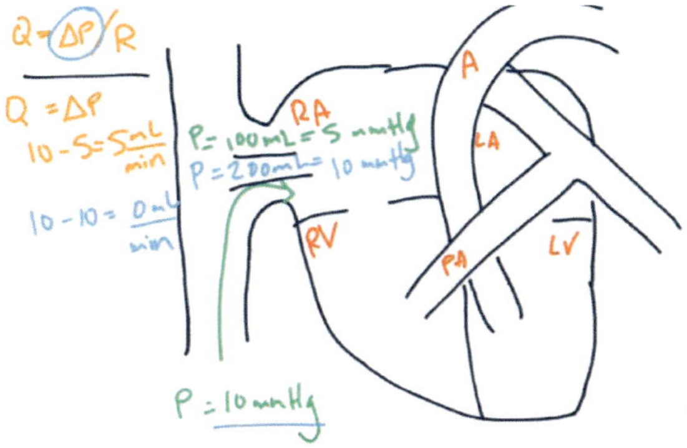

(1) Changes in blood volume result in changes in the MSFP and cause shifts in the venous return curve.

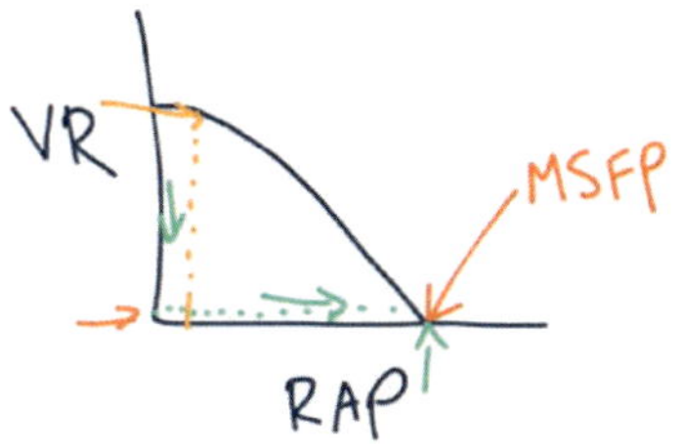

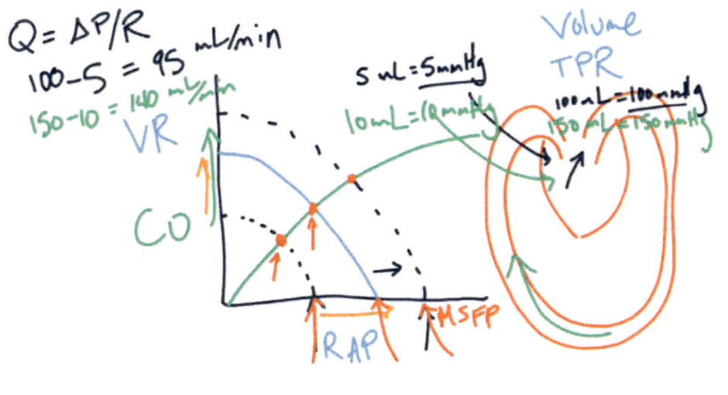

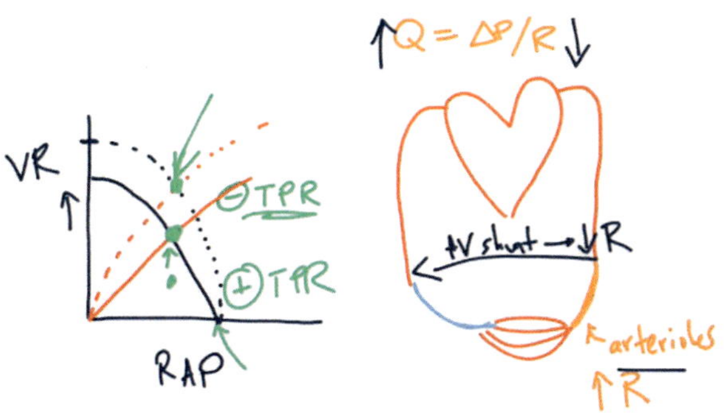

REVIEW QUESTIONS

1. How would an infusion of catecholamines alter the cardiac and vascular function curve?

- **Catecholamines → ↑ intracellular calcium → ↑ contractility/inotropy → ↑ cardiac output**
- **As cardiac output ↑, blood in the right atrium ↓ → ↑ pressure gradient between periphery and heart → ↑ venous return**

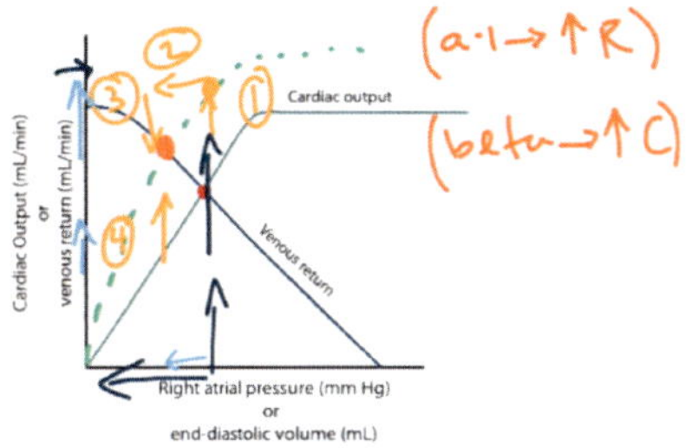

2. How would the cardiac and vascular function curve be altered in a patient with jugular venous distention and known congestive heart failure?

- **Decompensated CHF → ↓ cardiac output →↓ renal perfusion → ↑ RAAS → ↑ volume → ↑ preload and mean systemic filling pressure (MSFP)**
- **↑ right atrial pressure → ↓ pressure gradient from periphery to heart → ↓ venous return**

Compensation - normal CO
1) ↑ Sympathetic
2) ↑ Volume
3) Hypertrophy

decompensation
↓ CO

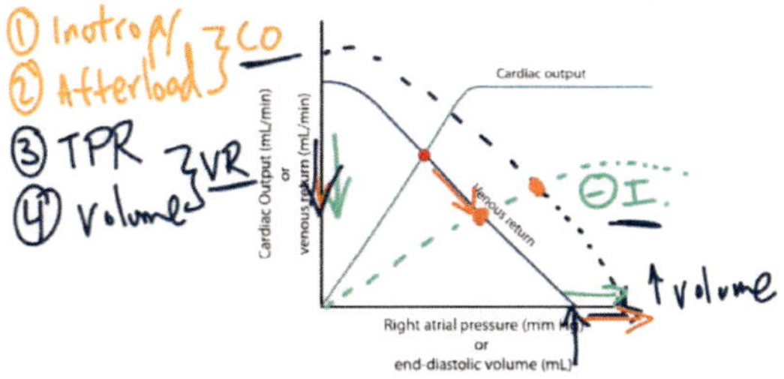

Section VII - Cardiac Pressure Tracings

I. Pressure Tracing (Figure 2.10)

A. Pressure tracings are a way to graphically measure the pressures in the left atrium, left ventricle, and aorta during a single cardiac cycle.

B. Pressure tracings are commonly used to examine valvular abnormalities.

1. Mitral regurgitation
2. Mitral stenosis
3. Aortic stenosis
4. Aortic regurgitation

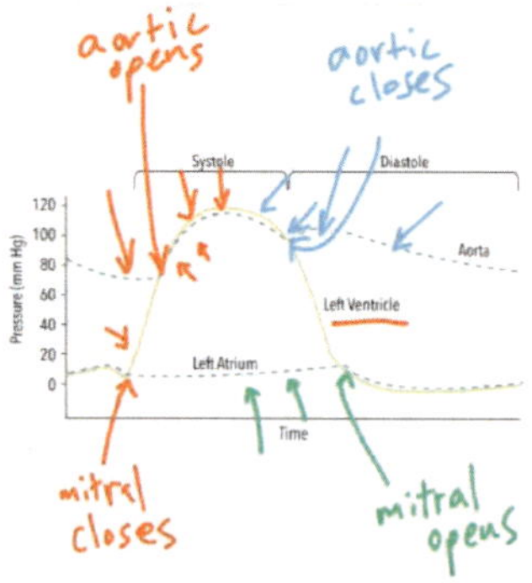

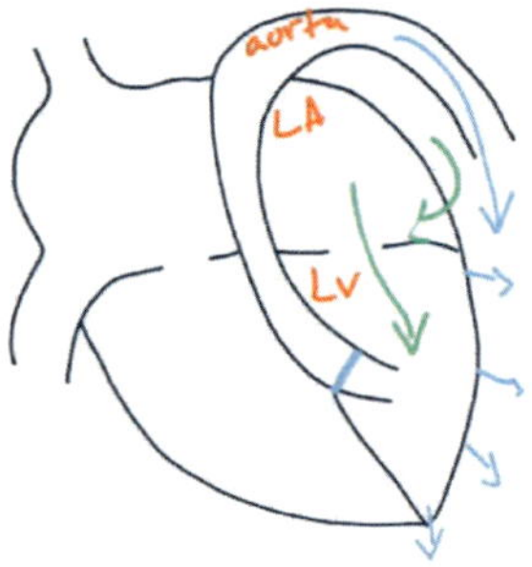

C. Jugular Venous Pulse (JVP)

1. The JVP is measured by placing the tip of a central line near the right atrium.
2. The central line can detect changes in pressure near this region and can produce a waveform known as the JVP.
3. Increases in pressure cause positive slopes on the JVP waveform.
4. Decreases in pressure cause negative slopes on the JVP waveform.

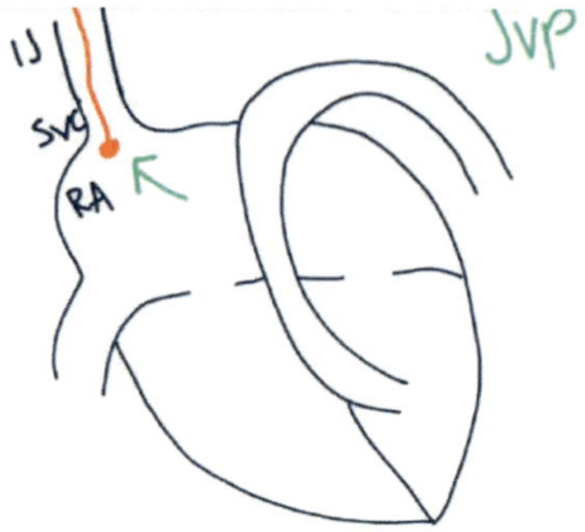

5. Waves
   a) The a wave is caused by right atrial contraction.
   b) The c wave is caused by closure of the tricuspid valve.
   c) The x wave is caused by right atrial relaxation.
   d) The v wave is caused by filling of the right atrium.

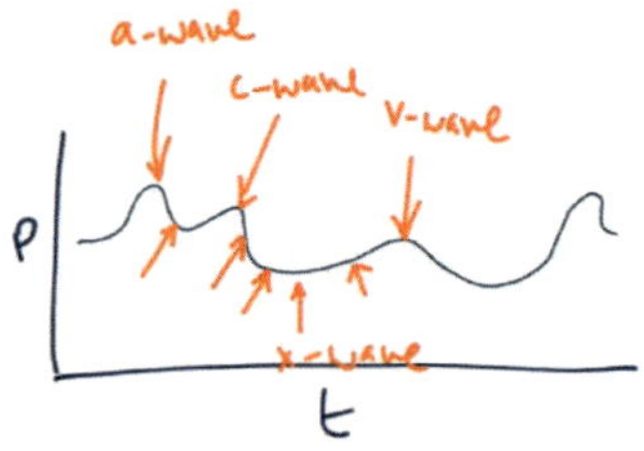

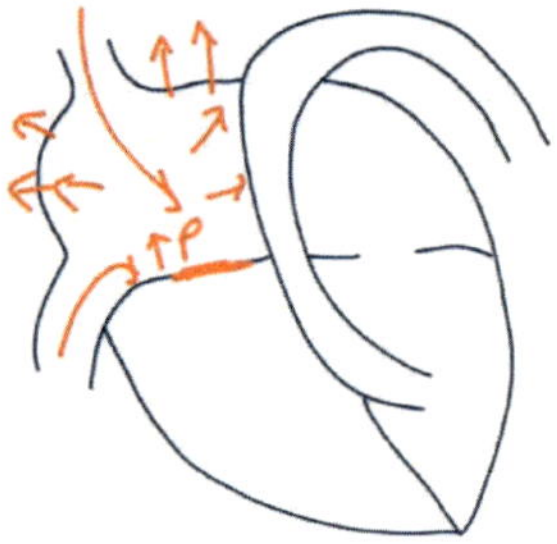

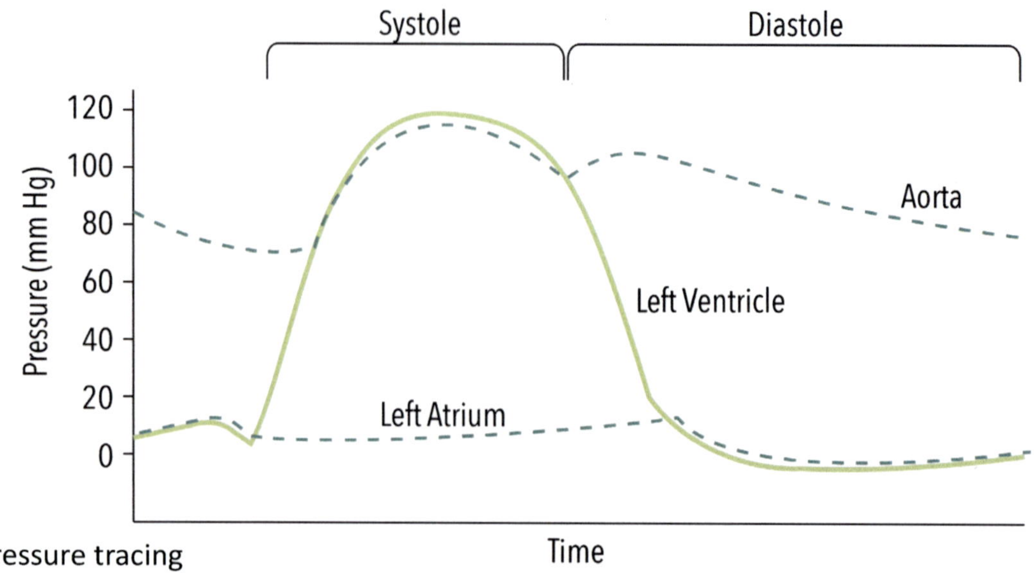

Figure 2.10 - Pressure tracing

e) The y wave is caused by emptying of the right atrium.

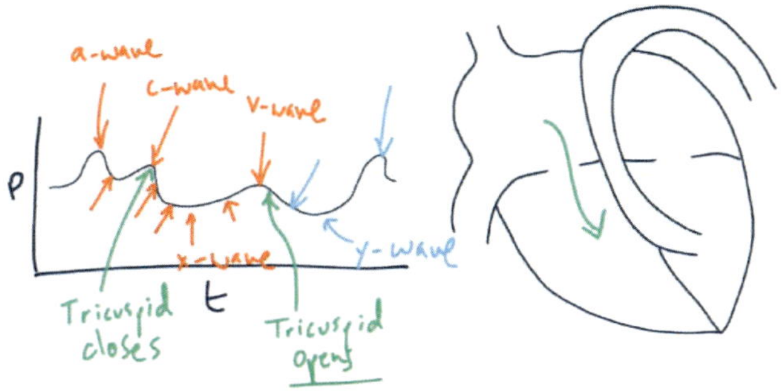

REVIEW QUESTIONS

1. How would the pressure tracing figure change in a patient with mitral regurgitation?

- **Mitral regurgitation → ↑ blood volume enters left atrium during systole → ↑ left atrial pressure during systole**

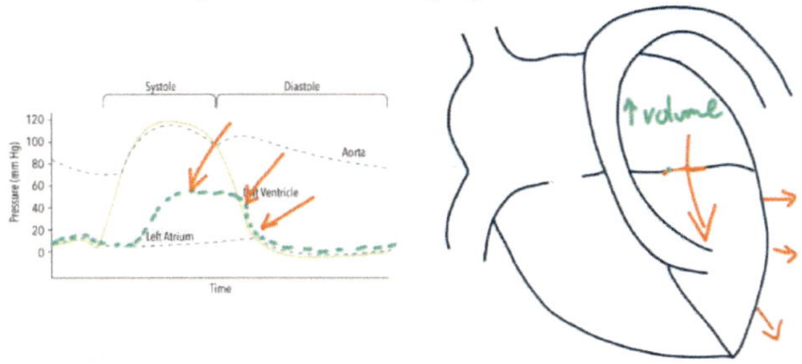

2. How would the pressure tracing figure change in a patient with mitral stenosis?

- **Mitral stenosis → ↓ blood moves from the left atrium to the left ventricle → ↑ blood/ pressure in left atrium during systole and diastole**

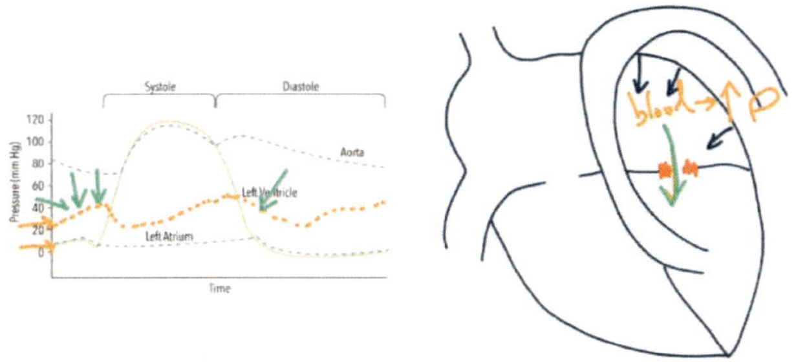

3. What microbe is most commonly associated with a pressure tracing indicating mitral stenosis?

- **Group A beta hemolytic streptococcus**
- **Early infection → mitral regurgitation**
- **Chronic infection → mitral stenosis**

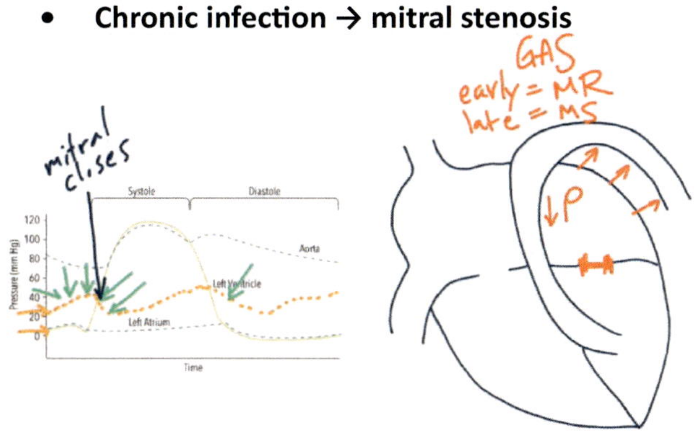

REVIEW QUESTIONS

4. How would the pressure tracing figure change in a patient with aortic regurgitation?

- **In aortic regurgitation, blood leaks from the aorta to the LV during diastole**
- **↓ blood in the aorta during diastole → ↓ aortic pressure during diastole**
- **↑ blood in the LV → ↑ LV pressure during diastole**

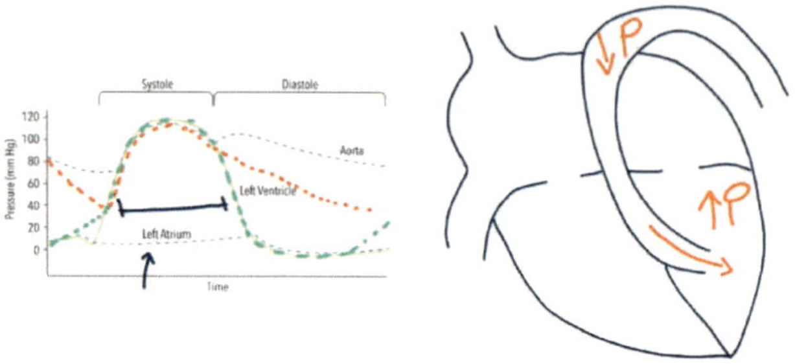

5. During what part of a pressure tracing figure indicating aortic regurgitation would you be able to hear the regurgitant murmur if you placed a stethoscope on the patient's left sternal border?

- **Aortic regurgitation → diastolic murmur → heard during diastole (refer to yellow line shown in image below)**

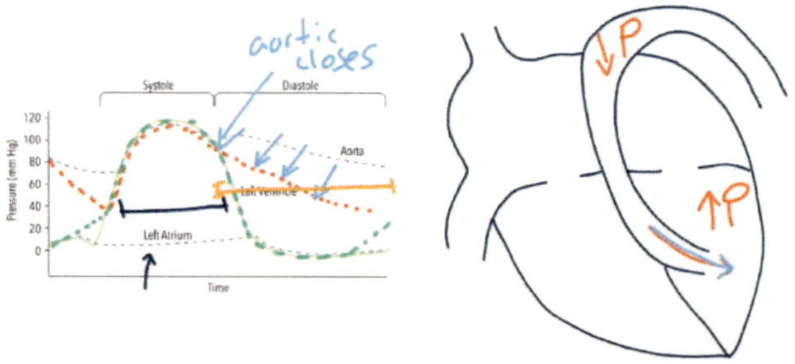

6. Why does head bobbing occur in patients with aortic regurgitation?

- **Blood leaks from aorta → LV**
- **↑ preload → ↑ stroke volume → ↑ blood volume entering carotid arteries → head bobbing**

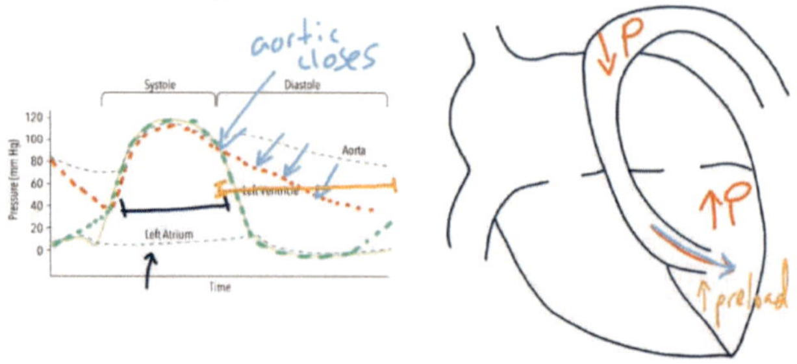

7. How would the pressure tracing figure change in a patient with aortic stenosis?

- **In aortic stenosis there is ↓ blood leaving the LV during systole**
- **With a stenotic aortic valve the pressure in the LV must ↑ more than normal to overcome the pressure in the aorta → ↑ LV systolic pressure**

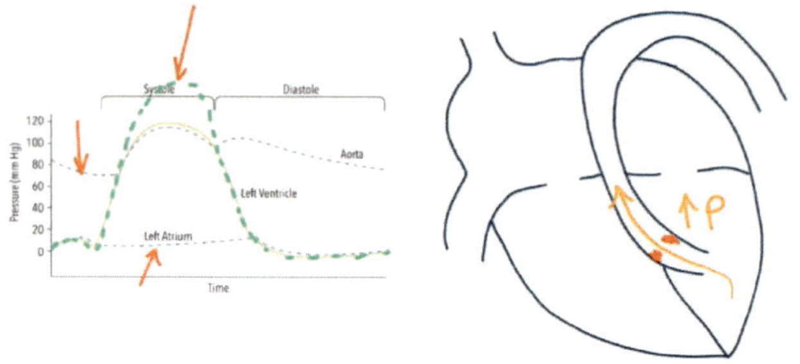

8. When would blood flow through the coronary arteries be the highest in a normal pressure tracing figure?

- **The blood flow equation is Q = ΔP / R**
- **The pressure is highest in the aorta just after the aortic valve closes. The pressure in the coronary arteries is lowest here because the blood has been emptying into the coronary sinus**
- **Thus, during diastole (just after the aortic valve closes) the pressure gradient is greatest → flow is greatest**

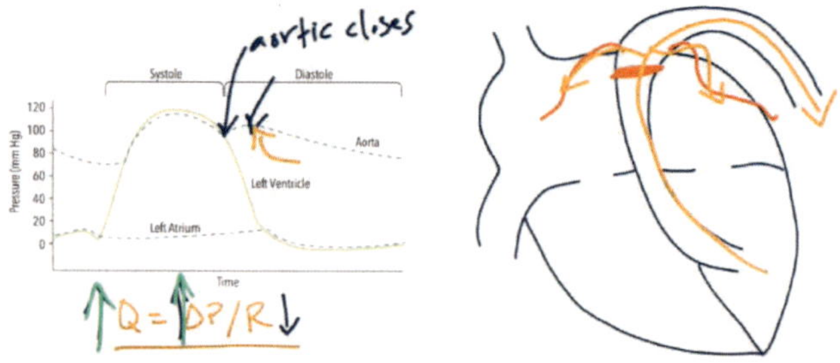

REVIEW QUESTIONS

9. How would pulmonary hypertension alter the JVP waveform?

- **Pulm HTN → right-sided hypertrophy → ↓ space within the heart → ↑ pressure and ↑ resistance**
- **↑ pressure during atrial contraction → ↑ A-wave**
- **↑ resistance → blood has a harder time emptying from the right atrium into the right ventricle → ↑ Y-wave**

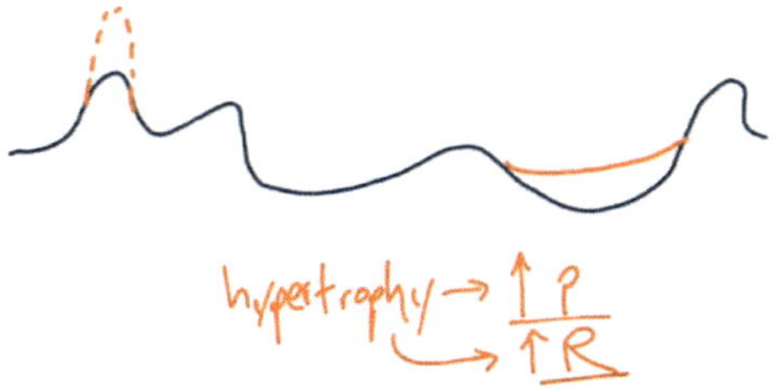

10. What electrical heart problem may result in a-waves similar to those seen in pulmonary hypertension?

- **Third degree heart block**
- **The atria and ventricles beat independently from one another.**
- **As the atria contracts against a closed tricuspid valve → ↑ pressure in the right atrium → cannon a-waves (green dotted drawing).**

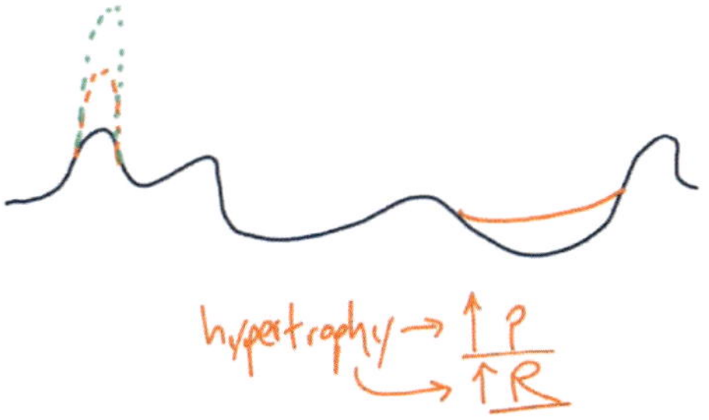

11. How would atrial fibrillation alter the JVP waveform?

- **A-fib → atria is not contracting → absent a-wave**
- **Atria is unable to relax properly → less steep x-wave**

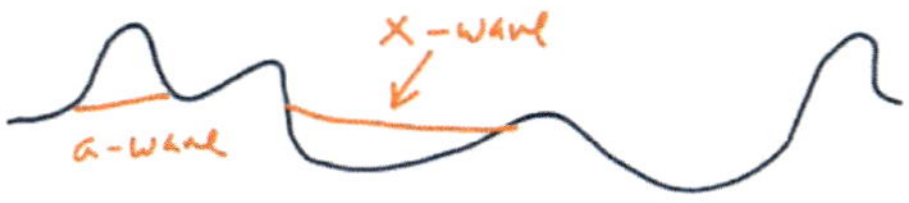

12. How would tricuspid regurgitation alter the JVP waveform?

- **C-wave represents closure of the tricuspid valve**
- **X-wave represents atrial relaxation.**
- **Tricuspid regurgitation → blood moves from RV to RA → ↑ blood/pressure in RA → ↑ x-wave**

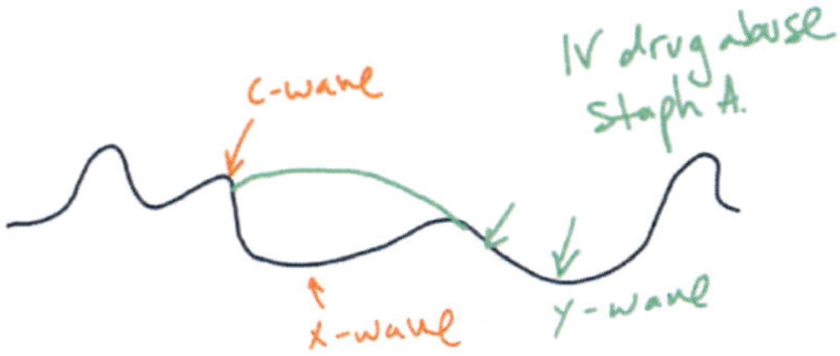

Section VIII - Baroreflex and Cardiovascular Changes

I. Baroreceptor Reflex

A. Responds to changes in blood pressure to help maintain a normotensive state

B. Composed of the carotid sinus (CN IX) and the aortic arch (CN X).

C. Considered upregulated when the efferent limb of CN IX and X are inhibited (e.g. decreased stimulation of CN X will increase heart rate and contractility. This is considered initiation of the baroreceptor reflex).

D. Increased blood pressure → increased firing of the afferent limbs of CN IX and X → increased stimulation of the nucleus tractus solitarius in medulla of brain → increased efferent firing of CN X → decreased sympathetic stimulation of the heart and vasculature throughout body

E. Decreased blood pressure → decreased stretching of vessels → decreased firing rate of the afferent fibers of CN IX and CN X → decreased stimulation of the nucleus tractus solitarius in the medulla of the brain → decreased medullary stimulation of efferent CN X → increased sympathetic firing to the heart and vasculature throughout body

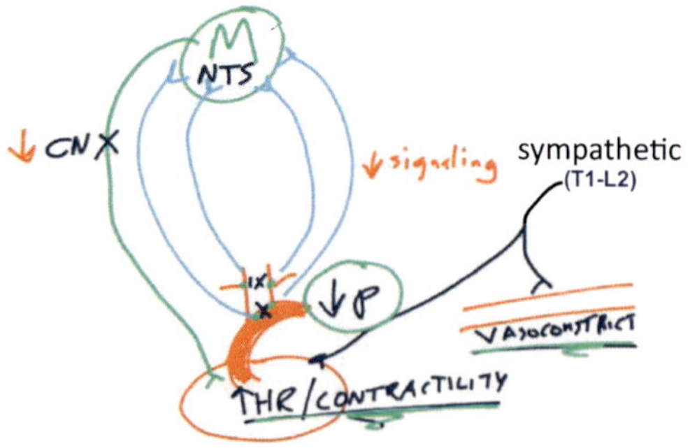

F. Responses to the supine position

1. Blood pools in the veins due to their high compliance. This increases the capillary pressure which can lead to edema.

2. The relaxation of skeletal muscles decreases the movement of blood from the venous system to the heart → decreased preload and cardiac output

G. Responses to standing

1. There will be a decrease in blood pressure → decreased carotid sinus afferent nerve firing → increased sympathetic response → vasoconstriction of arterioles and veins → increased blood pressure

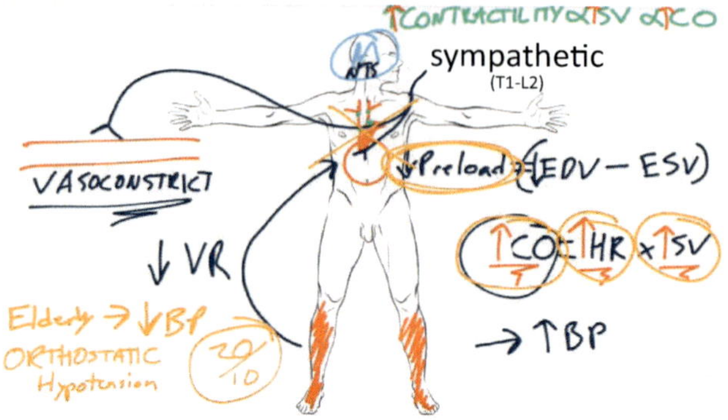

II. Chemoreceptor Reflex

A. Include central (ventrolateral medulla) and peripheral (aortic and carotid) chemoreceptors

B. Peripheral chemoreceptors

1. Stimulated by increased CO_2, decreased O_2, decreased pH → sympathetic stimulation of heart and vasculature (and lungs)

C. Central chemoreceptors

1. Stimulated by increased CO_2 and decreased pH → sympathetic stimulation of heart and vasculature (and lungs)

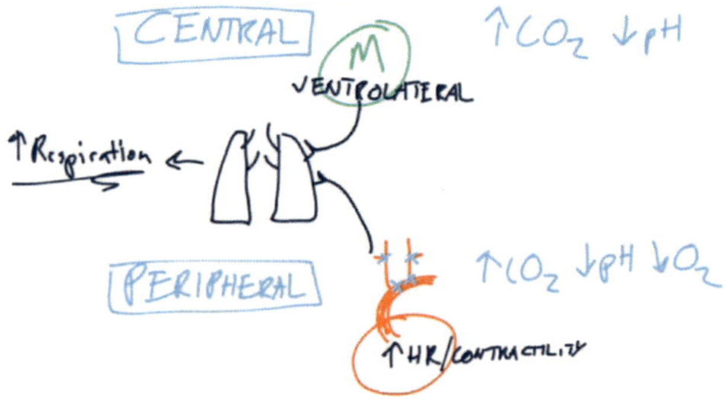

III. Cardiovascular Autonomics

A. Sympathetic

1. Heart: β_1 receptors on SA and AV nodes → increased heart rate and contractility

2. Arteries

a) Skeletal muscle arteries:

(1) α_1 receptor stimulation → vasoconstriction

(2) β_2 receptors stimulation → vasodilation

(3) At rest, α_1 receptors dominate → overall vasoconstriction

(4) During exercise, local metabolic factors inhibit α_1 receptors and dilate local arteries → overall vasodilation

b) Visceral arteries: α_1 receptor stimulation → vasoconstriction

3. Veins: α_1 receptor stimulation → vasoconstriction → increased venous return to right atrium
4. Visceral Vasculature and Skin: α_1 receptor stimulation → vasoconstriction → blood shunted away from visceral organs and skin
5. Sympathetic stimulation of the adrenal medulla → increased release of catecholamines → increased sympathetic response throughout body
6. Overall: increased total peripheral resistance (TPR) and increased heart activity

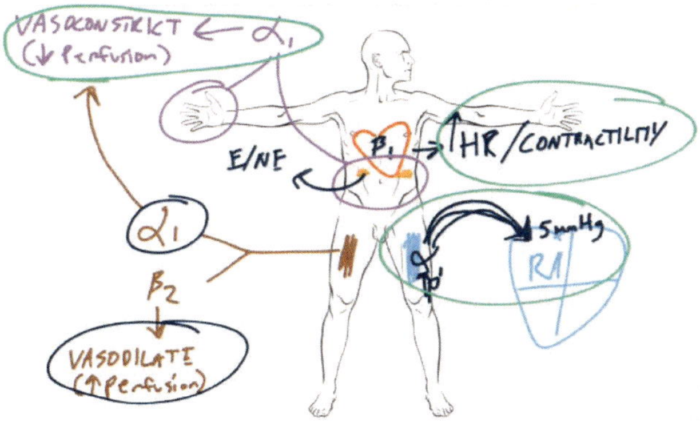

B. Parasympathetic

1. Heart: M_2 receptor stimulation → decreased heart rate and contractility
2. Visceral Vasculature: M_3 receptor stimulation → increased blood flow to internal organs

IV. Metabolic Demand

A. Increased metabolic demand

1. Means more ATP is being used up and is converted to adenosine → increased adenosine causes vasodilation
2. Lower levels of ATP → decreased Na^+/K^+ pump activity → increased extracellular K^+, which causes vasodilation
3. Glucose is being used for energy → CO_2 is produced → CO_2 then causes vasodilation
4. Insufficient O_2 → more glucose shunted to fermentation, producing lactate → increased lactate → increased vasodilation
5. Adenosine, K^+, CO_2, and lactate will increase vasodilation of surrounding vessels → more blood will flow to the tissue (active hyperemia) → increased oxygen consumption from tissues → cells able to keep up with increased metabolic demand

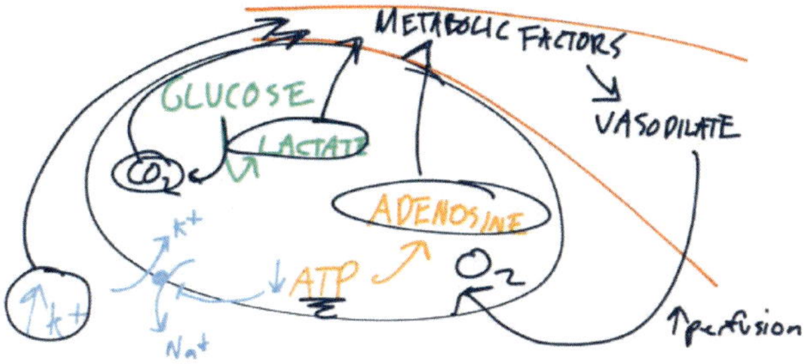

V. Hyperemia

A. Increase in blood flow to an organ

1. There are two types

a) Active: the blood flow to a given organ is determined by its metabolic demand (CO_2, adenosine, lactate, K^+).

b) Reactive: the blood flow to an organ is increased following an occlusive event (e.g. ventricular systole, skeletal muscle flexion).

VI. Circulations

A. Coronary circulation

1. Active hyperemia

a) Increased contractility → increased metabolic demand of myocardium → vasodilation of coronary arteries → increased perfusion of myocardium, especially in diastole when coronary vessels are not compressed

b) Adenosine and CO_2 are the most important metabolic factors.

2. Reactive hyperemia

a) Ventricular contraction during systole → increased ventricular pressure → compression of coronary arteries → decreased perfusion during systole → reactive hyperemia during diastole

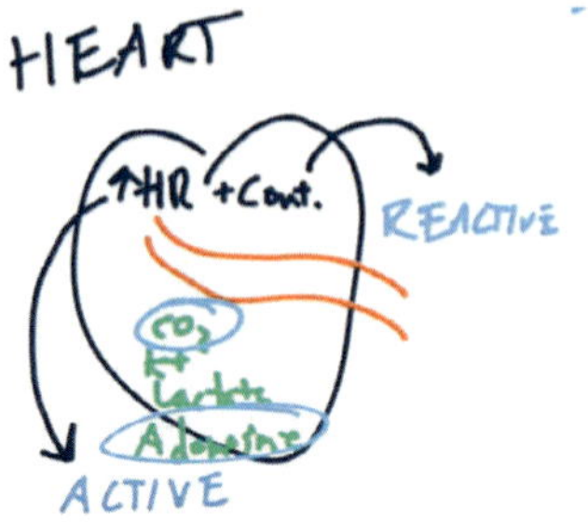

B. Cerebral circulation

1. Active hyperemia

    a) CO_2 is the most important metabolic factor.

        1. Decreased perfusion → syncope

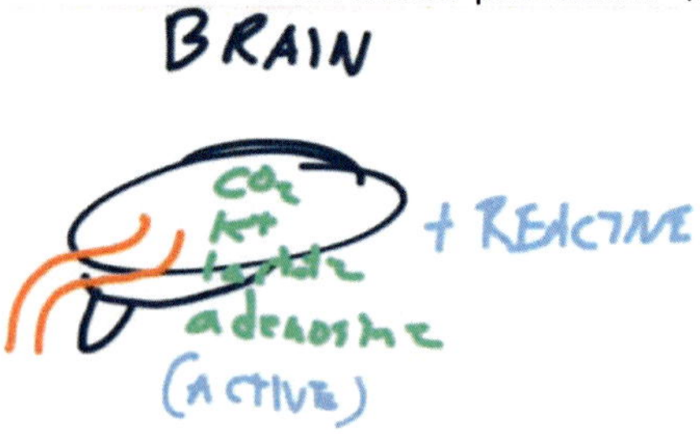

C. Skeletal muscle

1. Active hyperemia.
2. Reactive hyperemia.
3. Sympathetic stimulation of α_1 (constrict) and β_2 (dilate) receptors.

    a) β_2 receptor effect dominates during exercise → decreased TPR

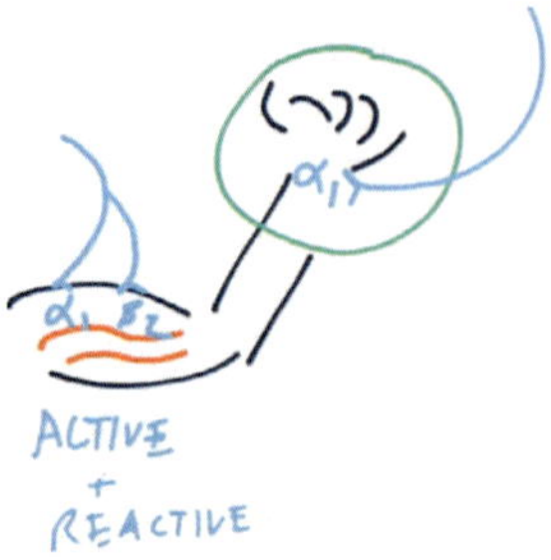

D. Skin

1. Sympathetic nerves play large role.
2. Trauma causes dilation from histamine release.

VII. Blood Alterations and Responses

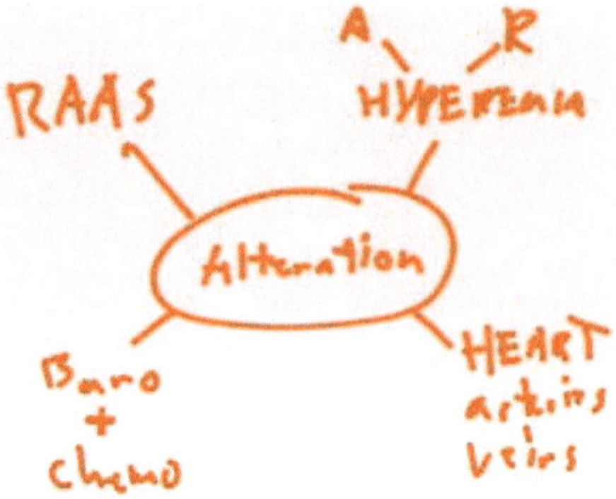

A. Exercise

1. Hyperemia

    a) Active

        (1) Increased metabolic demand of skeletal myofibers → increased K^+, CO_2, adenosine, and lactate → vasodilation → increased perfusion of skeletal muscle tissues and greater filtration of blood into lymph

    b) Reactive

        (1) During each contraction of the skeletal muscle, arteries feeding the muscle are momentarily occluded → reactive hyperemia

2. Heart and vasculature

    a) Increased sympathetic activity →

        (1) β_1 receptor stimulation of SA and AV nodes → increased heart rate and contractility

        (2) α_1 receptor stimulation of veins → vasoconstriction → increased venous return to heart → increased preload and cardiac output

        (3) β_2 receptor stimulation of arteries in the skeletal muscle → arteriole vasodilation → increased pressure reaches capillaries → increased skeletal muscle perfusion

3. Hormonal changes

    a) Hypoxia during exercise → upregulation of vascular endothelial growth factor (VEGF) from the endothelial cells → increased production of capillaries

4. Overall, exercise causes vasodilation of arteries feeding the skeletal muscles, which decreases total peripheral resistance.

B. Blood loss

1. Local changes

a) At the site of vessel damage, endothelin will be released → vasoconstriction to prevent further blood loss at the site

2. Baroreceptor reflex

a) Hypovolemia → decreased stretch on baroreceptor fibers → decreased stimulation of CN X and increased sympathetic firing to blood vessels and heart

(1) → increased heart rate and contractility (β_1 receptors) → increased CO

(2) → vasoconstriction of veins (α_1 receptor) → increased venous return

(3) → vasoconstriction of arteries (α_1 receptor) → increased TPR and more blood reserved for heart and brain → decreased perfusion of skin and visceral organs

3. RAAS

a) Increased activity of the Renin-Angiotensin-Aldosterone System (RAAS) → increased H_2O and Na^+ reabsorption → increased blood pressure

b) Increased release of ADH → increased H_2O reabsorption from collecting duct → increased blood pressure

c) ADH also causes vasoconstriction → increased blood pressure

C. Shock

1. Hypovolemic shock

a) Decreased blood pressure

(1) Decreased stretch on baroreceptors → decreased parasympathetic action on heart → increased sympathetic action→ increased CO, venous return and widespread arterial vasoconstriction

(2) Decreased renal perfusion → stimulation of RAAS.

2. Cardiogenic shock

a) Decreased CO

(1) Decreased stretch on baroreceptors → decreased parasympathetic action on heart → increased sympathetic action→ increased preload and afterload, venous return and widespread arterial vasoconstriction

(2) → stimulation of RAAS

REVIEW QUESTIONS

1. What would happen to the baroreflex in a patient with acute decompensated heart failure?

   - **Decreased CO results in decreased stretch of baroreceptors, resulting in decreased stimulation of the NTS in the medulla and decreased parasympathetic activity on the heart (i.e. decreased baroreflex)**
   - **Decreased parasympathetic activity results in a relative increase in sympathetic activity originating from spinal cord levels T1-L2**

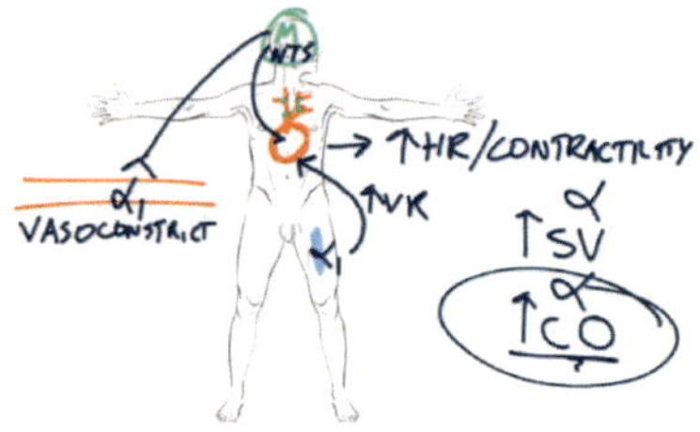

2. What would a carotid massage do to the baroreflex?

   - **Carotid massage mimics increased blood pressure on baroreceptors (specifically those located in the carotids: CN IX receptors and afferents)**
   - **NTS of medulla sends signal out through CN X, thereby decreases heart rate and contractility**

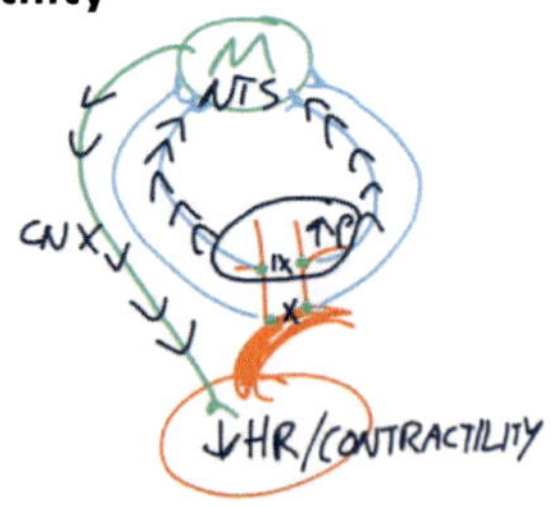

3. During repetitive weight lifting, does the muscle tissue receive blood from active or reactive hyperemia?

   - **Transient compression of the vessel during weight lifting results in reactive hyperemia**
   - **Exercise also creates metabolic byproducts which dilate the vessels (active hyperemia)**

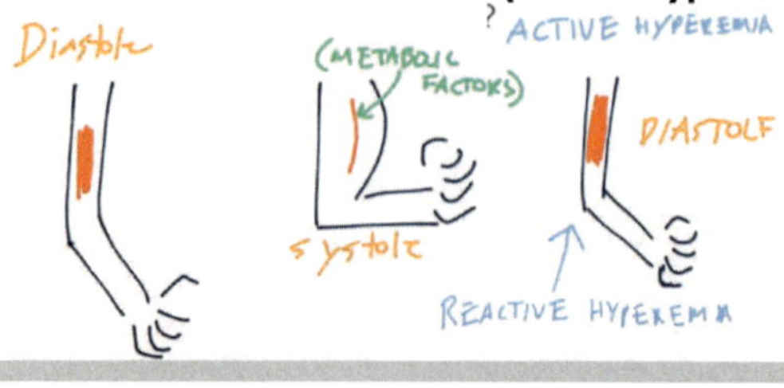

4. What would aortic stenosis do to the concentration of adenosine in the coronary arteries?

   - **Aortic stenosis results in increased stroke work, thereby increasing metabolic demand and release metabolic factors: adenosine and CO_2**

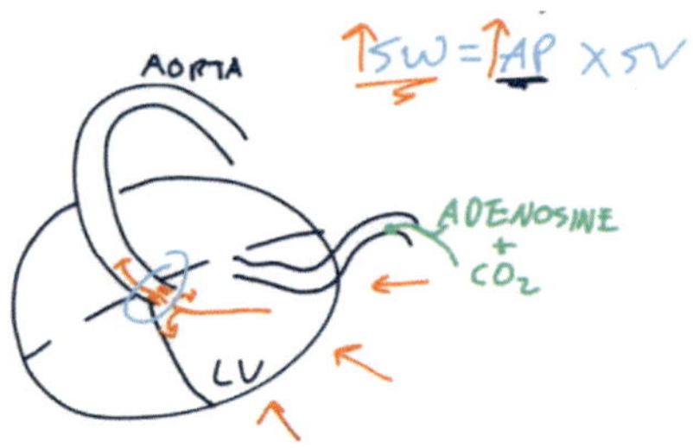

5. How could severe vomiting cause syncope?

   - **Severe vomiting increases pressure on baroreceptors**
   - **Sudden increased parasympathetic activity can decrease heart rate and contractility can cause decreased brain perfusion and syncope**
   - **Likewise, in moments of intense and sudden fear, the baroreflex can be extreme enough to cause syncope**

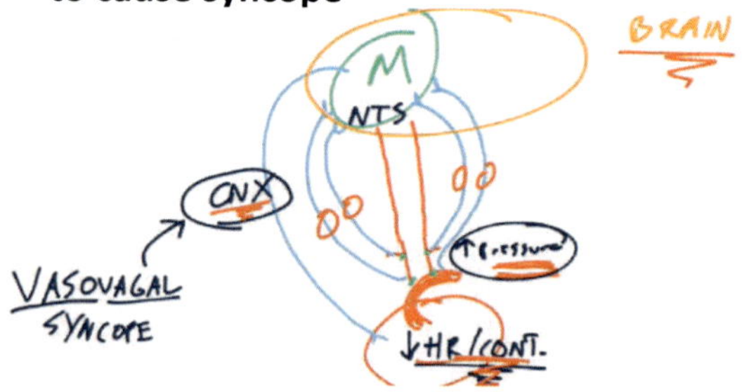

6. What would a large, rapid bolus of IV fluid do to heart rate? What would happen to HR if the IV fluid was administered slowly?

   - **A bolus is able to put pressure on the baroreceptors, decreasing heart rate. Slow administration is unable to do this.**

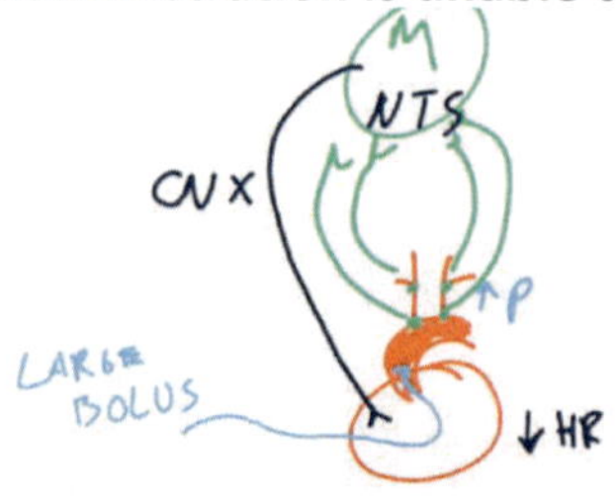

Section IX - Heart Sounds and Murmurs

I. Heart Sounds

Normal Heart Sounds

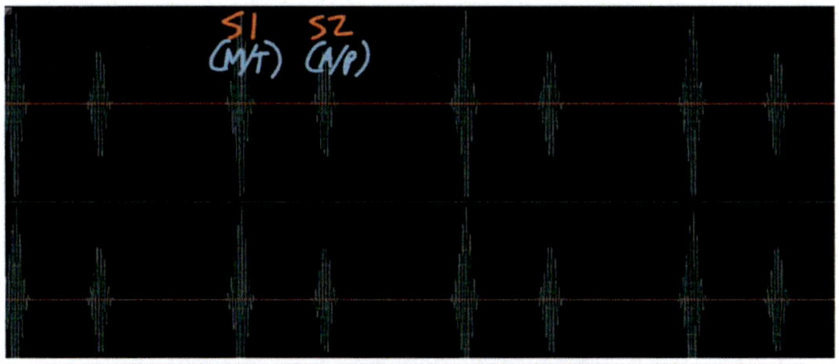

- S1 occurs when the mitral and tricuspid valves close
- S2 occurs when the aortic and pulmonic valves close
- S2 splitting can occur as the aortic and pulmonic valves close at different times

Pressue-Volume Loop

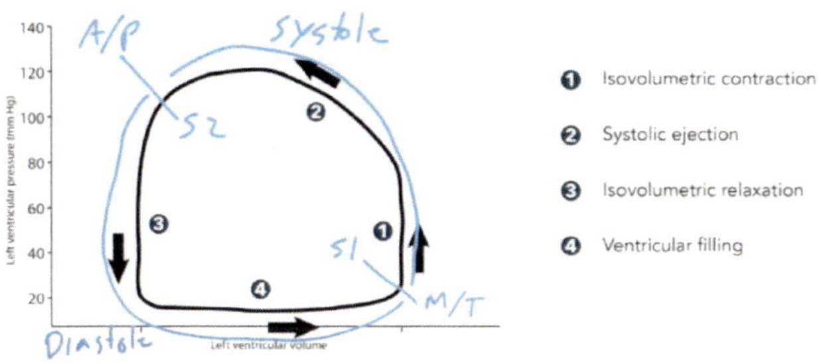

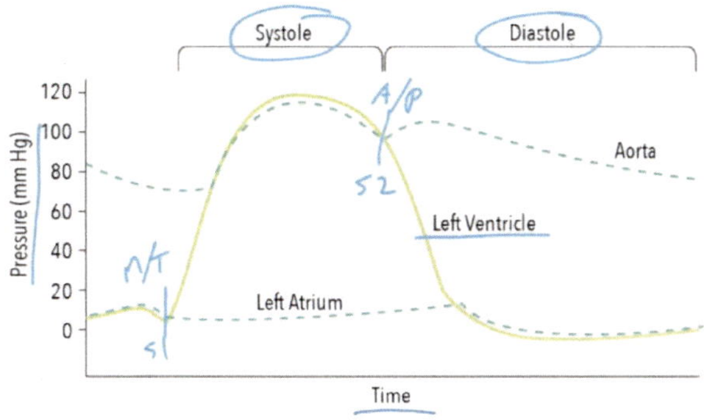

A. The first normal noticeable heart sound as the heart cycles through systole and diastole is referred to as S1. S1 is heard when the mitral and tricuspid valves close during systole as blood leaves the ventricles and pushes these valves shut.

B. The second normal noticeable heart sound as the heart cycles through systole and diastole is referred to as S2. S2 is heard when the aortic and pulmonic valves close.

S2 Splitting

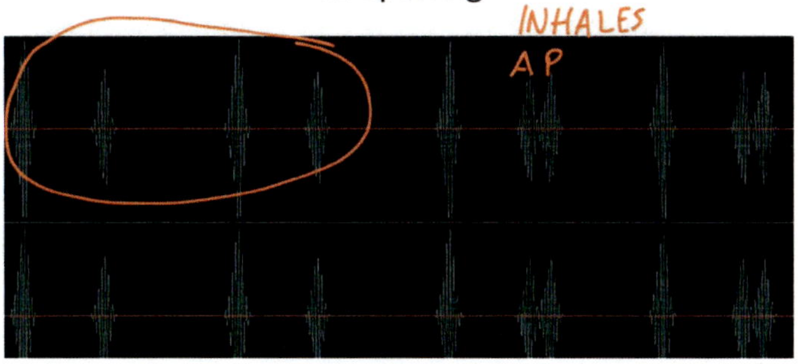

1. S2 can further be divided into A2 and P2. A2 refers to the aortic valve and P2 refers to the pulmonic valve.
2. S2 can normally be auscultated as two separate sounds upon inspiration due to the slight differences in time when the aortic and pulmonic valves close.

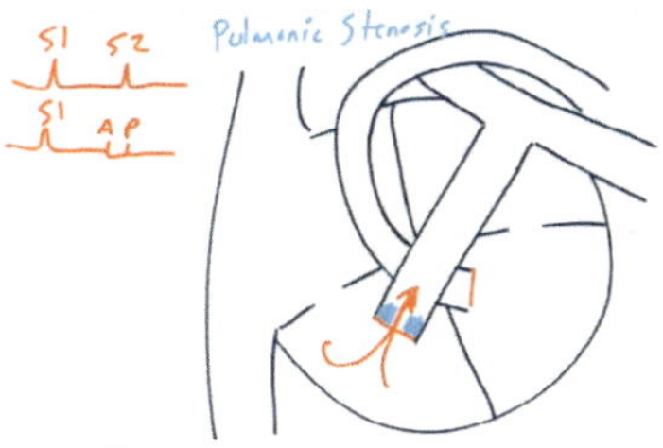

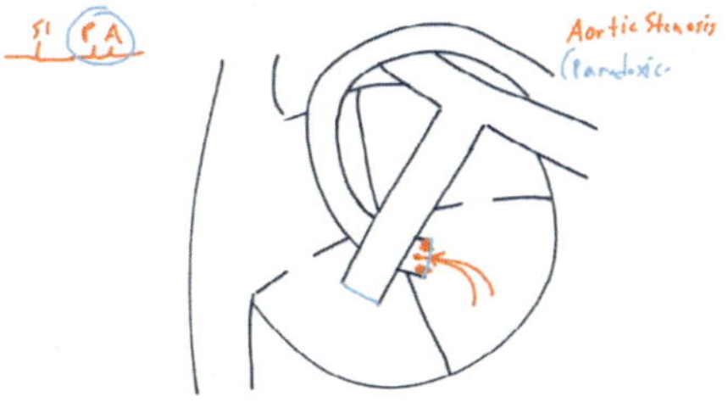

a) During inspiration the diaphragm moves downward resulting in increased space in the thoracic cavity → drop in intrathoracic pressure → vessels are compressed less allowing more blood to enter the right side of the heart → more blood must leave the RV compared to the LV so the pulmonic valve closes slightly after the aortic valve

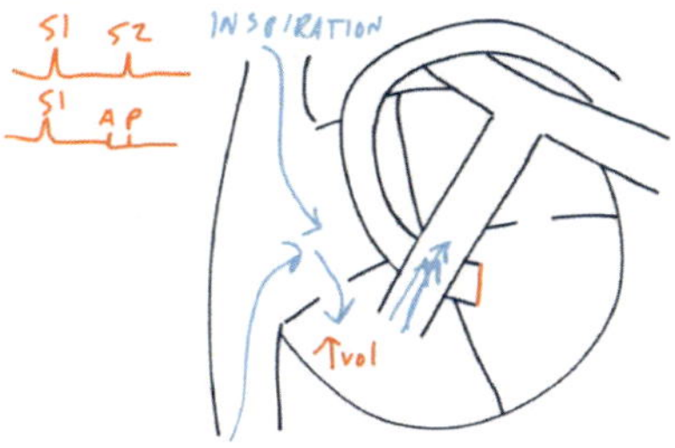

C. S3 is due to the ventricles reaching maximal compliance resulting in a sudden decrease in blood velocity and is pathologic in adults. Can be normal in children.

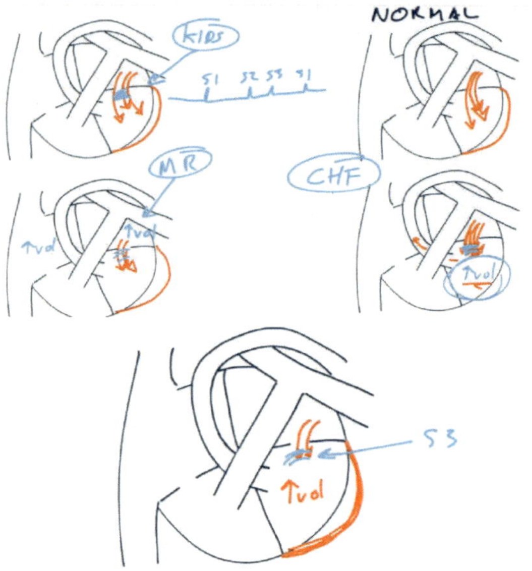

D. S4 is due to turbulent blood flowing against stiffened ventricles. It is commonly associated with chronic hypertension with resultant ventricular hypertrophy. Can be relatively benign in the elderly but is never normal, even in children.

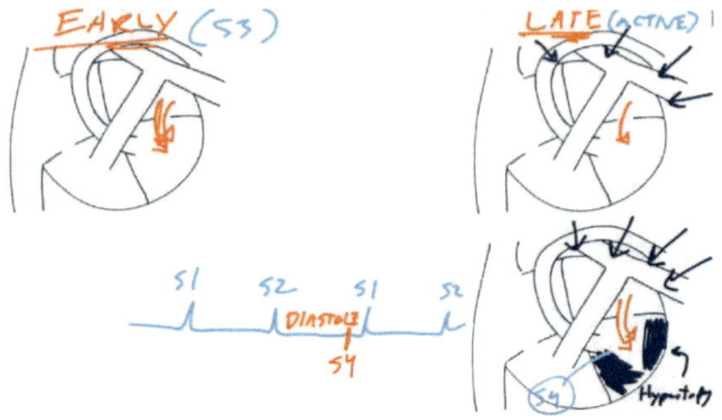

E. Systolic murmurs

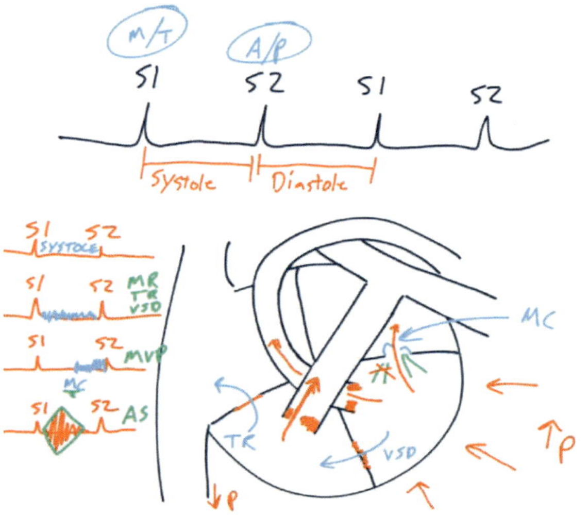

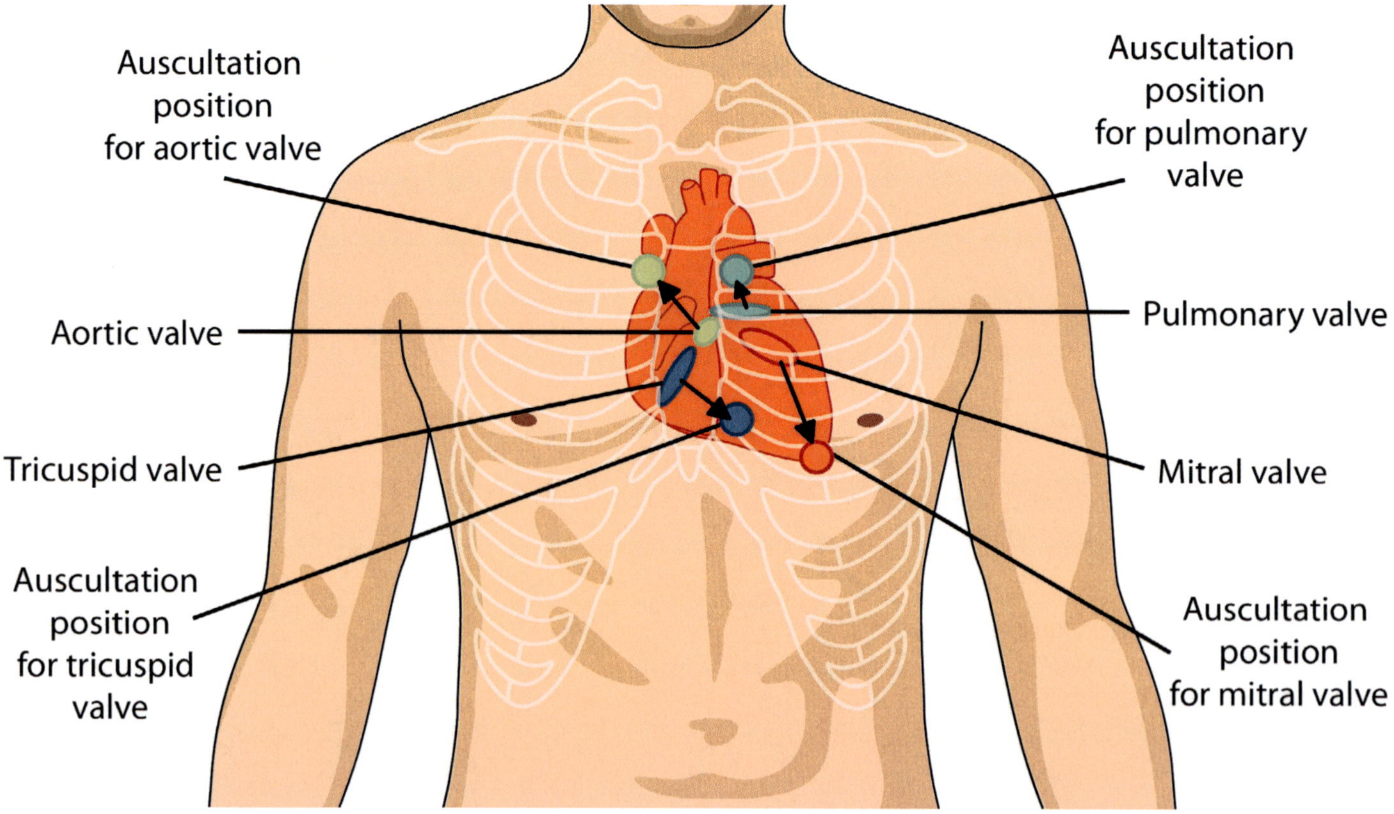

Figure 2.11 - Auscultation of the Heart

1. Ventricular septal defect
    a) A hole in the ventricular wall, usually congenital.
    b) Blood flows from high pressure to low pressure. So, from the left ventricle to the right ventricle during systole.
    c) Produces a holosystolic sound.
    d) Oxygen saturation of blood in the right ventricle will be higher than that of the right atrium.

Mitral and Tricuspid Regurgitation and VSD

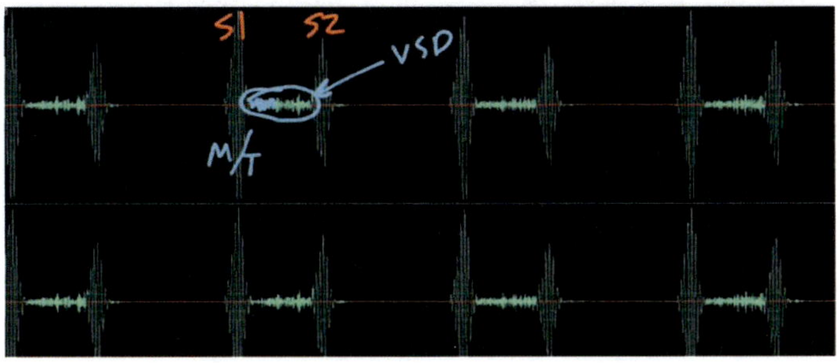

2. Mitral regurgitation
    a) During systole, blood re-enters the left atrium from the left ventricle → increased pressure in the left atrium in systole
    b) Typically a holosystolic murmur heard near the apex which radiates to the axilla.
3. Tricuspid regurgitation
    a) During systole, blood re-enters the right atrium from the right ventricle → increased pressure in right atrium during diastole
4. Mitral valve prolapse
    a) Blood regurgitates through mitral valve after a mid-systolic click.
    b) Increased pressure in left atrium.

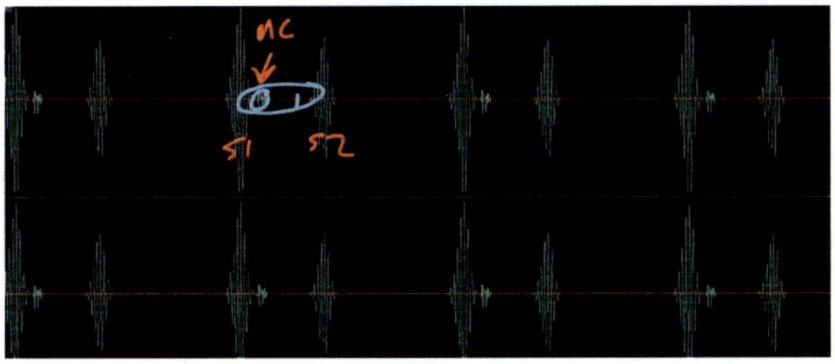

5. Aortic stenosis
    a) Greater resistance to the blood flow out of the left ventricle to the aorta → increased left ventricular pressure during systole; decreased systolic pressure
    b) The left ventricle becomes hypertrophied and less compliant. It is dependent upon left atrial contraction to maintain proper diastolic filling.

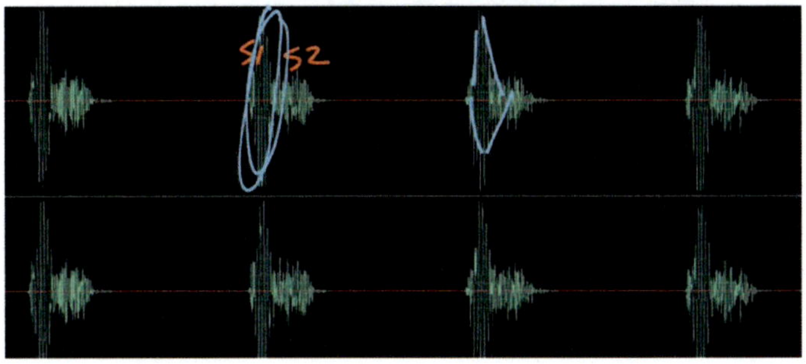

F. Diastolic

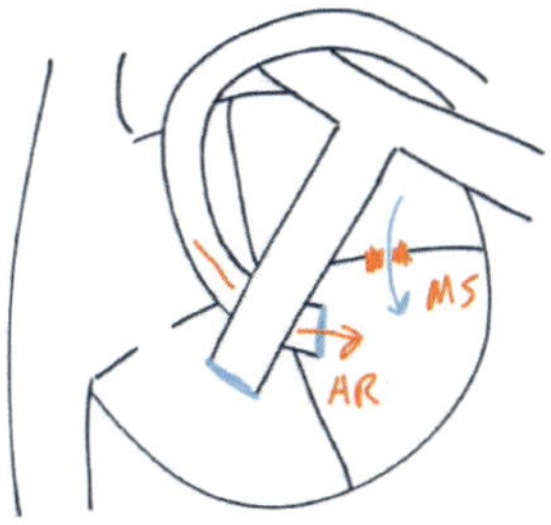

1. Aortic regurgitation

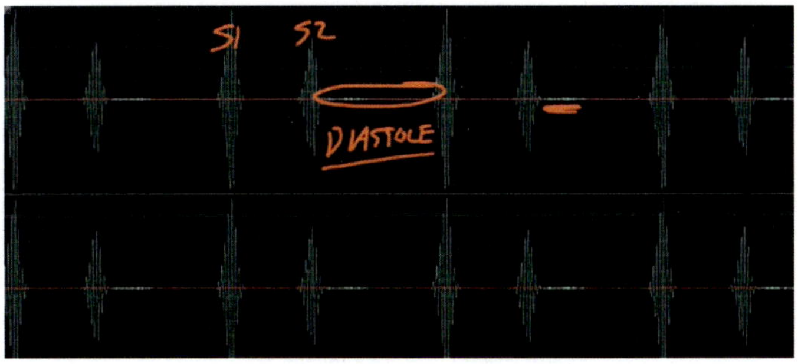

    a) Blood re-enters the left ventricle during diastole → decreased diastolic pressure. When systole begins, there is an increase in blood volume in the left ventricle → increased systolic pressure.
    b) Results in increased systolic pressure (more blood is being ejected from the LV due to large regurgitant volumes) and decreased diastolic pressure (the elastic recoil of the aorta is not pumping as much blood because some of it leaks back into the LV during diastole) thus widening the pulse pressure (pulse pressure = systolic - diastolic).

2. Mitral stenosis

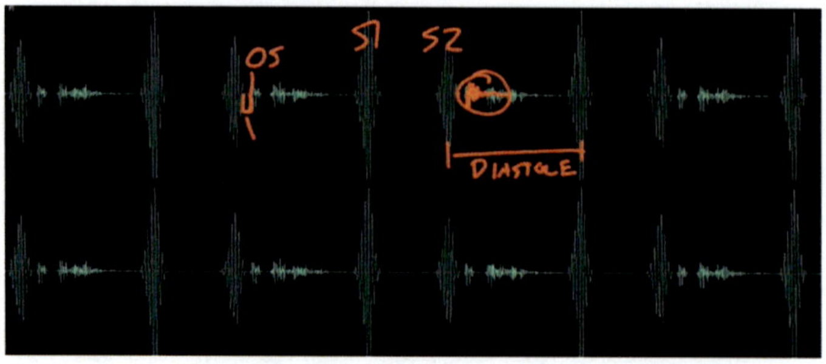

a) The mitral valve is stenotic making it difficult for blood to enter the left ventricle during diastole → greater volume of blood remains in the left atrium during systole → increased left atrial systolic pressure

G. Continuous

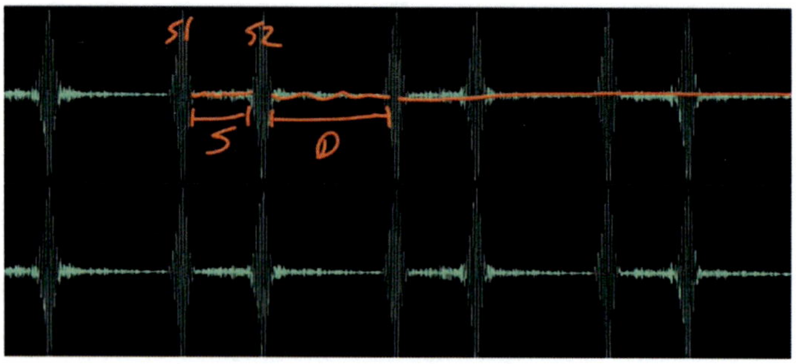

1. Patent ductus arteriosus

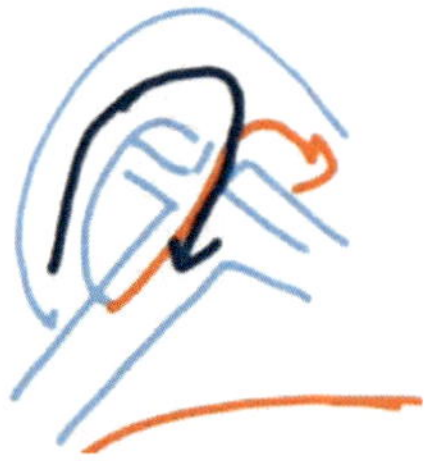

a) The murmur can be heard during systole and diastole. Heard best at the left sternal border just below the clavicle. Can close spontaneously several hours after birth.

H. Atrial septal defect

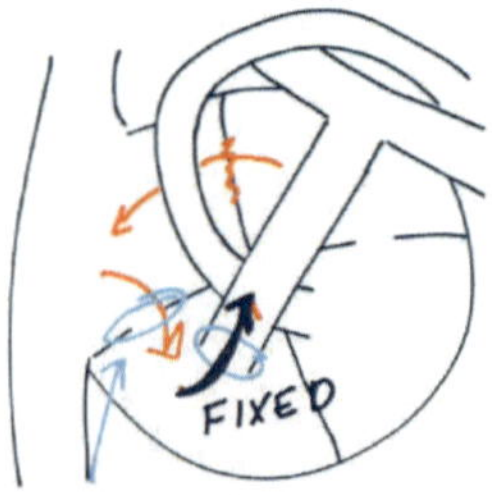

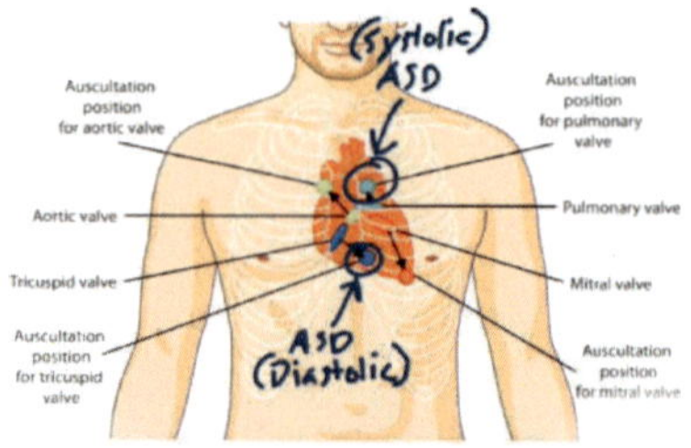

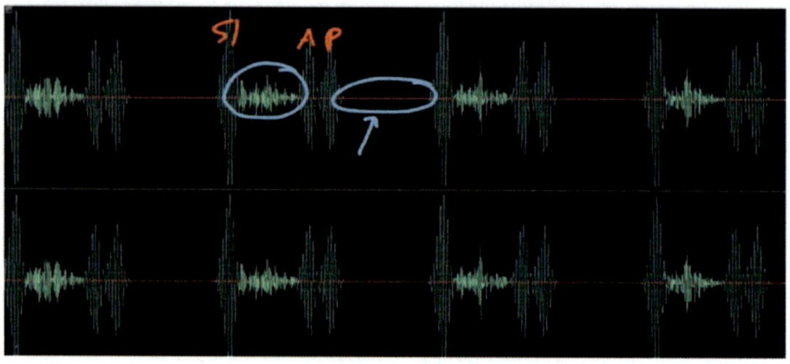

1. A hole is present in the interatrial wall.
2. Blood flows from left atrium to the right atrium during systole.
3. Produces a holosystolic sound.
4. Causes increased flow through the pulmonic valve, causing a fixed splitting of S2.

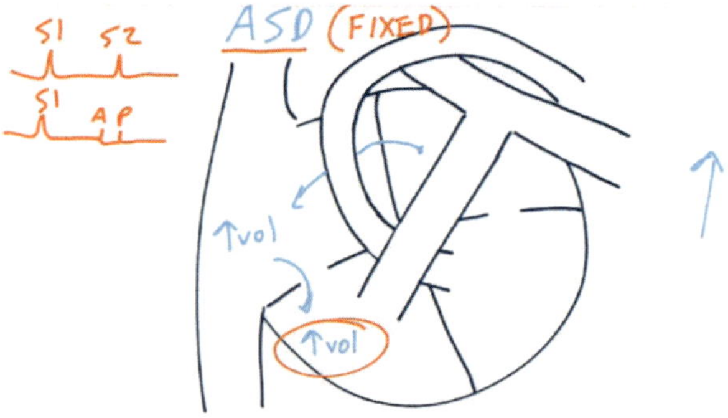

I. Heart sounds during Inspiration

1. Intrathoracic cavity expands → decreased pressure in right atrium → increased venous return → louder right-sided murmurs

J. Heart sounds during expiration

1. Increased pulmonary return to LA → increased volume in LA and LV → louder left-sided murmurs

REVIEW QUESTIONS

1. A patient has a murmur that increases during inspiration and occurs during systole. What is the likely cause?

    - **Inspiration increases the intensity of right-sided murmurs (tricuspid or pulmonic)**
    - **Since it occurs during systole it must be TR or PS (not TS or PR)**
    - **Upon learning it is best auscultated at the 5th intercostal space, TR the best answer**

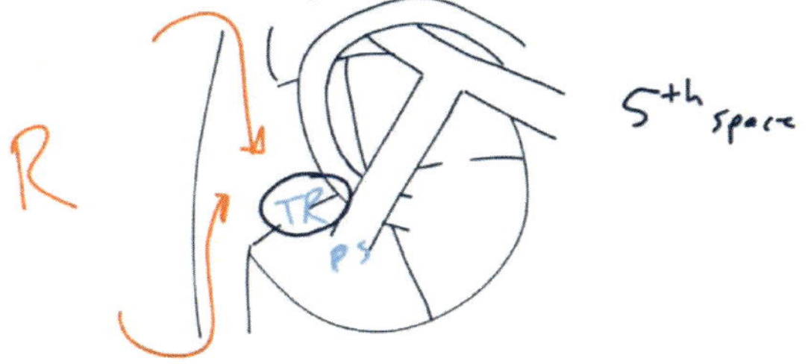

2. Where would this best be auscultated?

    - **Aortic Stenosis**

3. What would the murmur do to the PV loop?

    - **Prolonged AS would cause LV hypertrophy and decreased compliance**
    - **AS would also increase afterload (ESV moves right)**

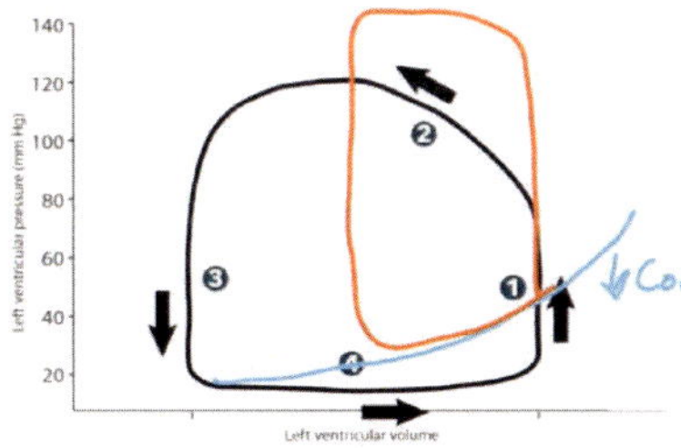

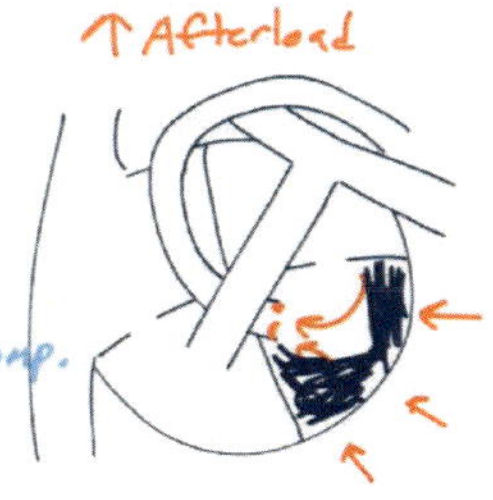

4. What would the murmur do to the pressure tracings graph?

    - **MR results in increased blood entering the LA during systole**

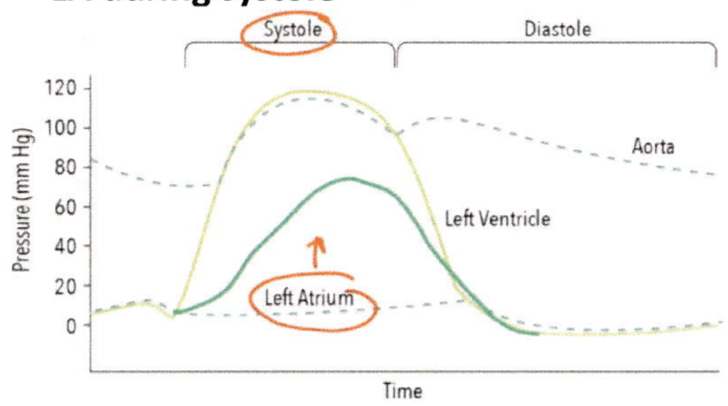

5. What would the murmur do to the pressure tracings graph?

    - **AR results in increased blood entering the LV during diastole**
    - **Aortic pressure would decrease during diastole and is either normal or higher during systole (increased EDV)**
    - **Pulse pressure will increase (PP=SBP-DBP)**

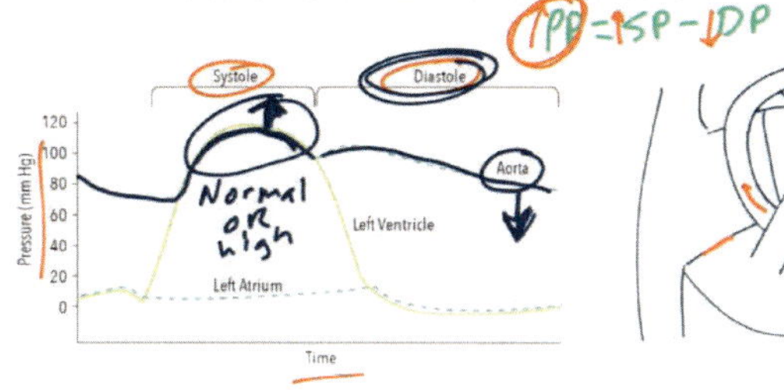

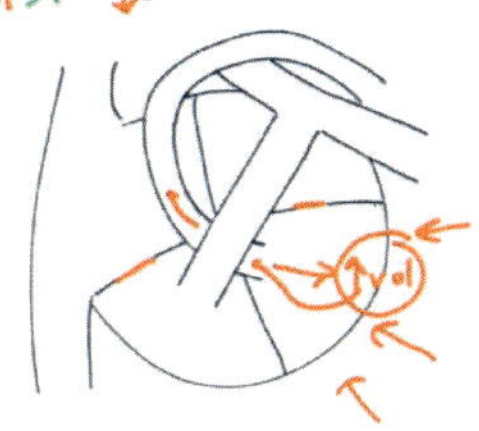

PULMONOLOGY

Section I - Pulmonary and Bronchopulmonary Circulation

I. Circulation

A. Bronchopulmonary circulation

1. Supplied by blood from the systemic circulation but drains into the left atrium.

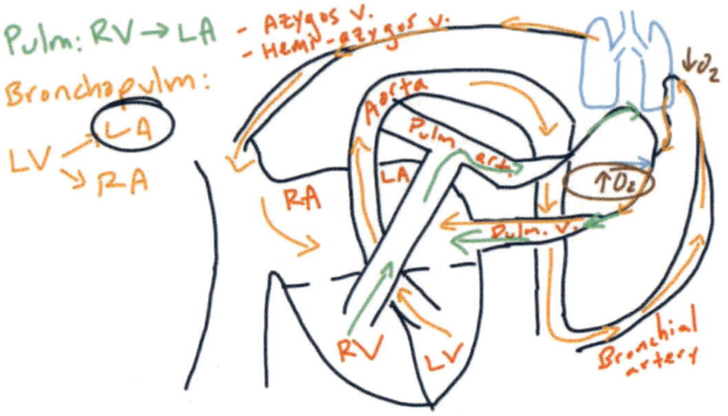

B. Pulmonary circulation

1. Supplied by blood from the right ventricle and drains into the left atrium.
2. Pressure in the pulmonary artery is around 15 mmHg.
3. Blood flow regulation
   a) Hypoxia in the alveoli cause vasoconstriction of adjacent pulmonary vessels → blood is directed toward alveoli with higher PaO_2

REVIEW QUESTIONS ?

1. A researcher is studying pulmonary tissue necrosis in mice. After surgically removing several pulmonary arteries she notices that the lungs are still adequately oxygenated. Why?

   - **The lungs receive a dual blood supply which includes the pulmonary arteries and the bronchial arteries**
   - **In this example tissue necrosis is unlikely to occur as the bronchial arteries will continue to provide sufficient oxygenation to the lungs**

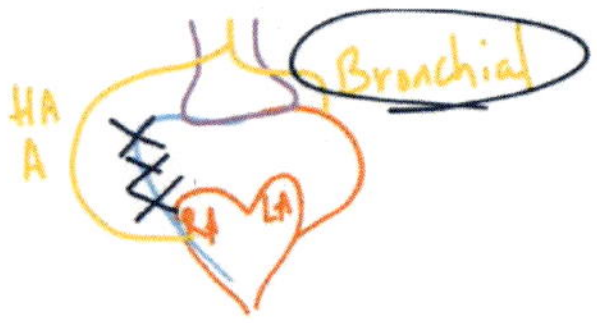

2. How would the resistance of the pulmonary vasculature of a patient at high altitude differ from that of a patient at sea level?

   - **High altitude → ↓ oxygen**
   - **Hypoxia causes vasodilation in most tissues**
   - **In the lungs, however, hypoxia → vasoconstriction → ↓ luminal radius → ↑ pulmonary vascular resistance**

↑R = 8ηl/πr⁴ ↓

↑ altitude → ↓ hypoxia → ↓ radius → ↑ R

Section II - Spirometry

I. Lung Volumes and Spirometry

A. Spirometry (Figure 3.1 - Normal Spirogram)

1. Measures lung volumes and capacities
2. Measures how fast one exhales (FEV_1)
3. Data from spirometry can be used to generate various graphs (spirogram, flow-volume loop, flow vs. volume, etc.)
4. Assesses lung function (PFT)
5. Cannot measure residual volume (RV)

B. Volumes

1. Inspiratory reserve volume (IRV)
2. Tidal volume (V_T)
3. Expiratory reserve volume (ERV)
4. Residual volume (RV)
   a) Cannot be measured by using spirometry
   b) Helium dilution and nitrogen washout
      (a) Used to determine functional residual capacity (FRC)
      (b) Once FRC is obtained, residual volume (RV) and total lung capacity (TLC) can be derived using other known values.
         (i) FRC is found
         (ii) FRC - ERV = RV
         (iii) FRC + IC = TLC

C. Capacities (2+ volumes)

1. Inspiratory capacity (IC)
2. Vital capacity (VC) or forced vital capacity (FVC)
3. Functional residual capacity (FRC)
4. Total lung capacity (TLC)

D. Obstructive Lung Diseases

1. Cannot fully exhale → ↑ RV
   a) ↑ FRC → ↑ TLC
   b) ↓ ERV
2. Less space to inhale → ↓ IRV and ↓ ERV → ↓ FVC
3. ↑ TV (aka VT)
4. ↓ RR
5. Significantly ↓↓ FEV1 + mildly ↓ FVC → FEV1/FVC ratio (< 70%)

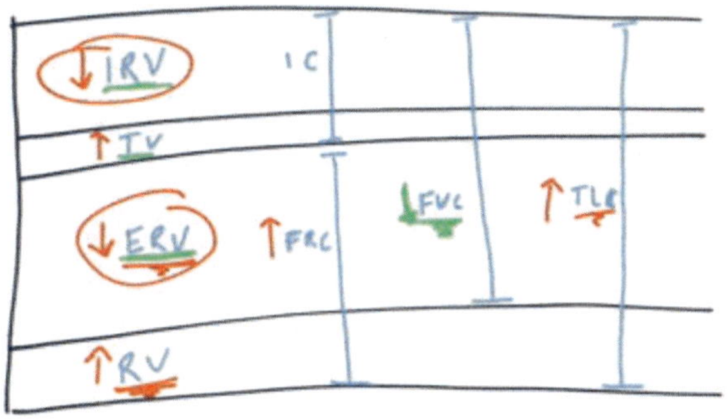

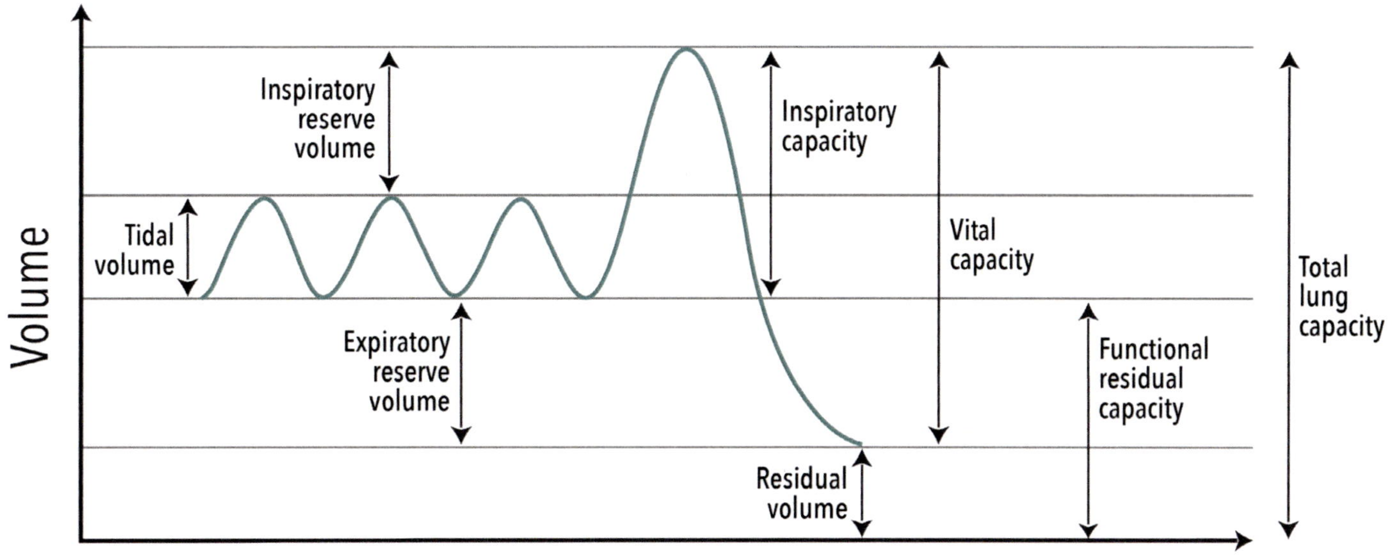

Figure 3.1 - Normal Spirogram

E. Forced expiratory volume (FEV_1)

1. The amount of air that can be expired in one second.
2. Significantly decreased in obstructive lung diseases

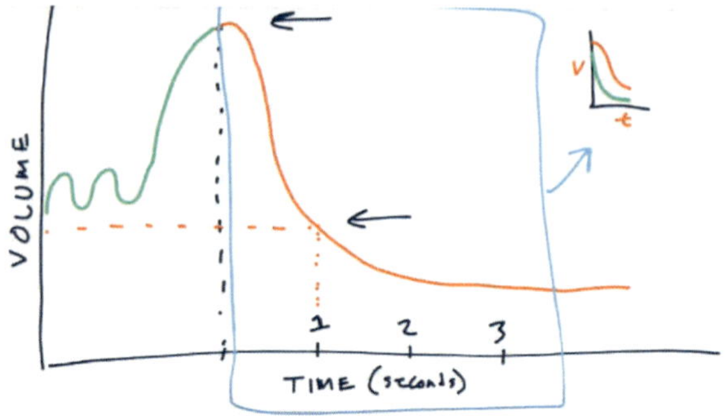

F. FEV_1/FVC ratio

1. Normally around 70%
2. The patient inhales as much as possible, then exhales as rapidly as possible (forced expiration test)
3. Decreased in obstructive lung diseases
   a) FEV_1 and FVC both decrease, but FEV_1 more significantly→ decreased ratio

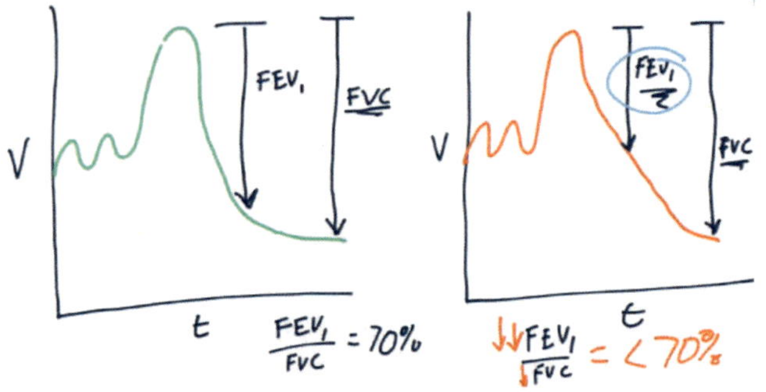

4. Restrictive Lung Diseases
   a) Cannot fully inhale → decreased IRV and TV
   b) Less air in lungs to exhale → decreased ERV→ decreased FRC
   c) Decreased IRV, TV, and FRC → decreased TLC
   d) Decreased IRV, TV, and ERV → significantly decreased FVC
   e) Decreased FEV_1 + significantly decreased FVC → increased FEV_1/FVC ratio (> 80%)

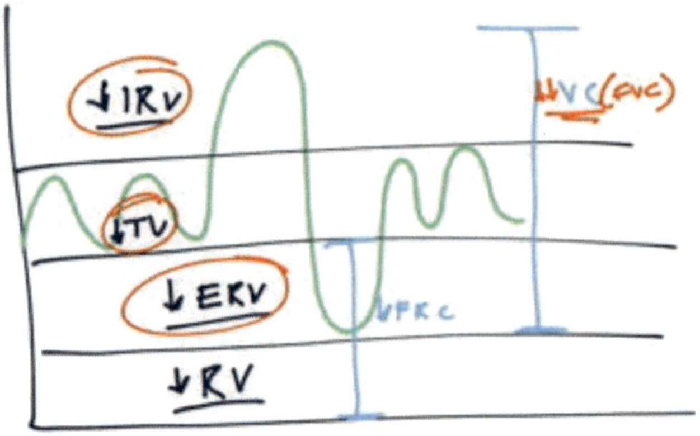

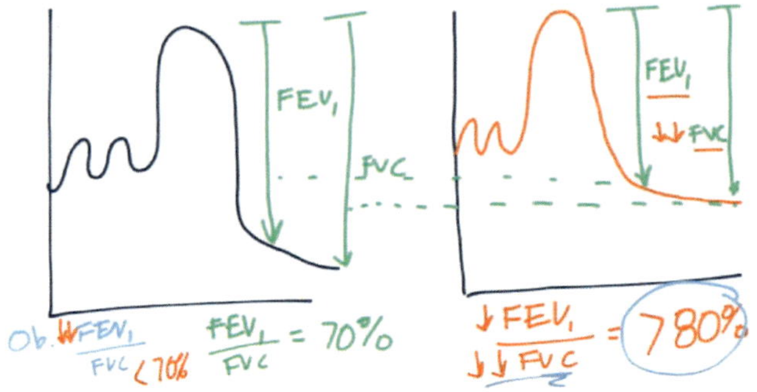

G. Flow-volume loops (See Figure 3.2)

1. Data gained from spirometry
2. Provides information on lung volumes as well as flow during inspiration and expiration
3. Used to identify respiratory pathologies (obstructive v. restrictive)

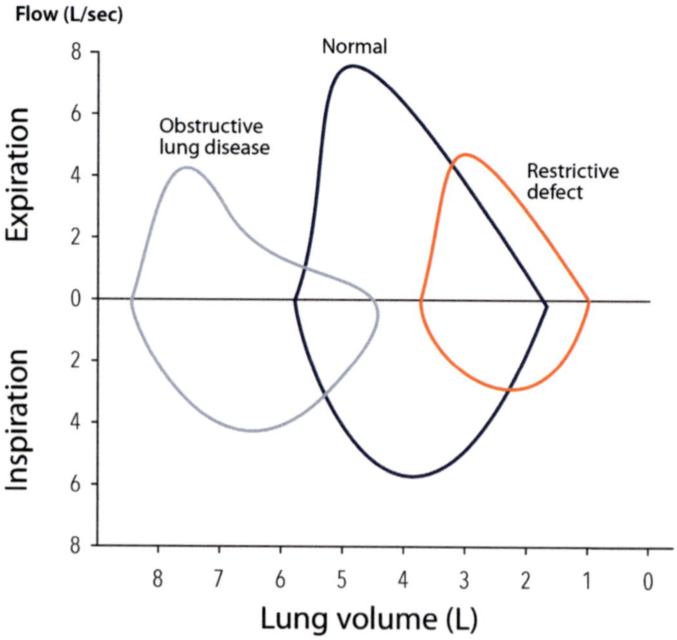

Figure 3.2 - Flow-Volume Loops

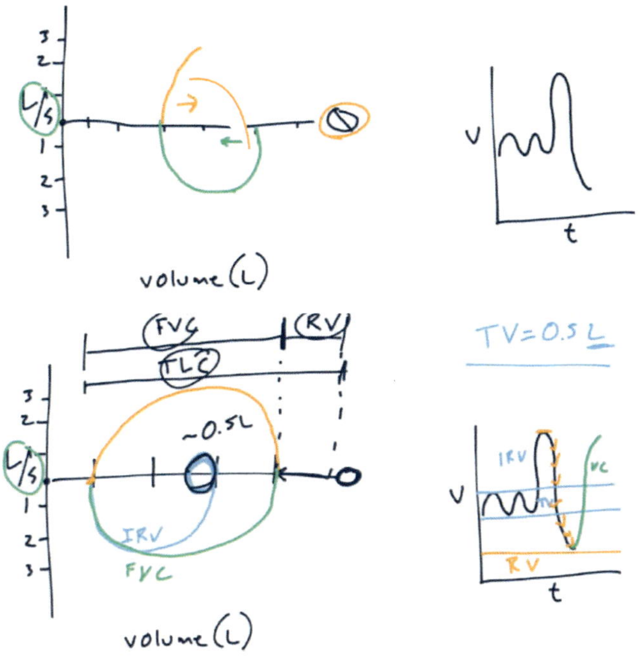

4. Flow-Volume Loop in Obstructive Diseases

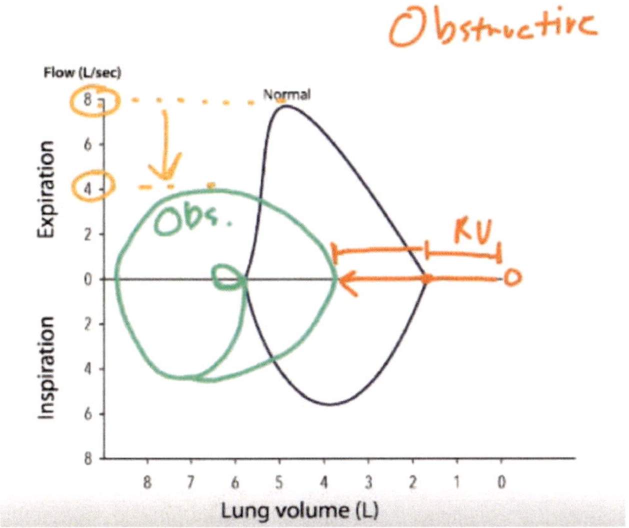

5. Flow-Volume Loop in Restrictive Diseases

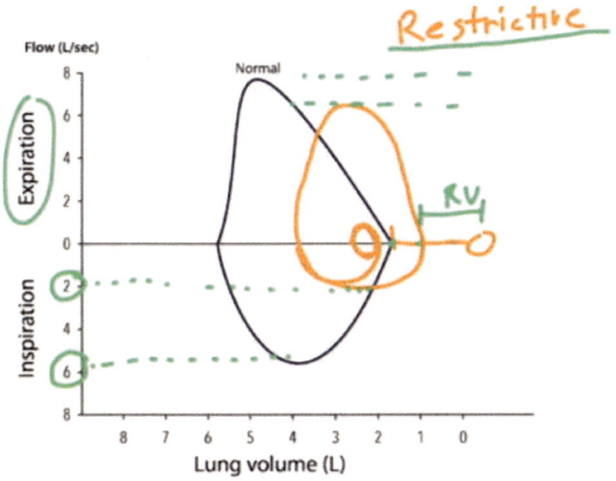

6. PEFR and MEFV on Flow-Volume Loops

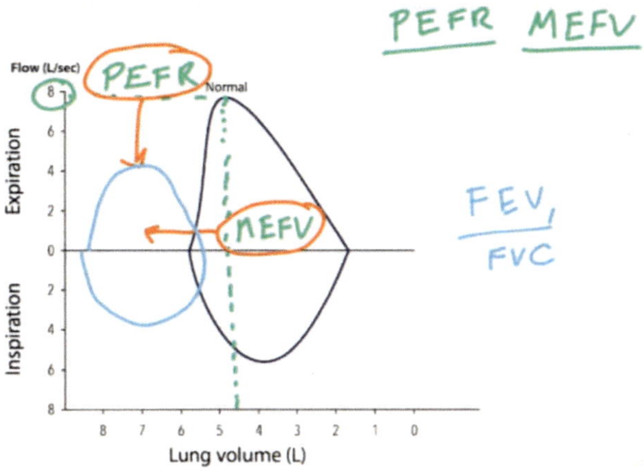

7. Peak expiratory flow rate (PEFR) is the highest peak
   a) Similar to maximum expiratory flow volume (MEFV)
   b) Tidal volume (V_T) is 500 mL
8. IV. FEV_1 in Obstructive Diseases

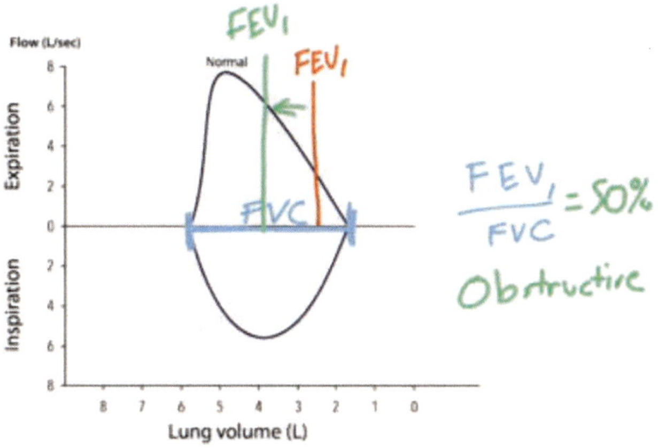

9. V. FEV1 in Restrictive Diseases

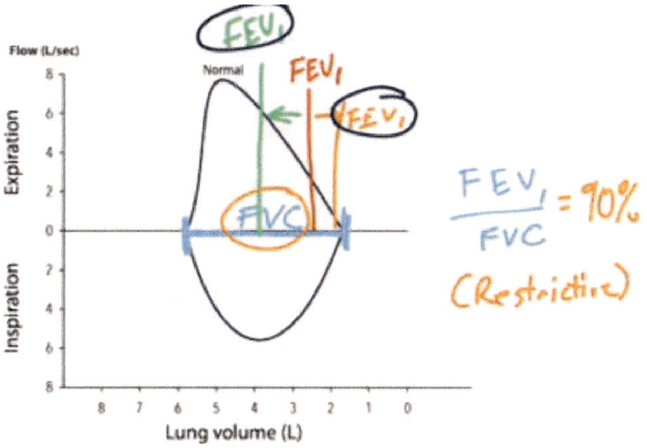

10. Ways you may be tested with diagrams on this topic

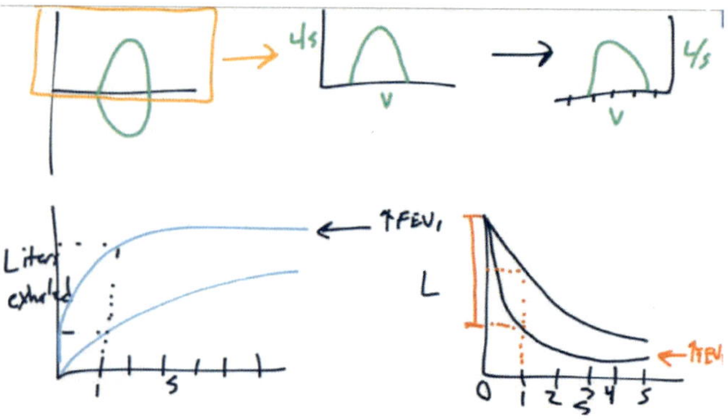

II. Radial traction and airflow

A. Airflow tends to collapse airways.

B. Elastic structure of airways prevents collapse (i.e. radial traction) while air is transferred.

C. Obstructive diseases decrease radial traction.

D. Restrictive diseases increase radial traction.

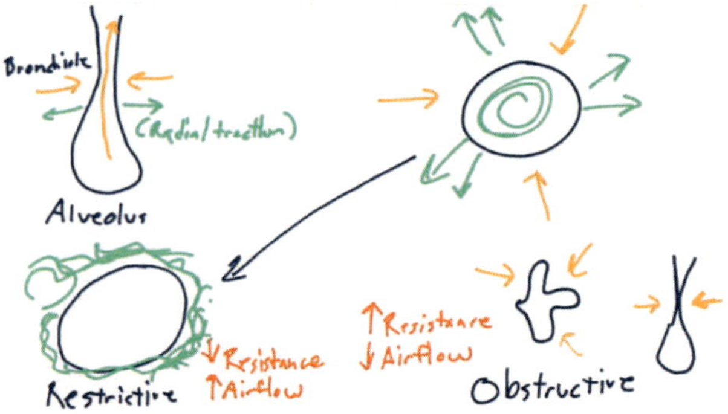

REVIEW QUESTIONS

1. What would happen to TLC and RV in a patient with chronic bronchitis?

- **Chronic bronchitis is an obstructive lung disease, resulting higher RV as well as TLC**
- **Although ERV may decrease slightly, it is negligible in this context**

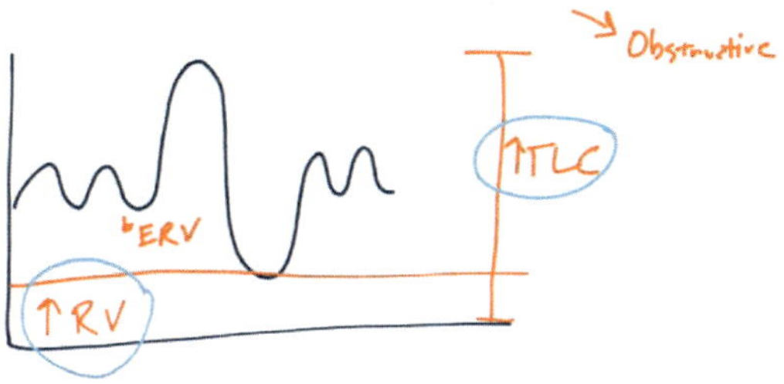

2. What would happen to VC and TLC in a patient with berylliosis?

- **Berylliosis is one of the pneumoconiosis (infiltrative/restrictive lung diseases)**
- **Restrictive diseases decrease the ability to inhale (low IRV, TV, ERV and VC)**
- **RV is normal or decreased (restrictive lung diseases don't retain air, as in obstructive)**
- **TLC is decreased. Note that ankylosing spondylitis is a restrictive pathology that has increased TLC. Other than this, think low TLC in restrictive.**

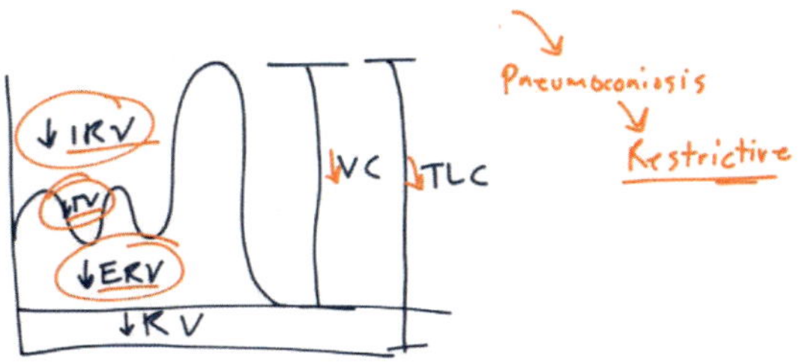

3. How do you find the FEV_1 in a flow volume loop?

- **Trick question. You cannot discern FEV_1 by simply looking at a flow-volume loop**
- **Note that the y-axis measures L/sec (flow), not L (FEV_1)**

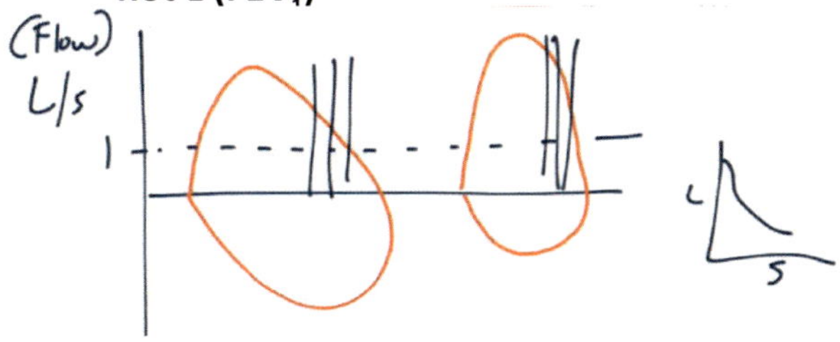

4. Conceptually identify the PEFR and MEFV for patient A and B. Why is MEFV greater in patient B?

- **Recall that L are higher as you move left on the x-axis**
- **Higher MEFV indicates higher air retention (i.e. obstructive pathology)**

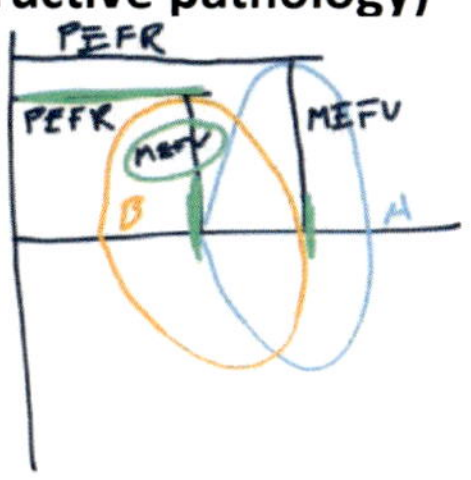

5. Two elderly patients (twins) have severe lung disease. One has restrictive pathology, the other obstructive. Which one can blow out the candles on their birthday cake?

↓FEV_1 in obstruction

6. FRC 4 L, ERV 1 L, VC 3.5 L, IC 2.5 L. What is the RV?

- **Plot given numbers on a spirograph to quickly determine how to get RV using simple math**
- **FRC (4 L) + IC (2.5 L) = TLC (6.5 L)**
- **TLC (6.5 L) - VC (3.5 L) = RV (3 L)**

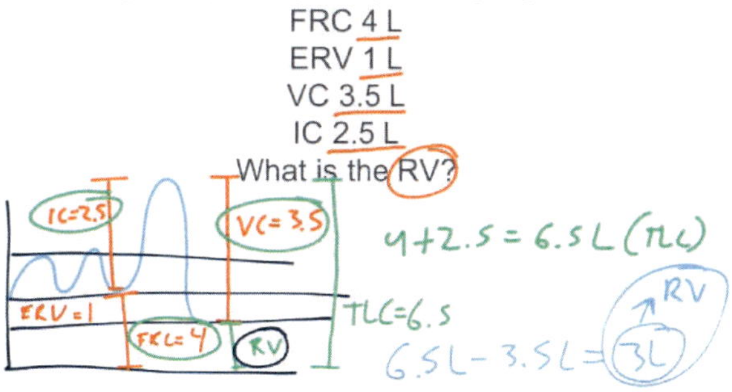

REVIEW QUESTIONS

7. If a patient exhales as normal and then inhales as much as possible, what was found? If the patient then exhales as much as possible, what lung volume/capacity was found?If we take the question a step further, how can we find the ERV?

- **From normal exhalation (lower part of TV), inhaling as much as possible reveals IC**
- **From top of spirograph to maximum exhalation is VC. Recall that RV is found using helium dilution or nitrogen washout)**

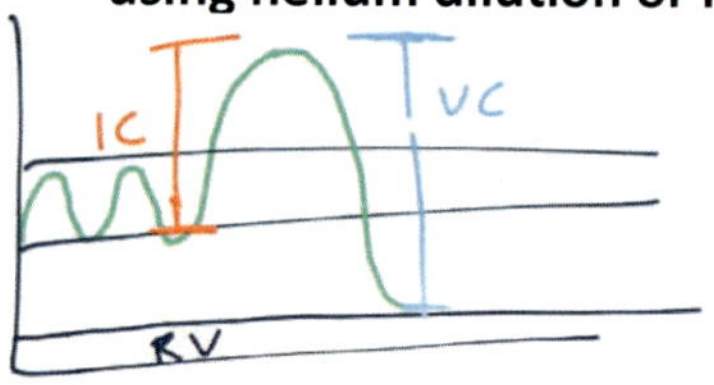

8. By looking at the flow-volume loop, what is the RV, FVC, TLC, and TV?

- **RV starts at 0 L and moves to right-most portion of loop (4 L)**
- **FVC (VC) is simply the extent of the loop on x-axis (4 L)**
- **TLC = FVC + RV**
- **TLC = 8**
- **TV is not shown but can be assumed to be 0.5 L**

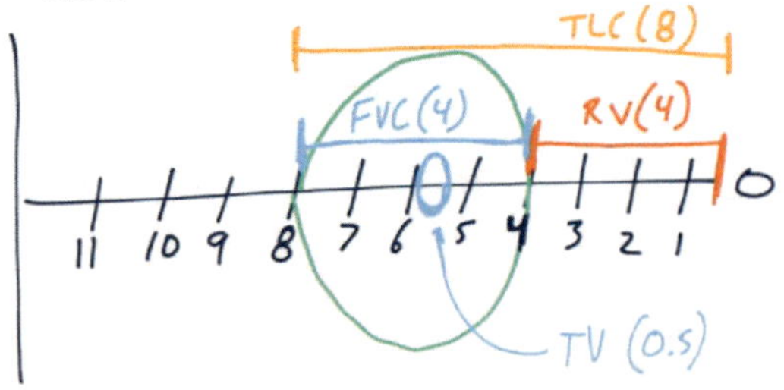

9. Which loop represents a person at rest?

- **Don't be confused by lack of expiratory portion of loop which would normally be the top half of the graph**
- **TV, unless otherwise stated, should be about 0.5 L (the innermost loop)**

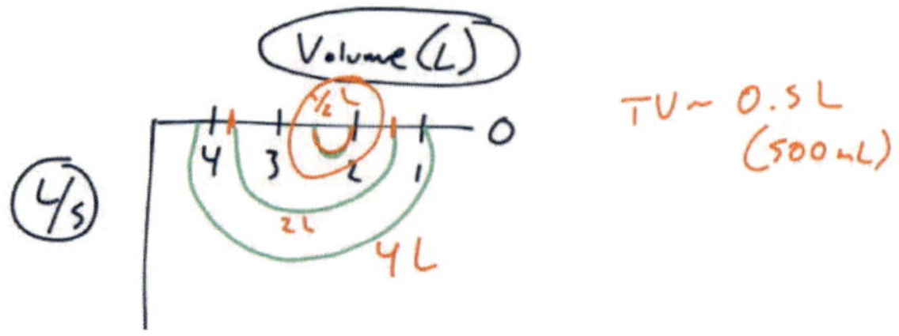

10. A clinic has the ability to perform only simple spirometry. What lung values will the clinicians be unable to obtain?

- **Normal (simple) spirometry cannot determine RV**
- **Without RV, one cannot obtain FRC or TLC (to obtain these values, nitrogen washout or helium dilution must be used)**

11. A patient undergoes spirometry with nitrogen washout. What is the TLC if FRC is 4.5 L and IC is 2 L?

- **TLC = IC + FRC. TLC = 6.5 L**
- **Note: This patient underwent nitrogen washout, allowing measurement of RV and FRC**

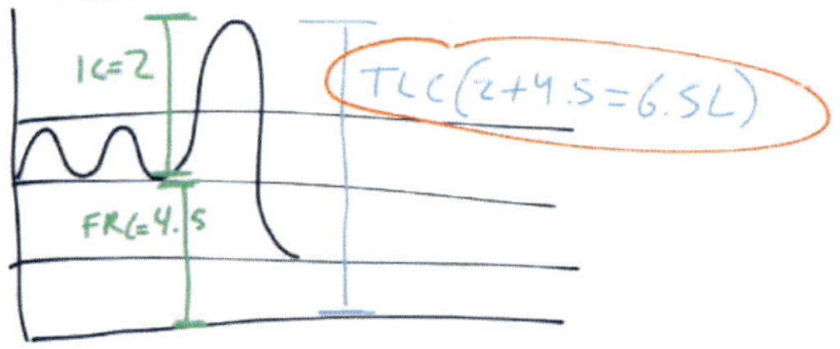

Section III - Pulmonology Equations

I. Equations

A. Minute ventilation

$$V_E = V_T \times RR$$

Where:
V_E = minute ventilation (mL/min)
V_T = tidal volume (mL/breath)
RR = respiratory rate (breaths/min)

1. Minute ventilation is the volume of air that enters the airways per minute.

B. Dead Space

$$V_D = V_T \times (P_ACO_2 - P_ECO_2 / P_ACO_2)$$

Where:
V_D = physiologic dead space (mL)
V_T = tidal volume (mL)
P_ACO_2 = partial pressure of CO_2 in the alveoli (mmHg)
P_ECO_2 = partial pressure of CO_2 in expired air (mmHg)

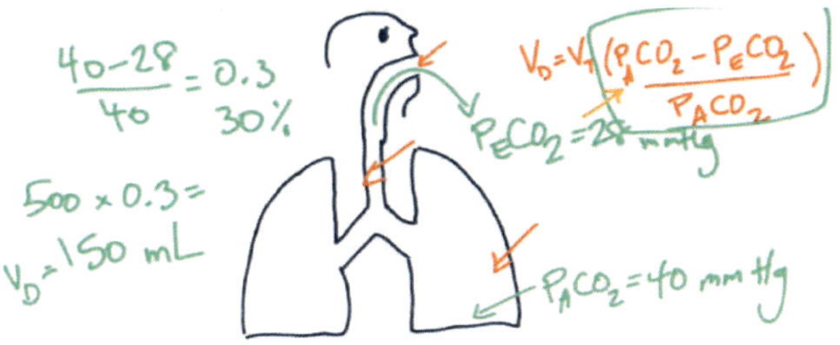

1. Physiologic dead space includes anatomic dead space and alveolar dead space.
2. Anatomic dead space is volume of air in the conducting airways in each breath. The gases here will not participate in gas exchange, hence the term anatomic dead space.
3. Alveolar dead space is the volume of air in each breath that resides in the alveoli and does not participate in gas exchange. Typically, most of the gases that enter the alveoli will participate in gas exchange. However, in some lung diseases, alveolar dead space can be significant.
4. In healthy people, anatomic dead space = physiologic dead space (alveolar dead space is negligible).

C. Alveolar ventilation

$$V_A = (V_T - V_D) \times RR$$

Where:
V_A = alveolar ventilation (mL/min)
V_T = tidal volume (mL/breath)
V_D = dead space (mL/breath).
RR = respiratory rate (breaths/min)

1. Alveolar ventilation is the volume of air that reaches the alveoli per minute.

D. Partial pressure of inspired oxygen equation (must first understand this to understand the alveolar gas equation)

$$PIO_2 = FIO_2 \, (Patm - PH_2O)$$

Where:
PIO_2 = partial pressure of inspired oxygen (mmHg)
FIO_2 = fraction of inspired oxygen
Patm = atmospheric pressure (mmHg)
PH_2O = partial pressure of water (mmHg)

1. Only 21% of the air is composed of oxygen. It is also composed of nitrogen and other molecules that do not contribute to FIO_2.
2. Patm is usually 760 mmHg (this is at sea level and will depend on the altitude).
3. PH_2O is usually 47 mmHg (water vapor is added to the air by the body before it reaches the lungs, which decreases the overall pressure of oxygen).

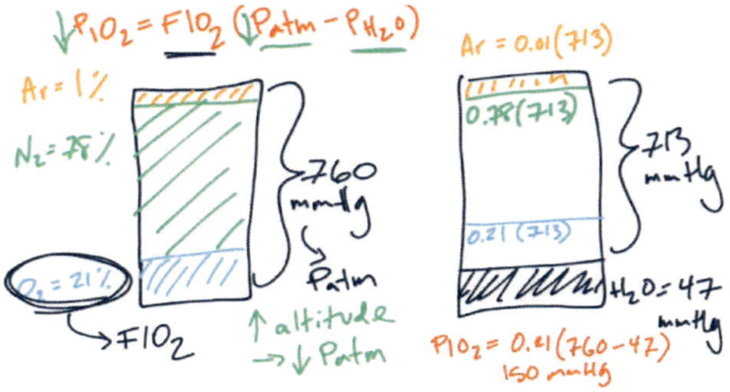

E. Alveolar gas equation

$$P_AO_2 = PIO_2 - (PaCO_2 / R)$$

Where:
P_AO_2 = partial pressure of O_2 in the alveoli (mmHg)
PIO_2 = partial pressure of inspired oxygen (mmHg)
$PaCO_2$ = partial pressure of CO_2 in the arterial blood (mmHg)
R = respiratory quotient (CO_2 produced / O_2 consumed)

1. The respiratory quotient varies depending on the concentration of fat vs glucose that is being metabolized.
2. The respiratory quotient decreases when fat is being metabolized and is increased when glucose is being metabolized.
3. If the respiratory quotient value is not provided, assume a value of 0.8.
4. Conceptually, ($PaCO_2$ / R) represents how much oxygen is leaving the alveoli and entering the blood.
5. Conceptually, PIO_2 represents how much oxygen is entering the airways.
6. The difference between PIO_2 and ($PaCO_2$ / R) represents the partial pressure of oxygen in the alveoli.

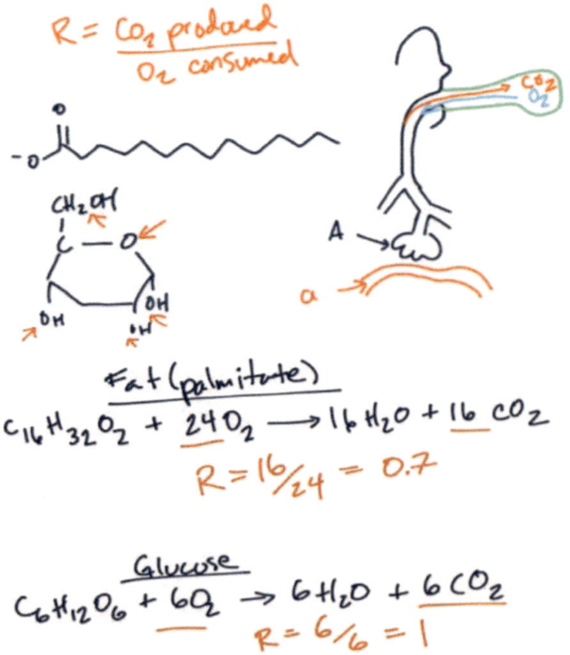

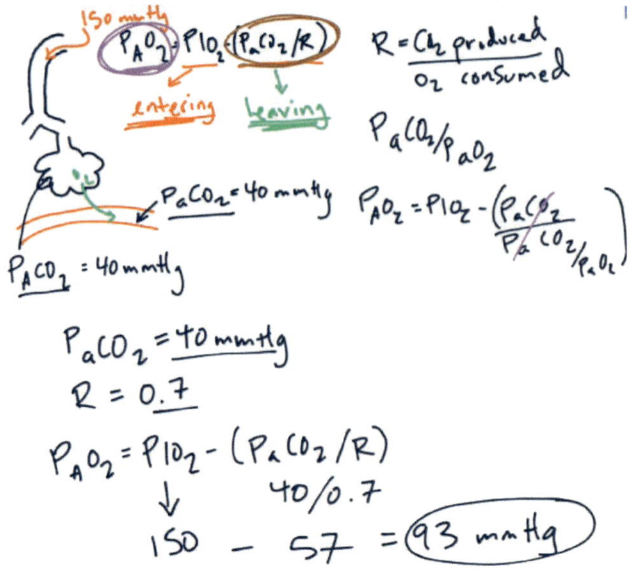

F. Resistance

$$R = 8\eta l / \pi r^4$$

Where:
R = resistance (mmHg ⊠ min/mL)
η = viscosity of the inspired gas
l = length of the airway
πr^4 = volume of a sphere

1. Hypoxia results in vasoconstriction of the pulmonary vasculature.
2. Resistance
   a) From the equation $R = 8L\eta / \pi r^4$ it would seem that the radius of the airway should have the greatest impact on the resistance to airflow. However, the smallest airways actually have the least resistance because the summated cross-sectional area is largest.

G. Compliance

$$C = V / P$$

Where:
C = compliance (mL/mmHg)
V = volume (mL)
P = pressure (mmHg)

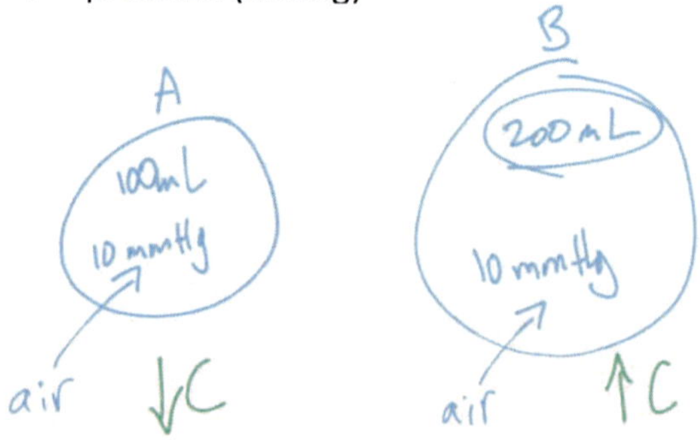

H. Laplace's law

$$P = 2T / r$$

Where:
P = pressure (mmHg)
T = surface tension
r = radius

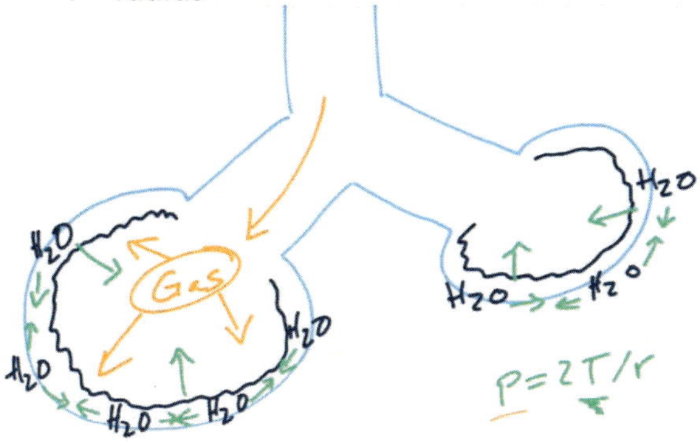

1. The pressure required to keep the alveoli distended is proportional to the surface tension and inversely proportional to the radius.

I. A-a gradient

$$\text{A-a gradient} = PAO_2 - PaO_2$$

Where:
PAO_2 = partial pressure of O_2 in the alveoli (mmHg)
PaO_2 = partial pressure of arterial O_2 (mmHg)

1. In healthy individuals, the PAO_2 is approximately 105 mmHg and the PaO_2 is approximately 100 mmHg.
2. A normal A-a gradient is 5-15 mmHg.

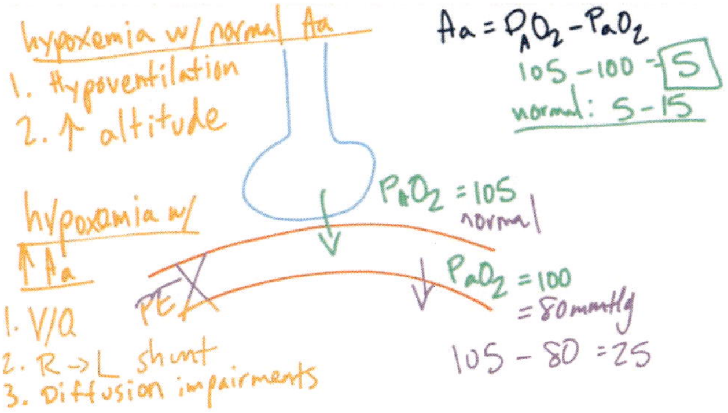

a) There are two major causes of normal Aa gradients in the presence of hypoxemia.
   (1) Hypoventilation
   (2) High altitude

b) There are three primary causes of increased Aa gradients in the presence of hypoxemia.
   (1) V/Q mismatch
   (2) Right to left shunt
   (3) Diffusion impairments

J. Oxygen content of the blood

$$O_2 \text{ content} = (1.34 \times Hb \times SaO_2) + (0.003 \times PaO_2)$$

Where:
1.34 = oxygen binding capacity of Hb (mL O_2 / g Hb)
Hb = hemoglobin concentration (g Hb/100 mL blood)
SaO_2 = % saturation of heme bound to O_2 (%)
0.003 = dissolvability of O_2 (mL O_2 / mmHg ⊠ 100 mL blood)
PaO_2 = partial pressure of arterial O_2 (mmHg)

1. The total oxygen content equation is informative because it describes how well the hemoglobin is oxygenated and how much dissolved oxygen is present in the arterial blood.

REVIEW QUESTIONS

1. How would minute ventilation be altered in a patient with a restrictive lung disease?

- **VE = VT X RR**
- **In a restrictive lung disease ↓ air can enter the lungs →↓ tidal volume (VT) →↑ respiratory rate (RR) as a form of compensation**
- **Minute ventilation (VE) is relatively normal.**

2. How would minute ventilation be altered in a patient with an obstructive lung disease?

- **VE = VT X RR**
- **In an obstructive lung disease (i.e. emphysema), the connective tissue surrounding the alveoli is damaged → loss of outward radial traction force → obstruction**
- **Patients compensate by ↑ tidal volume (VT) and ↓ respiratory rate (RR)**
- **This results in ↑ air within the bronchi which helps keeps the bronchi open in attempt to minimize airway obstruction,**
- **Thus minute ventilation (VE) stays relatively constant**

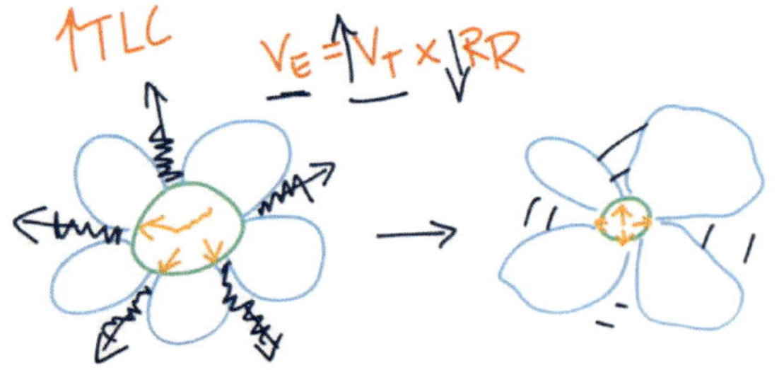

3. How would the physiologic dead space change in a patient with a pulmonary embolism?

- **In a PE ↓ blood reaches the alveoli → less oxygen within alveoli is able to participate in gas exchange →↑ physiologic dead space**

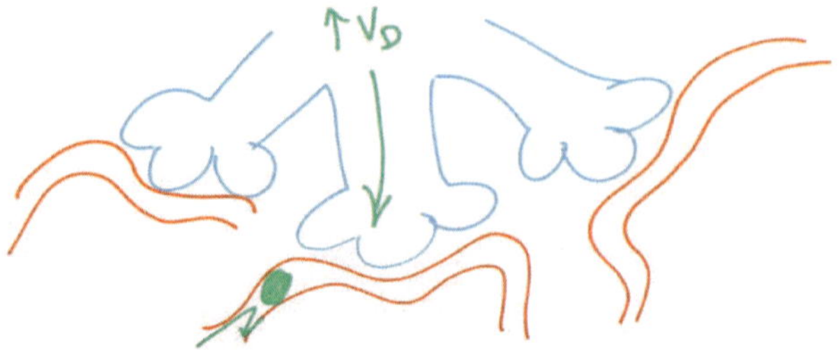

4. A 21-year-old presents with central macule & papule lesions surrounded by a ring of erythema. He is treated with azithromycin & his condition improves. What changes in V_D should you suspect during his initial presentation?

- **The patient has erythema multiforme due to mycoplasma pneumoniae**
- **Pneumonia →↓ function of alveoli →↑ physiologic dead space**

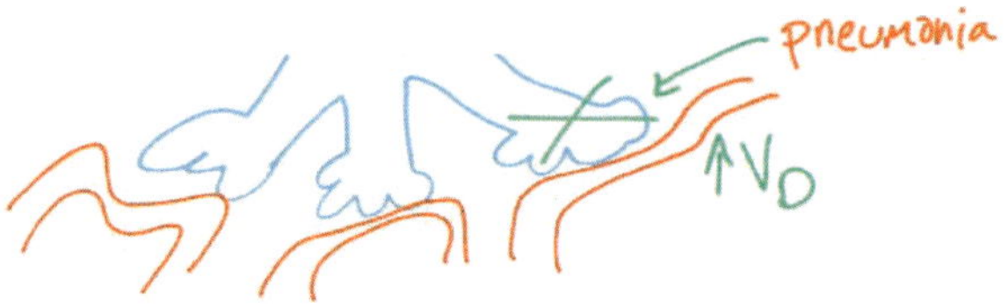

5. If the tidal volume is 500 mL/breath, the dead space is 150 mL/breath, and the respiratory rate is 10 breaths/min, then what is the alveolar ventilation?

- **Alveolar ventilation = 3,500 mL/min**
- **Minute ventilation = 5,000 mL/min (this includes dead space)**

$V_T = 500 \mid V_D = 150 \mid RR = 10 \mid V_A = ?$

$V_A = (V_T - V_D) \times RR$

$(500 - 150) \times 10 = 3{,}500 \text{ mL/min}$

$V_E = V_T \times RR$

$500 \times 10 = 5{,}000 \text{ mL/min}$

6. What part of the alveolar gas equation is altered in a patient on oxygen therapy?

- **FIO_2 (fraction of inspired oxygen)**
- **This is normally 21% of the atmosphere**
- **Oxygen therapy increases the FIO_2 →↑ PAO_2**

$\uparrow PAO_2 = \uparrow\uparrow PIO_2 - (P_aCO_2/R)$

$PIO_2 = FIO_2(P_{atm} - P_{H_2O})$ (P_{atm} = 760, P_{H_2O} = 47)

$0.21 \rightarrow 1.0$

$0.21(760 - 47) = 150$

$1(760 - 47) = 713$

REVIEW QUESTIONS

7. 45-year-old male presents to the Los Angeles ED w/ SOB. Arterial blood gas is drawn and the $PaCO_2$ is 50 mmHg (normal = 33-44 mmHg). What is the P_AO_2?

- **87.5 mmHg**
- **$P_AO_2 = PIO_2 - (PaCO_2 / R)$**
- **$PIO_2 = 150$**
- **R = 0.8**

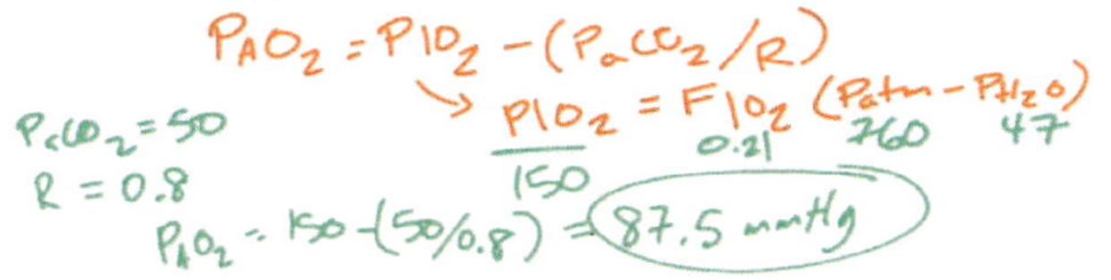

8. What is a chronic hypersensitivity disorder that alters the radius of the airways?

- **Asthma → ↑ constriction → ↓ radius → ↑ R**

9. What part of the airway is responsible for generating the most resistance?

- **The medium-sized airways**
- **Kinematic viscosity is greatest in the medium-sized airways due to turbulent airflow → ↑ resistance**

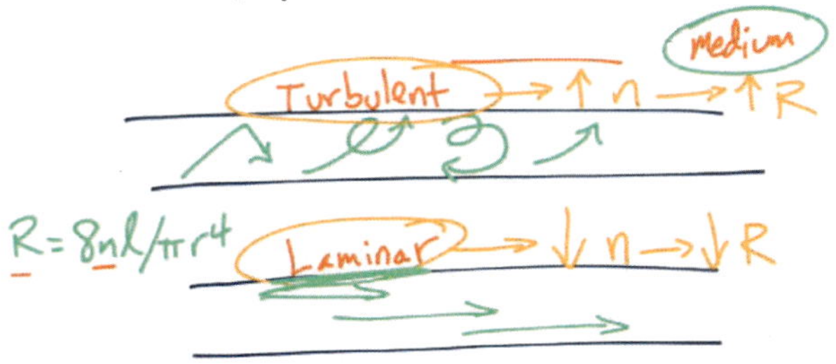

10. How would COPD alter the pulmonary vascular resistance?

- **COPD → airway obstruction → hypoxia → vasoconstriction → ↑ resistance**

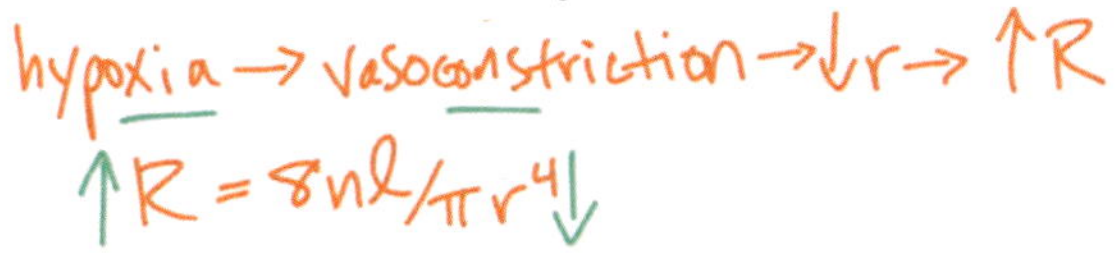

11. A patient with pulmonary hypertension is started on bosentan. How would the pulmonary vascular resistance be altered in this patient?

- **Endothelin-1 normally causes vasoconstriction**
- **Bosentan is an endothelin-1 antagonist → vasodilation → ↓ resistance**

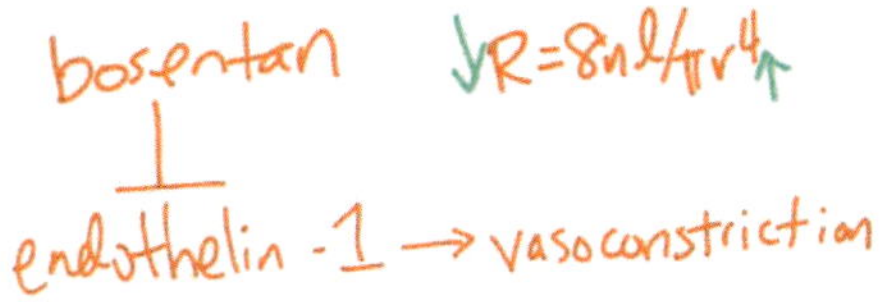

12. How does pulmonary vascular resistance change during the respiratory cycle?

- **Expiration: ↓ resistance**
- **Inspiration: ↑ resistance**
- **During expiration the thoracic cage collapses → ↑ pressure on the vasculature → ↓ radius**
- **During inspiration the thoracic cage expands → ↓ pressure → ↑ lengthwise expansion of the vasculature**

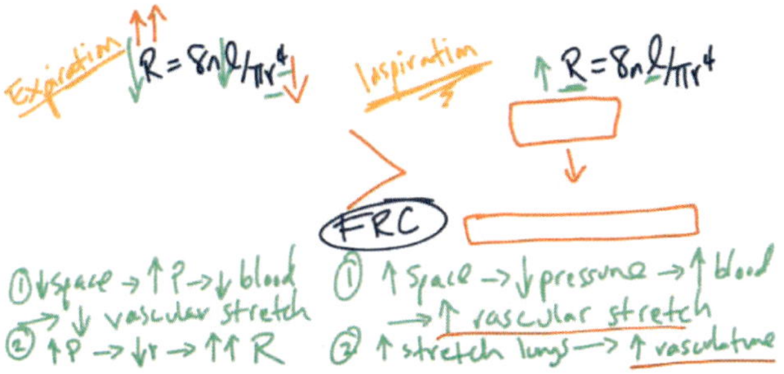

13. How could left sided heart failure alter pulmonary compliance?

- **Heart failure → ↑ volume in pulmonary vasculature → ↑ hydrostatic pressure → ↑ interstitial volume → ↓ pulmonary compliance**

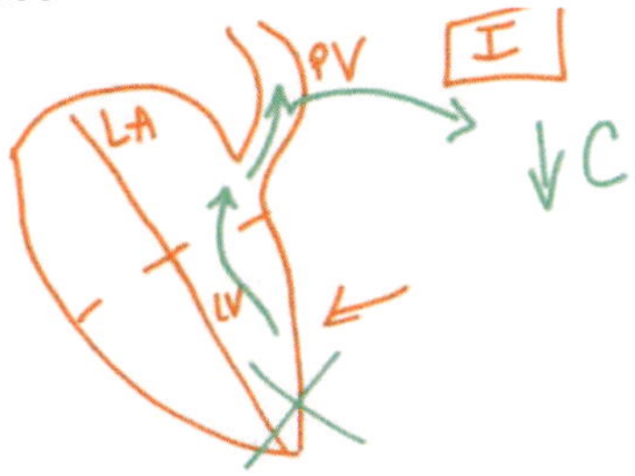

REVIEW QUESTIONS

14. What part of Laplace's law is altered by surfactant?

- **P = 2T / r**
- **Surface tension (T)**

$\downarrow P = 2T/r$

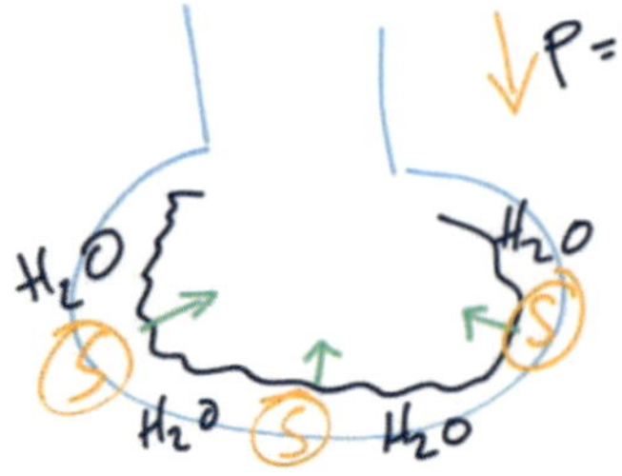

15. How does surfactant alter pulmonary compliance?

- **Surfactant reduces the surface tension such that less pressure is necessary to keep the alveoli open**
- **↓ pressure → ↑ compliance**

$\uparrow S \rightarrow \downarrow T \rightarrow \downarrow P \quad \uparrow C = V/P\downarrow$

16. A patient has a respiratory rate of 7, blood pH = 7.20 (normal = 7.35-7.45), $PaCO_2$ = 80 mmHg (normal = 33-45), PaO_2 = 43 mmHg (normal = 75-105). What is the Aa gradient and the likely diagnosis?

- **Aa = 7 (normal 5-15)**
- **Hypoxemia and a normal Aa gradient is most likely due to either hypoventilation or ↑ altitude**

$P_AO_2 = PIO_2 - (PaCO_2/R)$

$150 - (80/0.8) = 50$

① hypoventilation ② ↑ altitude

$Aa = P_AO_2 - PaO_2$

$50 - 43 = 7\ (5\text{-}15)$

17. What part of the total oxygen content equation is altered in a patient with anemia?

- **Hb**

$\downarrow O_2\ content = (1.34 \times \downarrow Hb \times SaO_2) + (0.003 \times PaO_2)$

18. What part of the total oxygen content equation is altered in a patient with a left ventricular myocardial infarction causing shortness of breath?

- **Left ventricular dysfunction → ↑ plasma in pulmonary interstitium → ↓ ability of O_2 to diffuse from alveoli into blood → ↓ PaO_2 and ↓ SaO_2**

$O_2\ Content = (1.34 \times Hb \times \downarrow SaO_2) + (0.003 \times \downarrow PaO_2)$

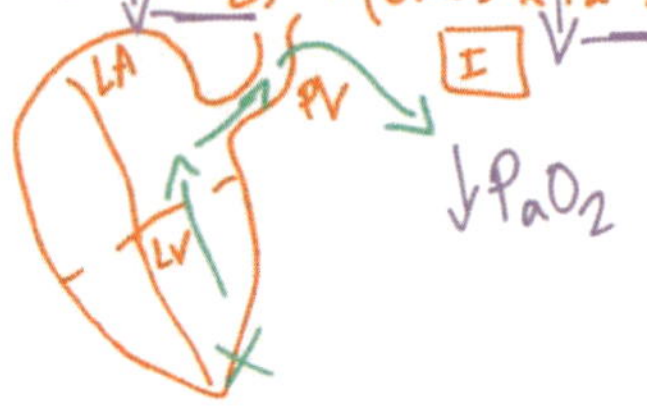

19. What part of the total oxygen content equation is altered in a patient with altitude sickness?

- **High altitude → ↓ Patm → ↓ PIO_2 → PAO_2 → PaO_2 and SaO_2**

$O_2\ Content = (1.34 \times Hb \times \downarrow SaO_2) + (0.003 \times \downarrow PaO_2)$

$\downarrow PIO_2 = FIO_2\ (\downarrow Patm - P_{H_2O})$

$\downarrow P_AO_2 = \downarrow PIO_2 - (P_aCO_2/R) \rightarrow \downarrow PaO_2 \rightarrow \downarrow SaO_2$

Section IV - Breathing Mechanics

I. Breathing Mechanics

A. Inspiration and expiration

1. Inspiration
   a) Diaphragm
   b) External intercostal muscles
   c) Accessory muscles
2. Expiration
   a) Abdominal wall muscles
   b) Internal intercostal muscles

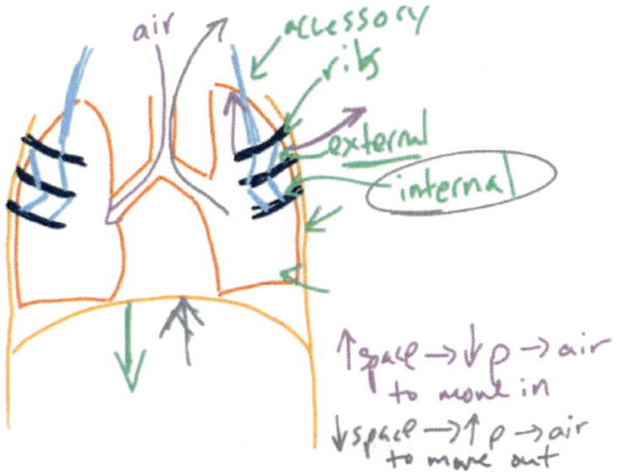

B. Lungs and Chest Wall

1. Figure 3.3 shows the compliance of the lungs and chest wall.
2. The lungs tend to collapse inward due to elastic recoil.
3. The chest tends to expand outward due to muscles and connective tissue.

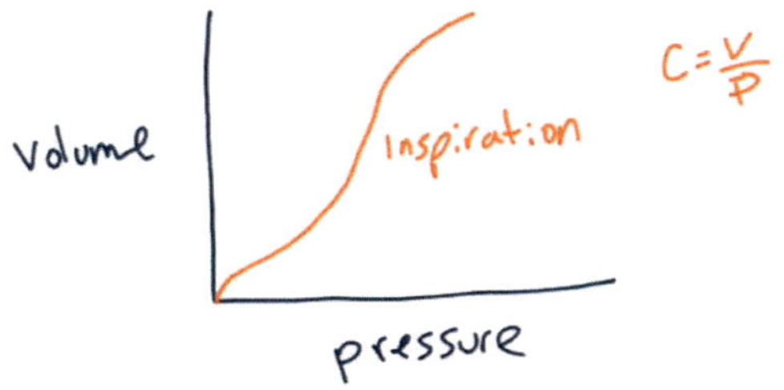

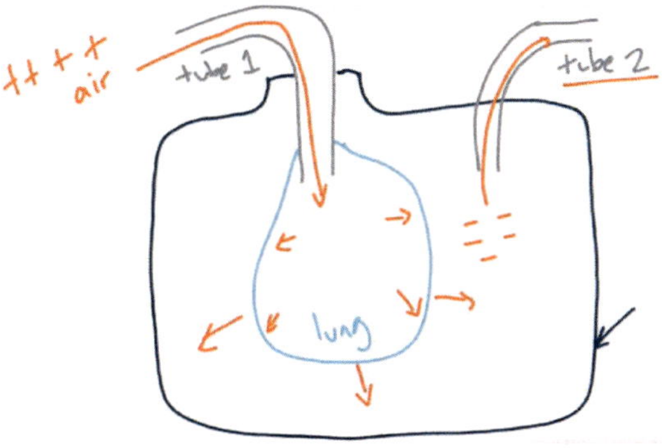

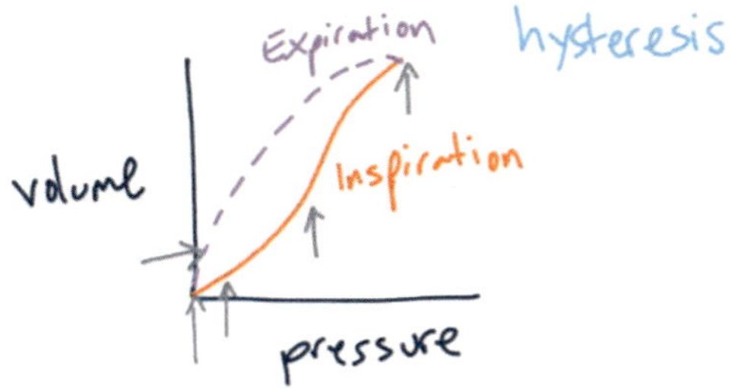

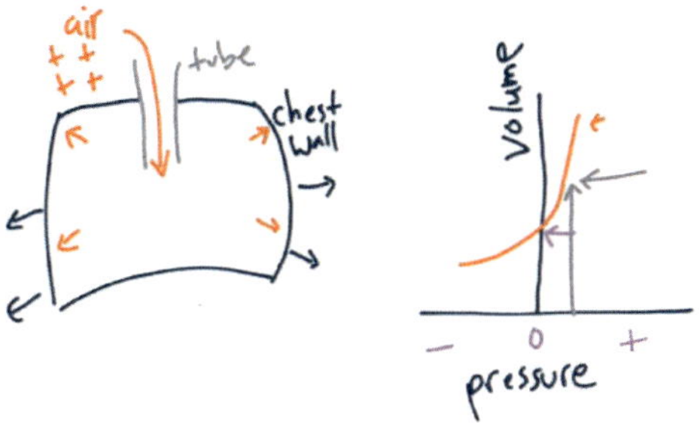

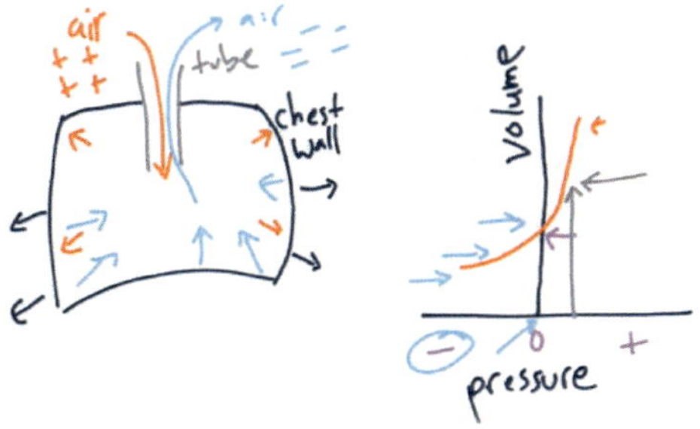

C. Pulmonary pressures

1. Figure 3.4 shows the alveolar and pleural pressures during inspiration and expiration.
2. Alveolar pressure

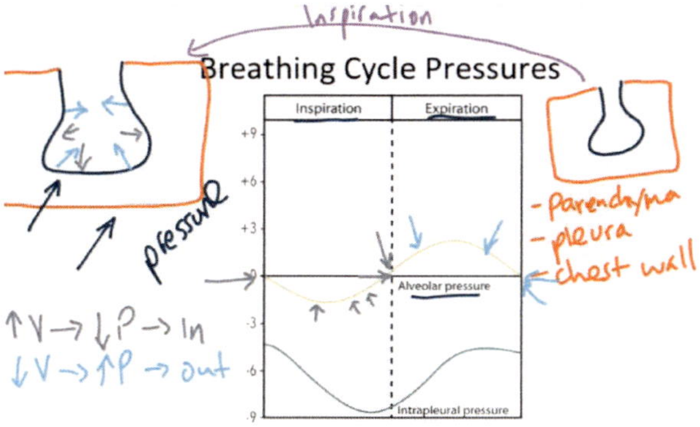

   a) Inspiration
      (1) During inspiration the space in the thorax increases and the alveoli expand.
      (2) The increased volume in the alveoli causes the pressure to decrease below atmospheric pressure.

(3) The pressure gradient allows oxygen to move from the atmosphere into the alveoli.

(4) As air enters the alveoli it exerts a pressure on the alveolar walls which causes the pressure in the alveoli to increase and eventually return to atmospheric pressure.

(5) When the pressures are equal air no longer moves in or out of the alveoli.

b) Expiration

(1) The space in the thorax decreases and the alveoli collapse inward.

(2) The decreased volume in the alveoli causes the pressure to increase above atmospheric pressure.

(3) The pressure gradient allows oxygen to move from the alveoli into the atmosphere.

(4) As air leaves the alveoli there are less molecules colliding with the alveolar walls which allows the pressure in the alveoli to decrease back to atmospheric pressure.

3. Intrapleural pressure

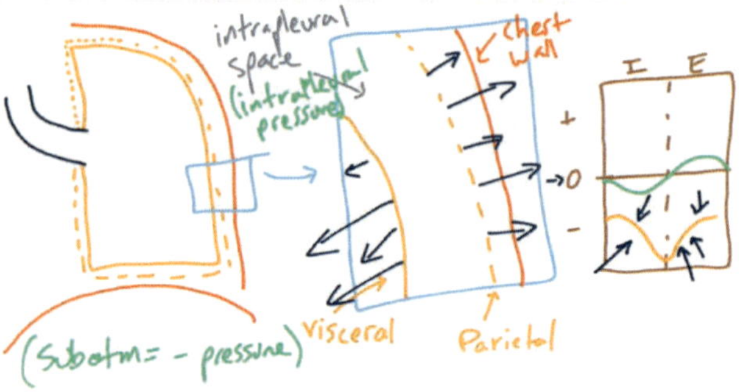

a) The pressure in the space between the visceral and parietal pleura.

b) In utero, the pleural cavity grows faster than the lungs which results in a subatmospheric pressure in the intrapleural space.

c) The subatmospheric pressure in the intrapleural space is like a vacuum that pulls the visceral and parietal layers of the lungs inward, as if trying to collapse the space.

d) Inspiration

(1) During inspiration the intrapleural space is stretched and the elastic property of the lungs pull the visceral pleura inward.

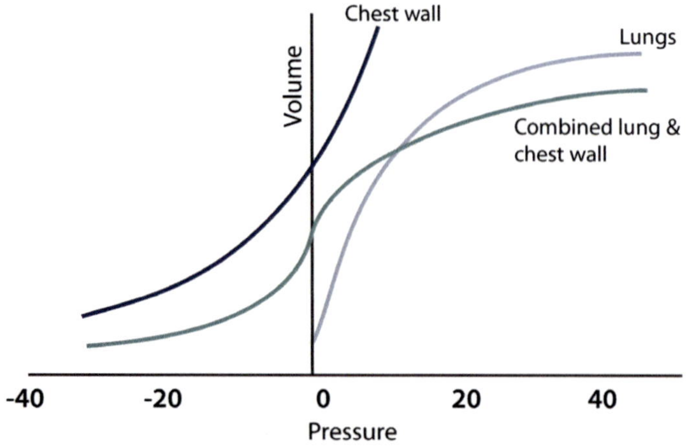

Figure 3.3 - Lung and chest wall compliance

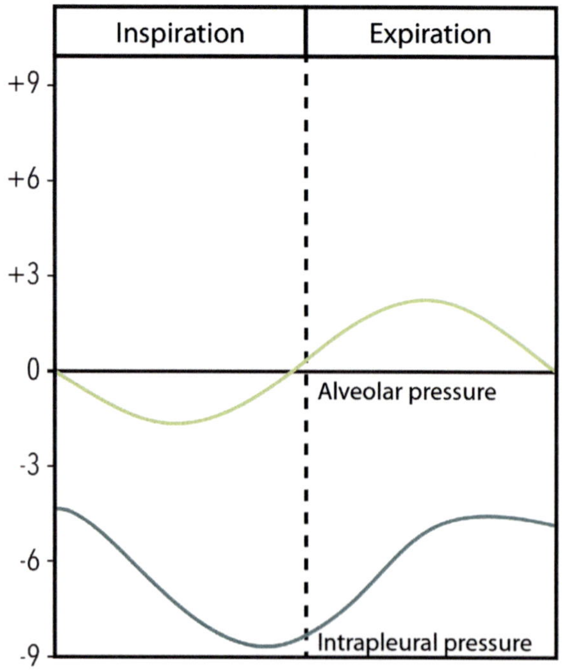

Figure 3.4 - Alveolar & Intrapleural Pressures

   (2) The outward expansion of the chest wall pulls the parietal pleura outward.
   (3) The increased pull in opposite directions increases the stretch-like forces on the intrapleural space, making the pressure become even lower than before, and creates a stronger vacuum-like force inside the space.
   (4) The increased negative pressure in the intrapleural space holds the lungs to the chest wall, allowing the lungs to expand.

e) Expiration
   (1) During expiration the stretch on the visceral and parietal pleura is decreased.
   (2) The decreased stretching forces causes the pressure to increase such that it is less negative compared to inspiration.

4. Transmural pressure
   a) The pressure across a wall, or several walls.
   b) Transmural pressure is simply the alveolar pressure minus the intrapleural pressure.
   c) Physiologically it is always positive and relatively constant throughout the breathing cycle.
   d) Conceptually, transmural pressure refers to an outward force that contributes to the expansion of lungs.

REVIEW QUESTIONS

1. How would the compliance curves of the chest wall and lungs be altered in an elderly patient?

- **Aging → calcifications of ribs from osteoarthritis and osteoporosis → ↓ compliance of chest wall**
- **Aging → ↓ lung elasticity → ↑ lung compliance**

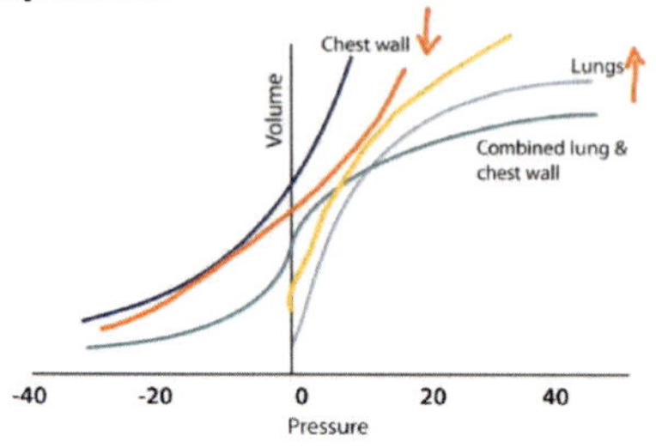

2. What is the alveolar pressure, intrapleural pressure, and transmural pressure at functional residual capacity (FRC)?

- **FRC represents the lungs at rest (atmospheric pressure = pressure inside lungs)**
- **Alveolar pressure = 760 mmHg**
- **Intrapleural pressure = 756 mmHg**
- **Transmural pressure = 4 mmHg**

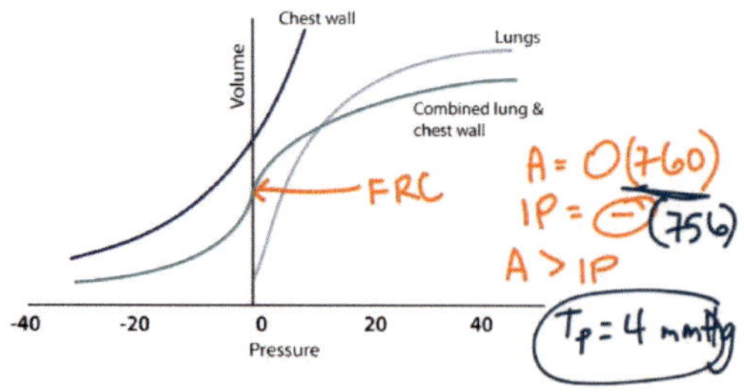

3. How would α1-antitrypsin deficiency alter the curve seen in figure 3.5?

- **α1-antitrypsin deficiency → ↓ elastin → ↑ lung compliance**

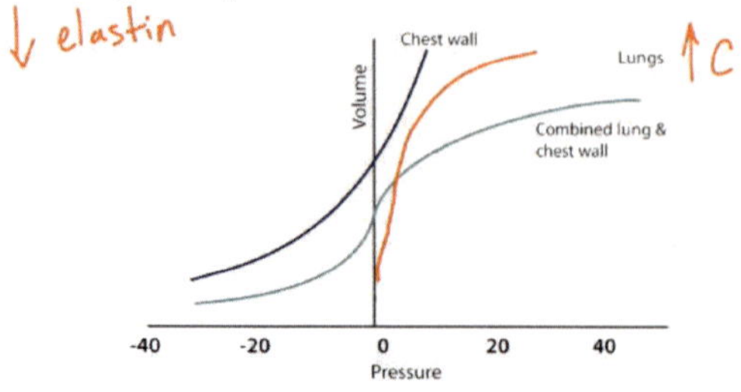

4. How could bleomycin toxicity alter the curve seen in figure 3.5?

- **Bleomycin → pulmonary fibrosis → ↓ lung compliance**

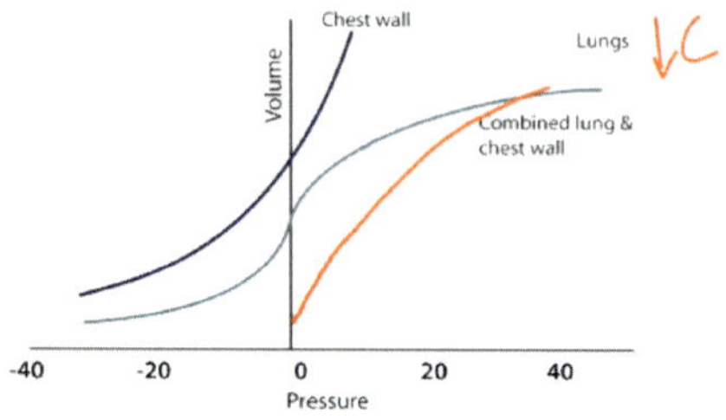

5. How does the pressure in the intrapleural space change during a pneumothorax?

- **Pneumothorax → intrapleural space is exposed to atmosphere and pressure equilibrates → outward pulling force of intrapleural space is lost → lung collapses**

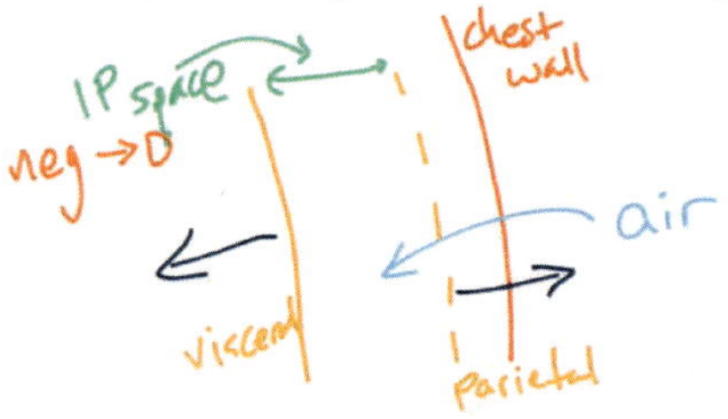

6. Why does a pneumothorax result in hyperresonant percussive sounds and diminished breath sounds?

- **Solid structures → dull percussion**
- **Hollow structures → hyperresonant percussion**
- **Lung collapse → lung is further away from chest wall → diminished breath sounds**

Section V - Gas Exchange

I. Gas Exchange

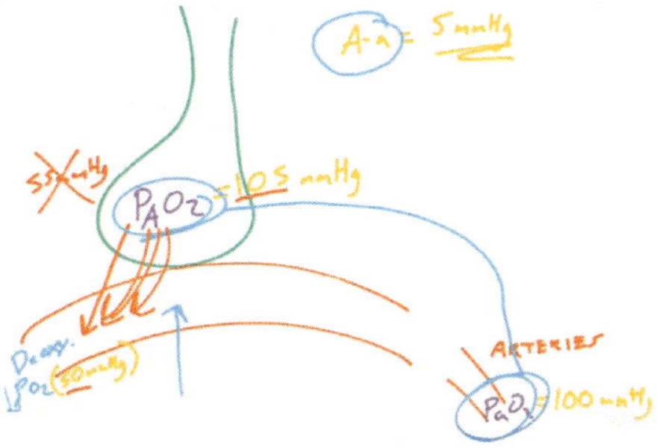

A. Hypoxemia

1. Decreased PaO_2

2. O_2 content equation = 1.34 × Hb × SaO_2 + (0.003 × PaO_2)

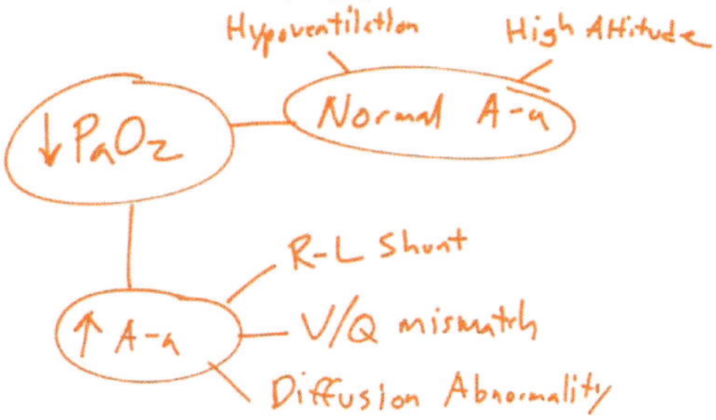

B. Hypoxia

1. Decreased O_2 delivery to the tissues.

2. O_2 delivery to tissues = O_2 content × CO.

C. A-a gradient

1. A-a gradient = PAO_2 - PaO_2

2. PAO_2 is the pressure of O_2 in the alveoli.

   a) Normally higher than PaO_2 (~105 mmHg).

3. PaO_2 is the pressure of O_2 in the arterial blood.

   a) Normally lower than PAO_2 (~100 mmHg).

   b) O_2 is driven from the alveolus to the capillary via a pressure gradient.

4. A normal A-a gradient is 5-15 mmHg.

   a) An increase in PaO_2 or a decrease in PAO_2 would decrease the A-a gradient.

   b) A decrease in PaO_2 or an increase in PAO_2 would increase the A-a gradient.

5. Hypoxemia + increased A-a gradient (>15 mmHg)

   a) V/Q mismatch

   b) Right to left shunt (e.g. VSD) → decreased PaO_2 reaching pulmonary circulation → decreased perfusion (Q) → increased V/Q ratio (V/Q mismatch)

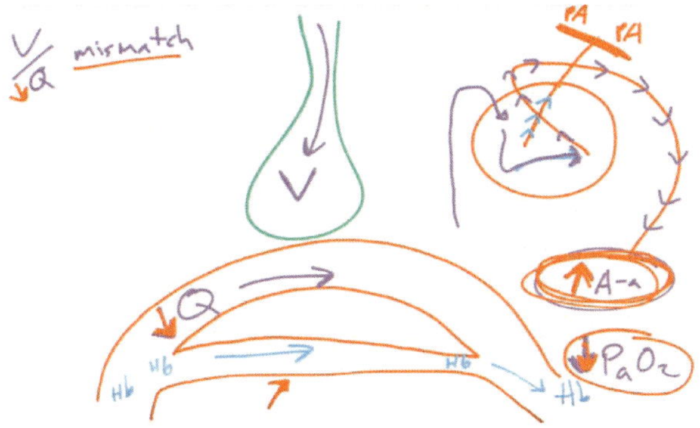

   c) Diffusion limitations

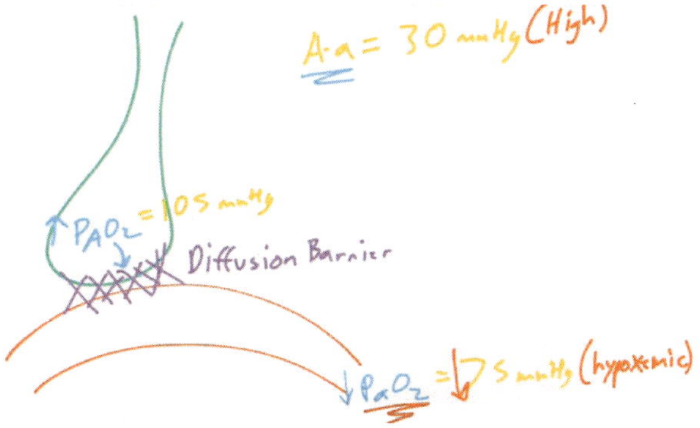

6. Hypoxemia + normal A-a gradient (5-15 mmHg)

   a) Hypoventilation

   b) High altitude

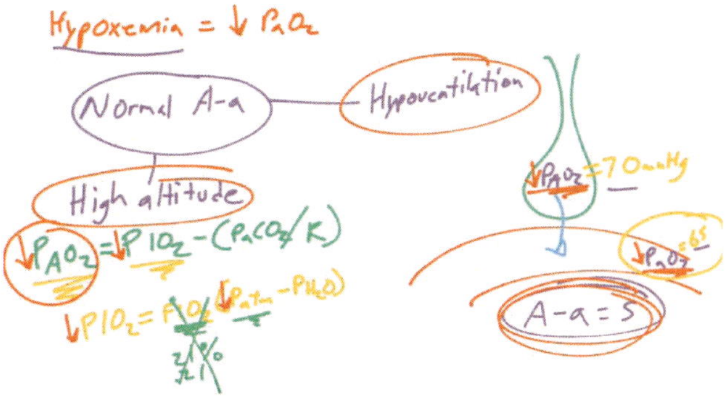

D. Hemoglobin-oxygen dissociation curve (Figure 3.5)

E. Right shifts

   a) ↑PCO_2

   b) ↑Temperature

   c) ↑2,3-DPG

d) ↓pH

e) ↑ altitude

1. Left shifts

   a) ↓PCO_2

   b) ↓Temperature

   c) ↓2,3-DPG

   d) ↑pH

   e) ↓ altitude

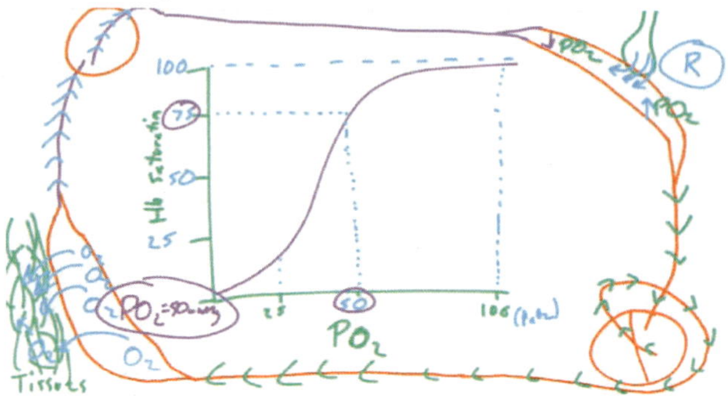

F. Perfusion-limited & diffusion-limited gas exchange

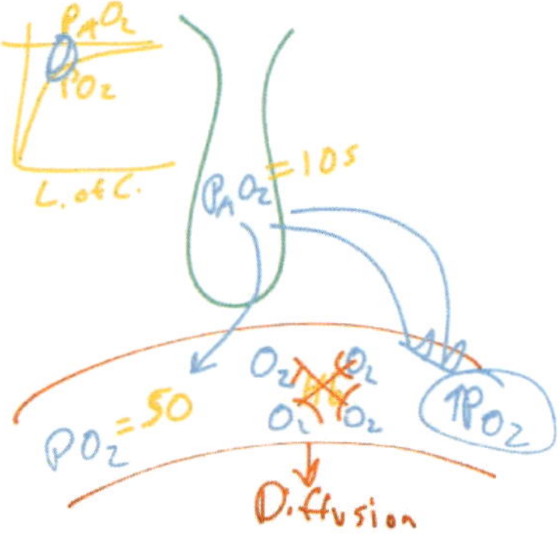

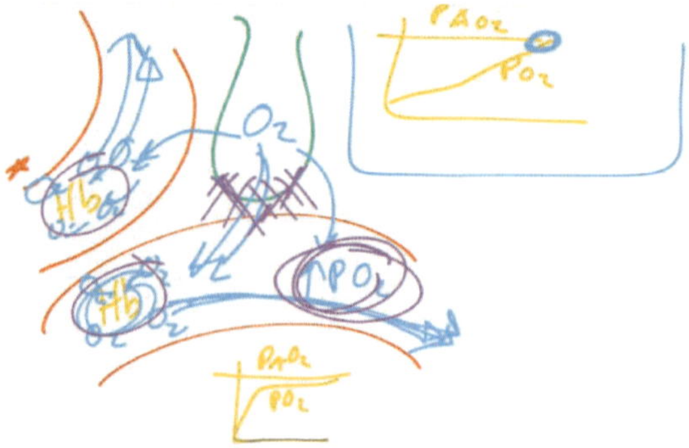

1. Perfusion-limited

   a) CO_2, N_2O, and O_2 (under normal conditions) are all perfusion limited gases.

   b) Gas is transferred as a result of a concentration gradient.

      (1) High PaO_2 (or PaN_2O) and low PO_2 (or PN_2O) causes O_2 (or N_2O) to leave the alveolus and enter the capillary.

      (2) High PCO_2 and low $PaCO_2$ causes CO_2 to leave the capillary and enter the alveolus.

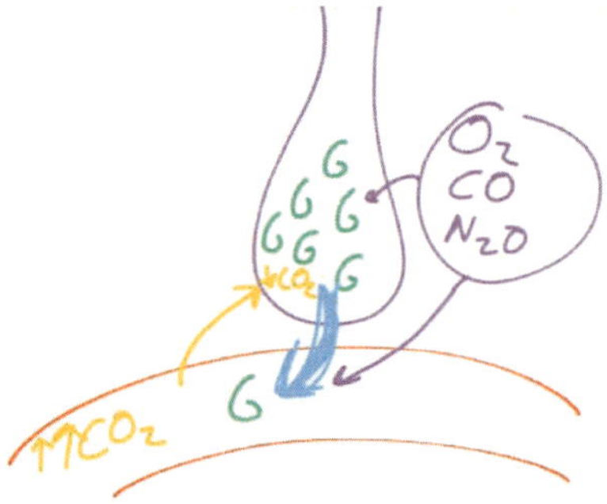

   c) Decreased concentration gradient → decreased transfer of gas

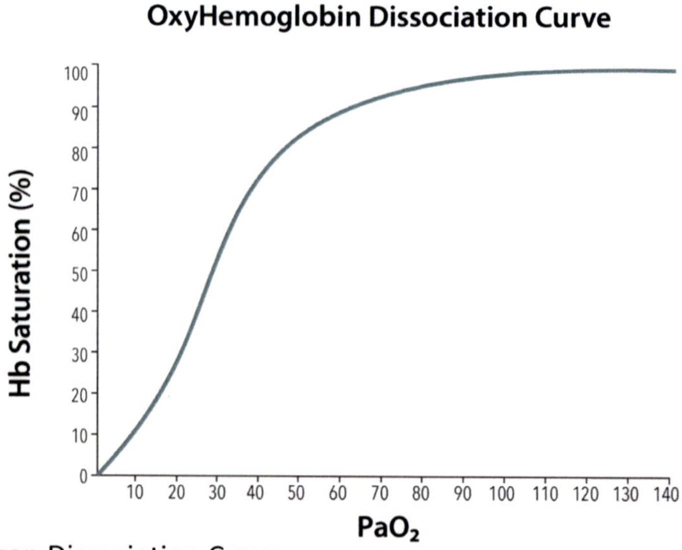

Figure 3.5 - Hemoglobin-oxygen Dissociation Curve

(1) The alveolar-capillary gradient relies on continued perfusion of the capillary to remove the gas that enters.

(2) Decreased capillary perfusion (e.g. pulmonary embolism) → increased PO_2 (or PN_2O) → decrease concentration gradient → decreased transfer of gas (hence the term perfusion-limited)

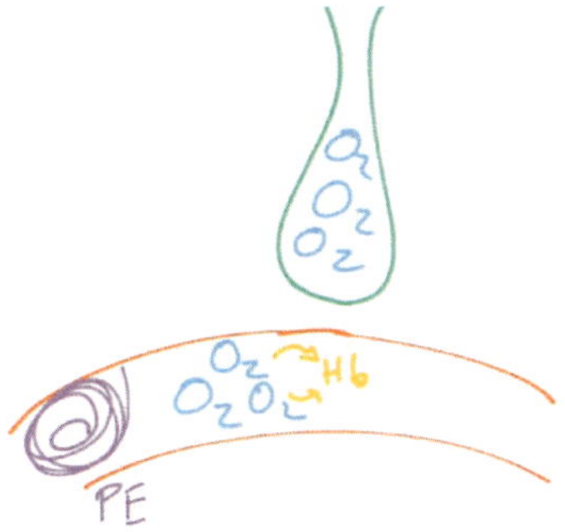

(3) Increased capillary perfusion → decreased PO_2 (or N_2O) → increased gradient → increased transfer of gas

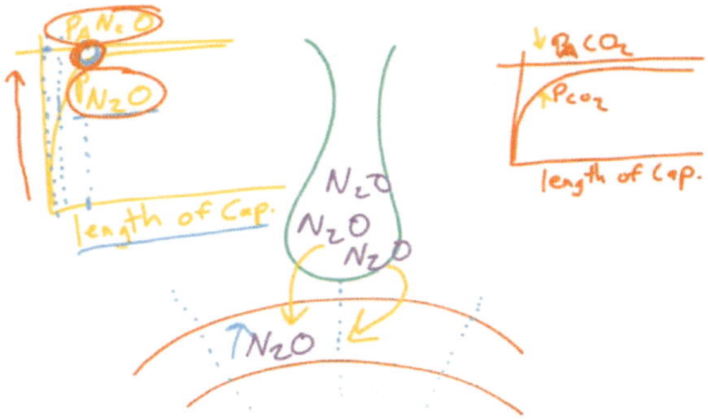

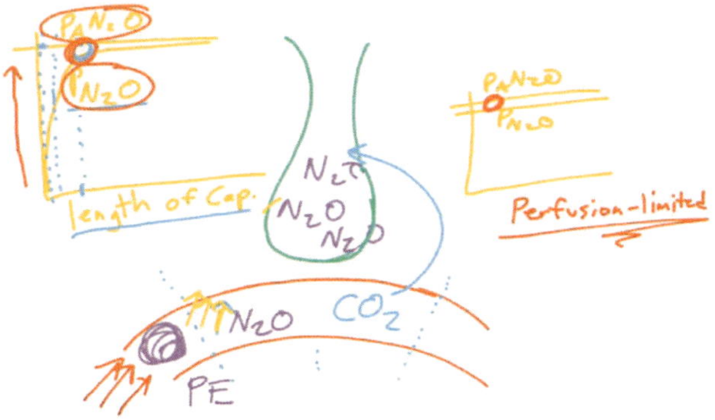

2. Diffusion-limited

a) CO and O_2 during exercise are diffusion-limited gases.

b) Gas is transferred as a result of a concentration gradient.

(1) High P_ACO and low PCO causes CO to leave the alveolus and enter the capillary.

(2) Hb avidly binds CO → PCO (free, unbound CO) is kept low → concentration gradient is continually favored

c) Decreased perfusion does not significantly alter concentration gradient.

(1) If perfusion is limited (e.g. pulmonary embolism), Hb will continue to bind up CO → PCO (free, unbound CO) continues to be low → concentration gradient is maintained → CO is continually transferred.

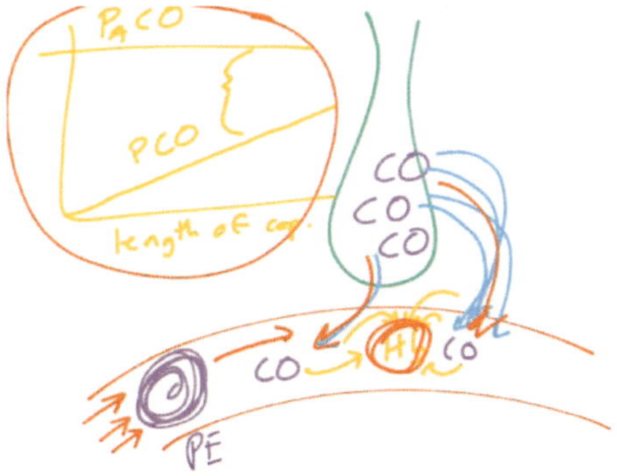

d) Diffusion barrier will decrease transfer of gas.

(1) Damaged or dysfunctional alveolar surface (e.g. emphysema, interstitial lung disease) → decreased diffusion of gas into the capillary (hence the term diffusion-limited)

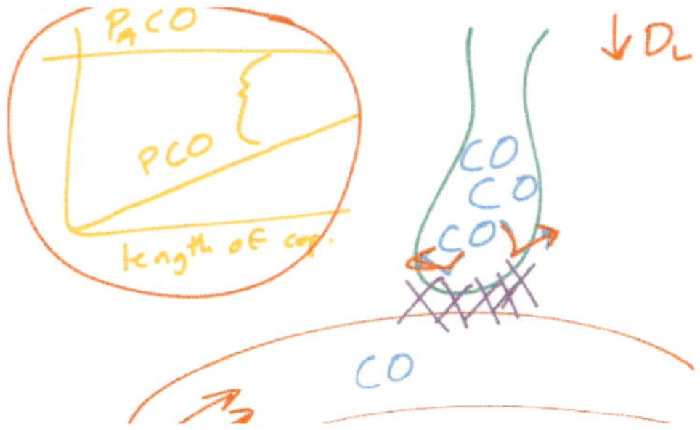

G. Gas delivery and exchange

1. Oxygen (O_2)

a) Arteries bring O_2 to the tissues.

b) The tissues take the O_2 and release CO_2 into the blood.

(1) CO_2 can cause vasodilation and promotes O_2 unloading from hemoglobin (favors T form of Hb).

(2) CO_2 is produced as a by-product of cellular respiration and rapidly diffuses into the plasma and RBCs.

(3) Within RBCs the following reaction occurs via the enzyme carbonic anhydrase: $CO_2 + H_2O \rightarrow HCO_3^- + H^+$

(4) The HCO_3^- is transported out of the cell in exchange for a chloride ion which enters the cell.

(5) CO_2 will decrease the pH of the blood by generating carbonic acid.

c) Veins return CO_2 to heart → deoxygenated blood enters the pulmonary vasculature → CO_2 is transferred to the alveoli in exchange for O_2 and the process starts over again

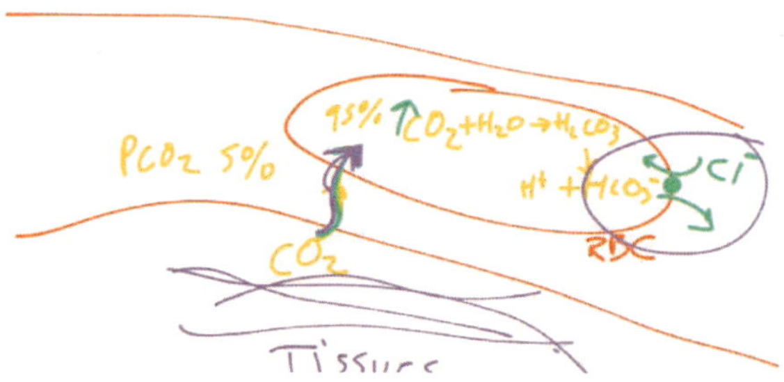

d) O_2 released into arteries

(1) PaO_2 normally ~100 mmHg

(2) $PaCO_2$ normally ~40 mmHg

e) At tissue/capillary level, O_2 is removed from blood

(1) CO_2 released into veins

(2) PvO_2 normally ~35 mmHg

(3) $PvCO_2$ normally ~45 mmHg

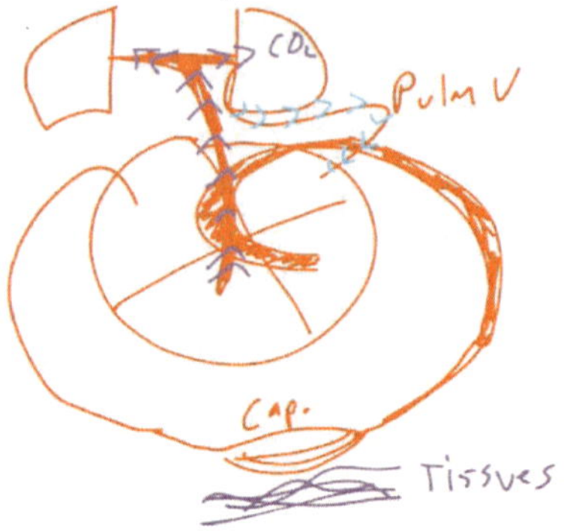

REVIEW QUESTIONS

1. What would happen to the PAO_2, PaO_2, and A-a gradient in a restrictive lung disease patient if given 100% supplemental O_2?

- **Interstitial lung diseases create a barrier to diffusion**
- **Recall $PIO_2 = FIO_2(Patm-PH_2O)$ and $PAO_2 = PIO_2 - (PaCO_2/R)$**
- **Increased FIO_2 causes increased PIO_2 and PAO_2, although the diffusion will block PaO_2 from receiving the increased alveolar O_2 (PAO_2) → increased A-a gradient.**

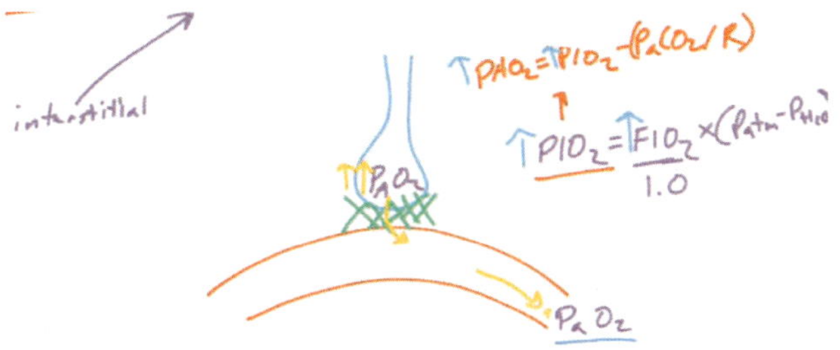

2. What would happen to the PaO_2, pH and A-a gradient in a pt with heroin intoxication?

- **Heroin intoxication can cause respiratory depression (hypoventilation/low PAO_2).**
- **Low PAO_2 leads to lower PaO_2.**
- **There is no alteration to diffusion, so A-a will remain the same.**
- **Lack of ventilation increases retention of $PaCO_2$, thereby decreasing serum pH.**

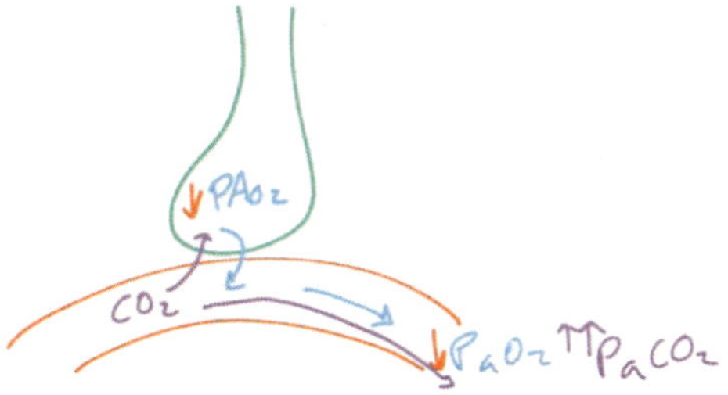

3. A pt has severe iron deficiency anemia. What does this do to PaO_2 and SaO_2?

- **Decreased Hb causes decreased O_2 content via equation**
- **PaO_2 has not changed, so neither will SaO_2 which relies on PaO_2 (not Hb)**
- **For remember that SaO_2 does not rely on Hb, think of SaO_2 as a single Hb molecule**

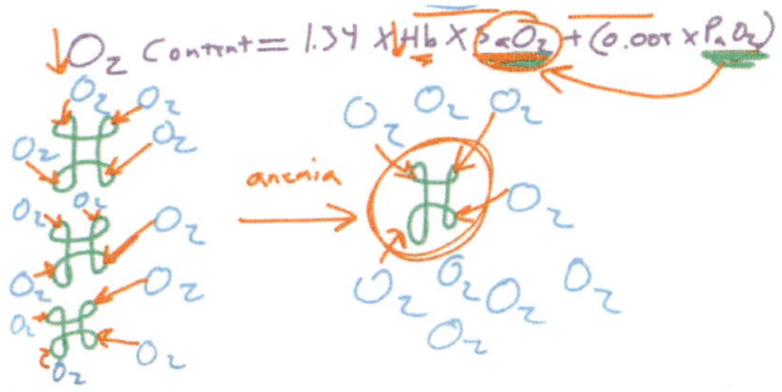

4. What form of Hb would be favored in a pt with very decreased 2,3-BPG?

- **2,3-BPG normally causes a right shift, facilitating O_2 unloading (T form)**
- **Low 2,3-BPG favors O_2 retention (R form)**

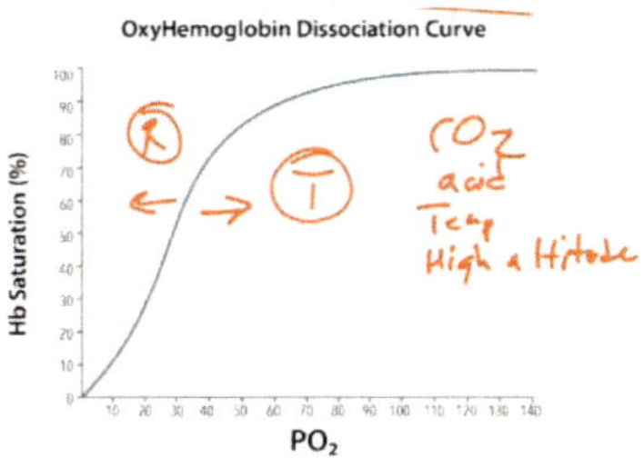

5. HbF has higher affinity for **O_2**. How would its curve appear compared to normal?

- **Increased affinity for O_2 can be thought of as a left shift**

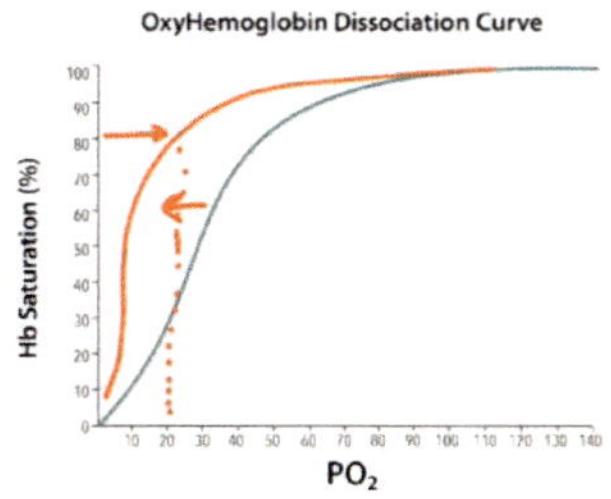

REVIEW QUESTIONS

6. A pt with a hypercoagulation disease takes an 8 hour flight and develops shortness of breath. What is the A-a gradient?

- **Suspect a PE in this scenario**
- **PE will impair perfusion leading to rapid saturation of hemoglobin with O_2, diminishing the gradient from the alveolus to the pulmonary capillaries (this is NOT the A-a gradient)**
- **Decreased O_2 entering the pulmonary capillary leads to decreased PaO_2, thus an increased A-a gradient**
- **Note: CO_2 will stop being delivered to the alveolus, leading to rapid equilibration at the interface, causing higher serum CO_2 and lower $PACO_2$**

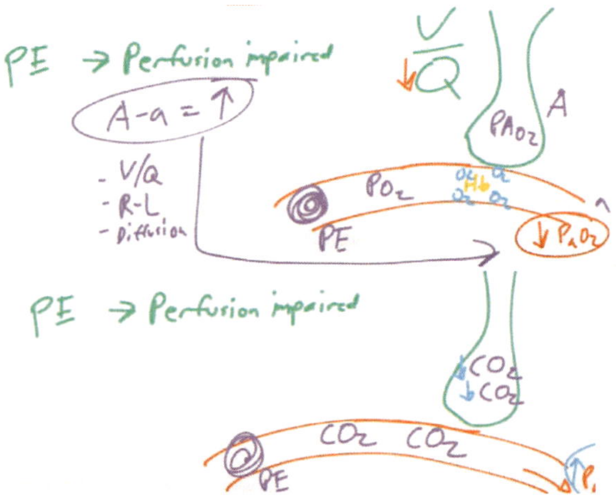

7. A pt moves into a new apartment and develops dizziness, weakness and nausea when he wakes up. What curve represents the gas causing the symptoms and why?

- **Suspect CO poisoning**
- **CO will bind to Hb with such high affinity that it will never equilibrate (the right graph)**
- **Note: in a patient with emphysema (diffusion barrier), there will be decreased diffusion of CO into the pulmonary capillaries (decreased DLCO)**

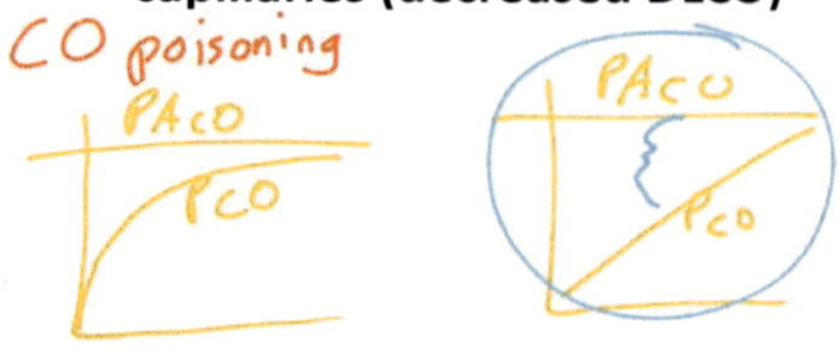

8. The blood of a healthy pt at rest is drawn and demonstrates a PO_2 of 130 mmHg and a PCO_2 of 10 mmHg. Was this drawn from the artery or vein or did something else happen?

- **PvO_2 should be <100 mmHg**
- **$PvCO_2$ should be >40 mmHg**
- **PaO_2 should be ~100 mmHg**
- **$PaCO_2$ should be ~35 mmHg**
- **An O_2 of 130 mmHg is too high for an artery and a CO_2 of 10 is too low**
- **Note that the atmospheric PO_2 is ~160 mmHg (higher than blood) and PCO_2 is ~0 (lower than blood). Thus, blood exposed to the atmosphere explains the labs levels**

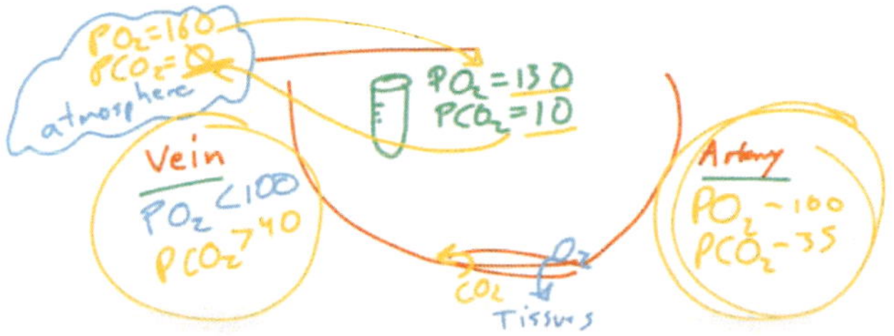

9. What would happen to extracellular chloride in a pt performing heavy dynamic exercise?

- **CO_2 is normally taken into RBC from tissues and converted to HCO_3^-**
- **HCO_3^- is exchanged at the RBC surface for Cl^-**
- **Exercise increases CO_2 and ultimately increased Cl^- entering the RBC, leading to low venous/extracellular Cl^-**
- **Note: Cl^- in the arteries would not have changed**

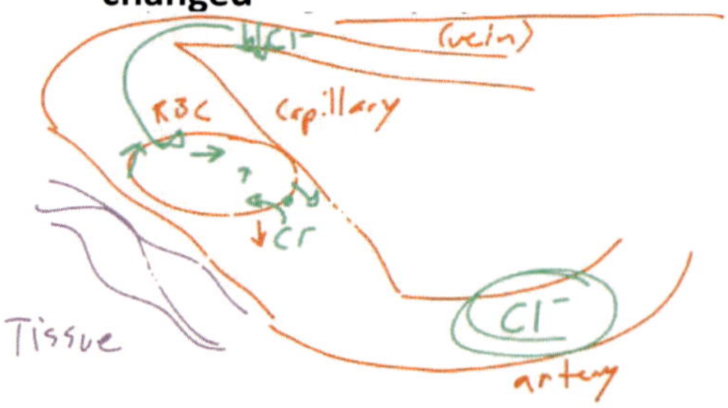

Section VI - V/Q Mismatch and Integrated Respiration

I. V/Q Mismatch

A. V = alveolar ventilation.

1. CO_2 diffuses from high concentration in the capillaries to the alveoli where concentration is low. Atmospheric CO_2 is quite low (~ 0 mmHg).

2. O_2 diffuses from a high concentration in the alveoli to a low concentration in the capillaries. Atmospheric O_2 is much higher than capillary O_2 concentration.

B. Q = pulmonary blood flow

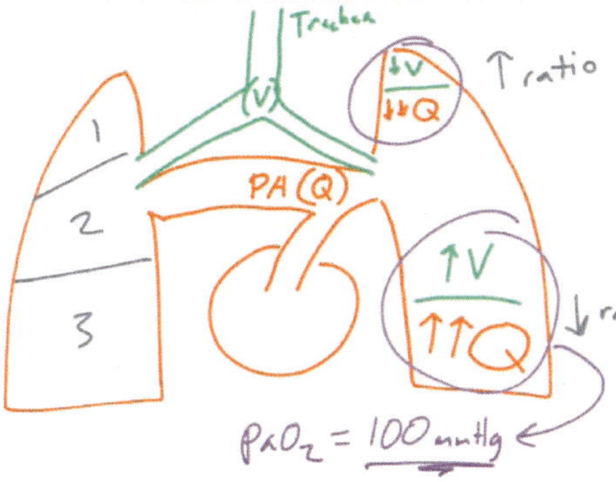

C. Ventilation to perfusion (V/Q) defects occur for a variety of reasons.

1. Decreased ventilation will cause a V/Q mismatch.

a) Foreign body obstruction → decreased ventilation → decreased V/Q ratio (V/Q mismatch)

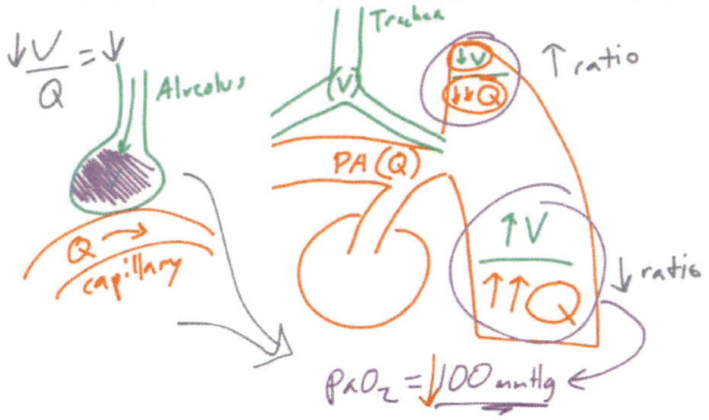

2. Decreased perfusion will cause a V/Q mismatch.

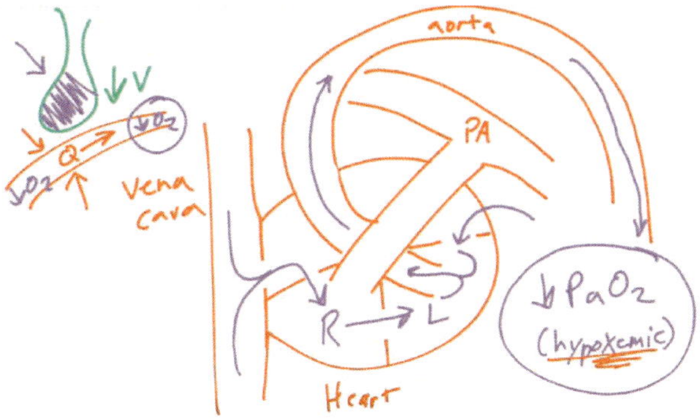

D. Regional differences in ventilation and perfusion

1. The base of the lungs have an increased ventilation and perfusion compared to the apices.

2. At the base the perfusion increase is much greater than the ventilation so the V/Q ratio decreases from the apices to the base.

E. Pulmonary embolism

1. Hypoxia increases ventilation and heart rate through the chemoreceptor reflex.

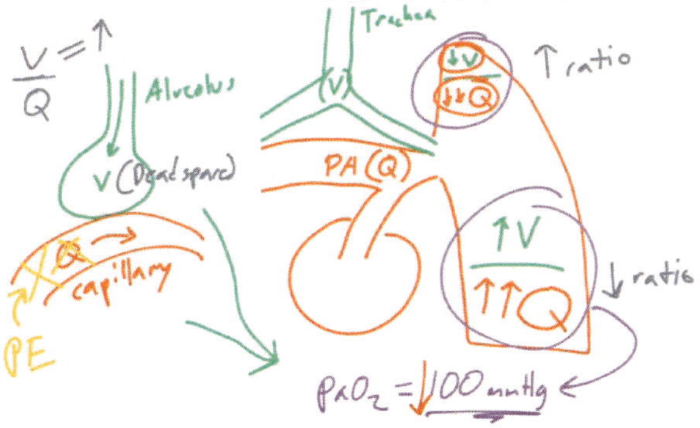

II. Respiration Integrated

A. Control of breathing

1. Respiratory center is the pons and medulla.

   a) The medulla stimulates the respiratory muscles (i.e. diaphragm and intercostal muscles) to increase or decrease respiration.

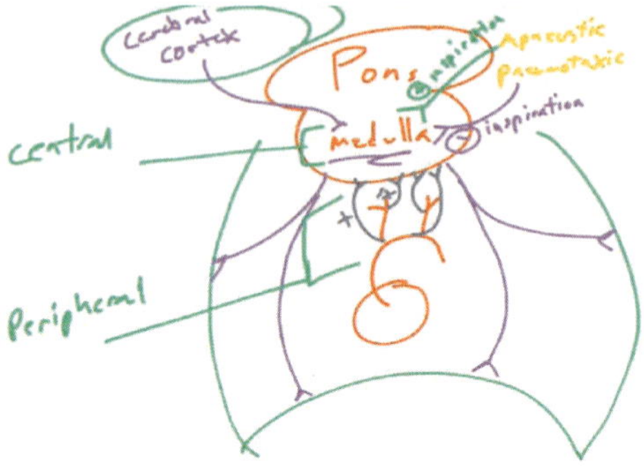

2. The respiratory center can be modulated unconsciously by the central and peripheral chemoreceptors and consciously by the cerebral cortex.

   a) Chemoreceptors

      (1) Central: Located in the medulla. Stimulated by increased [H^+].

         (a) Indirectly stimulated by increased CO_2 (CO_2 becomes H^+) → increased respiration.

      (2) Peripheral: Located in the aortic and carotid bodies.

         (a) Stimulated by increased CO_2, [H^+], or decreased O_2 → increased respiration.

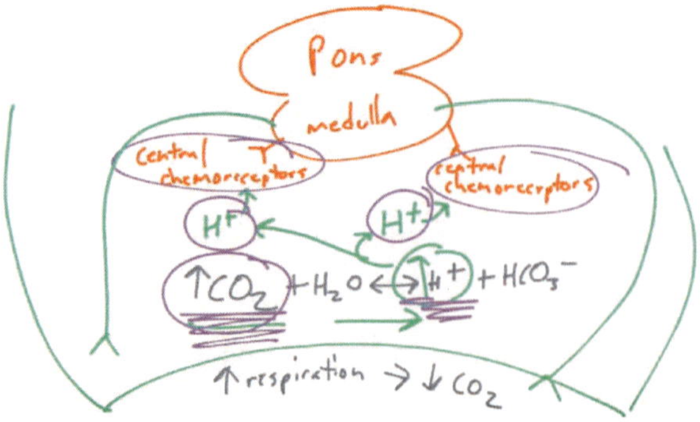

3. Hypoventilation

   a) The lungs and airways are not expanding fully.

      (1) Central hypoventilation → problem with the breathing centers or nervous system

      (2) Peripheral hypoventilation → structures impede the full expansion of the lungs such as kyphoscoliosis or severe obesity

      (3) Hypoventilation from metabolic compensation.

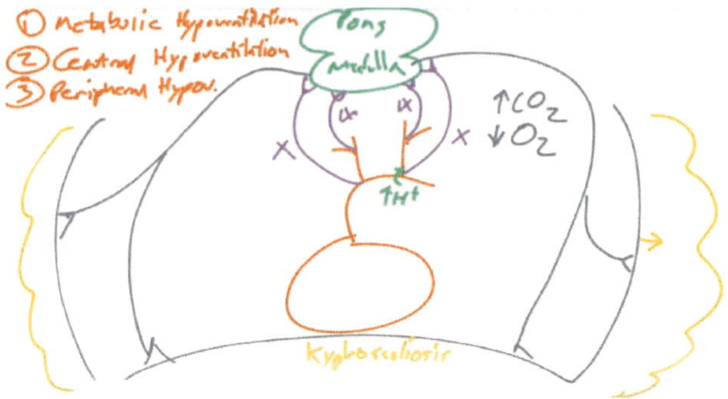

4. Hyperventilation

   a) Can occur for a variety of reasons (e.g. metabolic compensation, panic attack, etc).

B. Bronchoconstrictors and Bronchodilators

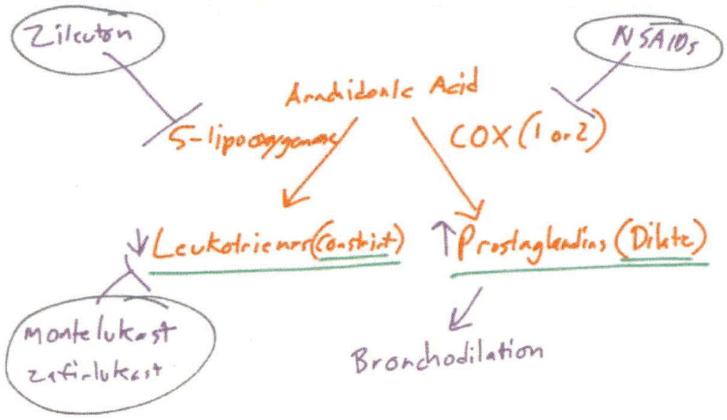

1. Dilation

   a) Prostaglandins

   b) β_2 receptors (sympathetic)

2. Constriction

   a) Leukotrienes

   b) Bradykinin

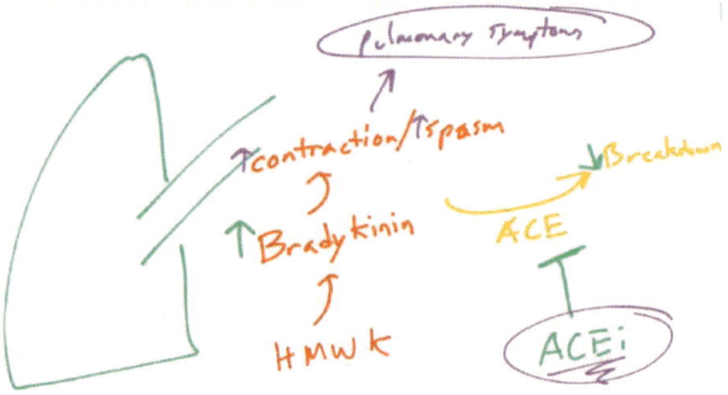

c) M_3 receptors (parasympathetic)

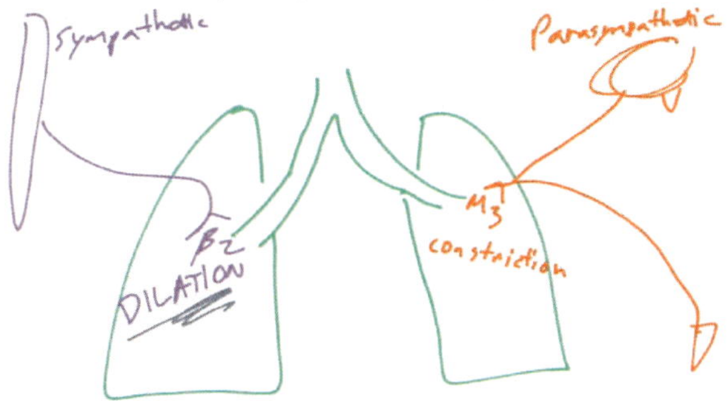

C. Vasoconstriction and Vasodilation

1. Dilation
   a) Nitric oxide
2. Constriction
   a) Ca^{2+}
   b) Endothelin
   c) α_1 receptors

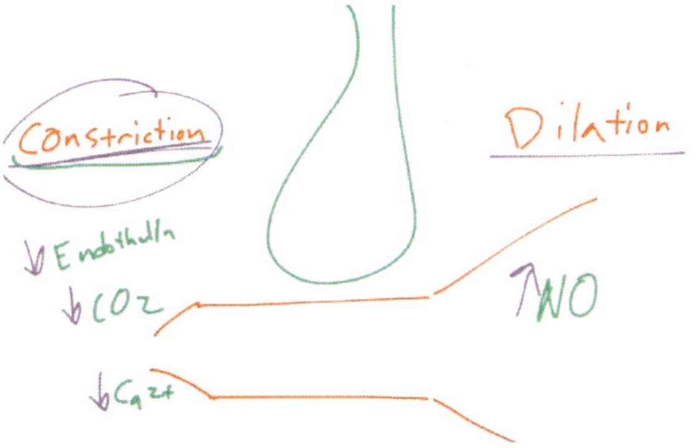

REVIEW QUESTIONS

1. An elderly woman has lobar pneumonia. What will happen to shunting?

- **Ventilation will decrease at this part of the lung, decreasing capillary O_2 in these regions → Hb will pass by lungs without getting oxygenated (intrapulmonary R-L shunt)**
- **Decreased O_2 will cause local vasoconstriction of pulmonary vessels, thereby decreasing the impact of the R-L shunt**

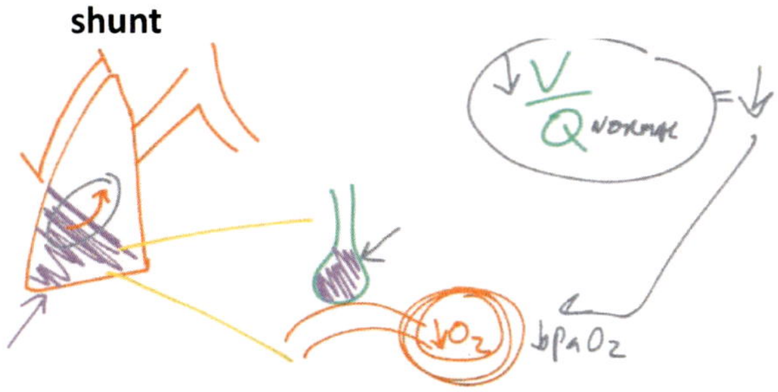

2. How would a pulmonary embolus affect pH?

- **Decreased perfusion results in decreased O_2 transfer from alveolus, leading to low PaO_2 (hypoxemia)**
- **Decreased PaO_2 will stimulate the peripheral chemoreceptors to increase respiration, leading to hyperventilation, decreased CO_2, and increased pH**

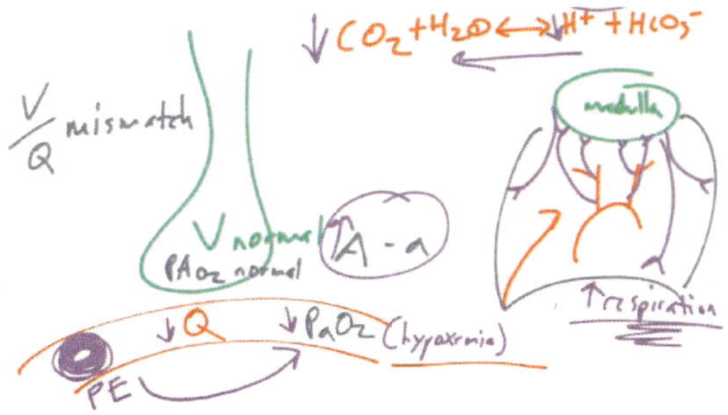

REVIEW QUESTIONS

3. A young boy inhales a peanut that blocks off the left bronchus. What will happen to the chemoreceptors and V/Q ratio?

   - **V/Q mismatch results in hypoxemia, stimulating peripheral chemoreceptors to increase respiratory rate**

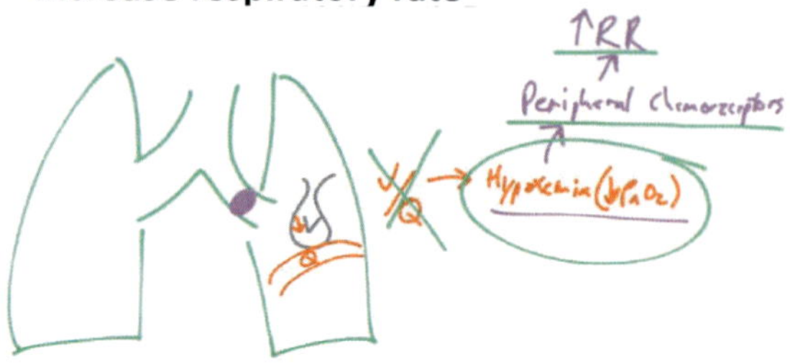

4. A patient has severe chronic bronchitis. Compared to normal, what would you expect to happen to levels of NO, Ca^{2+}, endothelin, PCO_2, and PO_2 in this patient?

   - **In a state of hypoxic vasoconstriction, expect higher levels of vasoconstrictors (CO_2, endothelin, and Ca_2^+)**

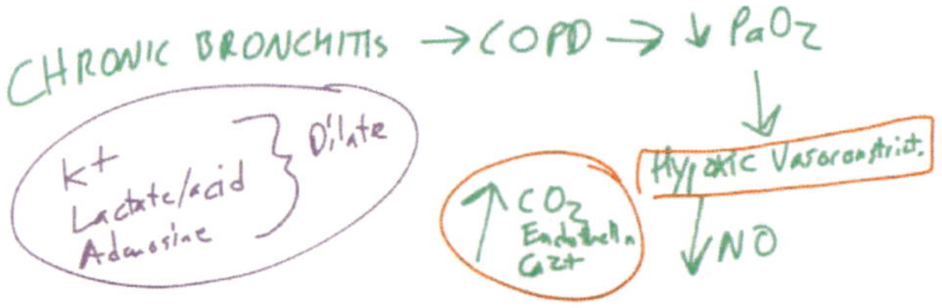

5. A pt has obstructive sleep apnea, what alterations occur?

   - **OSA can cause a V/Q mismatch at the alveolus, causing hypoxemia and hypercarbia (high $PaCO_2$)**
   - **Hypercarbia dilates cerebral vasculature but constricts pulmonary vasculature and stimulates chemoreceptors**

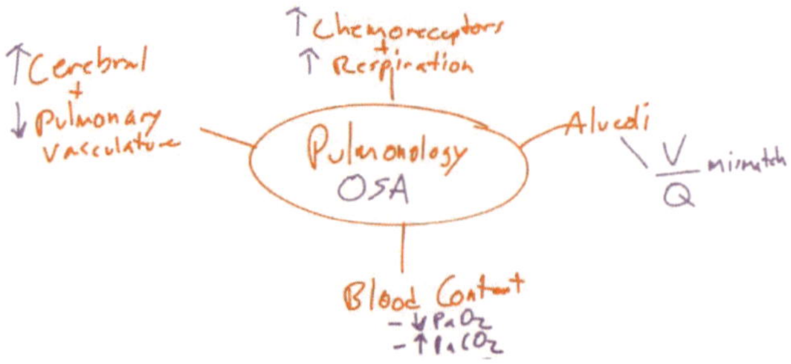

6. A pt is hyperventilating from a panic attack, what alterations occur?

   - **Hyperventilation would cause decrease $PaCO_2$ and increased PaO_2, leading to decreased chemoreceptor stimulation (although respiration would remain high since the pt is hyperventilating)**
   - **Low CO_2 would cause a relative constriction of cerebral vasculature (dizziness, syncope) and dilate pulmonary vasculature**

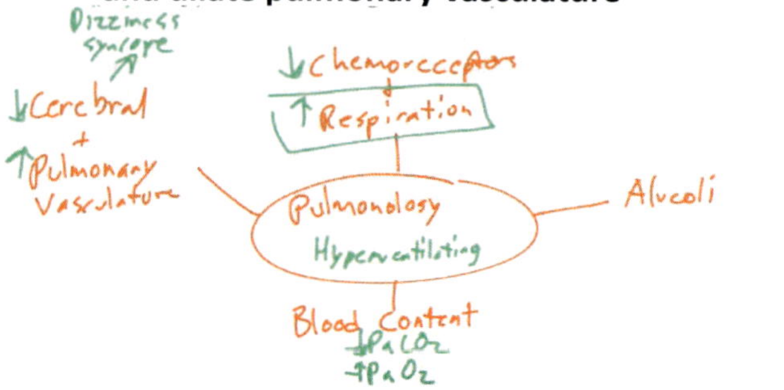

NEPHROLOGY

Section I - Introduction to Nephrology

I. Basic Principles

A. Primary functions of the kidneys

1. Removal of waste products (drugs, urea, etc.)
2. Electrolyte homeostasis
3. Acid-base regulation
4. Blood volume homeostasis
5. Regulation of erythropoiesis
6. Regulation of blood pressure
7. Regulation of bone health (vitamin D, calcium, and phosphorous)

II. Fluid Compartments

A. Distribution of water

1. The total body water (TBW) comprises 60% of body weight.
2. The intracellular space comprises 40% of body weight (⅔ of TBW).
3. The extracellular space comprises 20% of body weight (⅓ of TBW).

B. The measured volume of fluid compartments

1. Tritiated water can be used to measure TBW, because it is disbursed in all body compartments.
2. Mannitol can be used to measure the extracellular compartment, because the large size prevents it from crossing cellular membranes.
3. Evans blue can be used to measure the plasma volume, because it tightly binds to albumin.
4. A known mass of one of these substances can be injected into a patient, allowed to equilibrate, and then measured again to determine the volume of the compartment of interest using the following equation:

volume = amount / concentration

C. Redistribution of water between compartments

a) Osmolarity is the concentration of a solution.

b) NaCl, potassium, urea, and glucose are major physiologic contributors to osmolarity.

c) NaCl cannot cross the cellular membrane.

d) Water freely shifts between the compartments in response to changes in osmolarity.

e) The osmolarity of the extracellular fluid (ECF) is normally equal to the osmolarity of the intracellular fluid (ICF).

REVIEW QUESTIONS

1. How would anaphylaxis alter the volume in the intracellular and extracellular compartments?

   - **Anaphylaxis is a severe allergic reaction → antigen binds to IgE which activates mast cell to release histamine**
   - **Histamine dilates smooth muscle cells of arterioles → vasodilation. Also causes contraction of pericytes**
   - **↓ plasma volume, ↑ interstitial volume, unchanged extracellular fluid compartment volume**

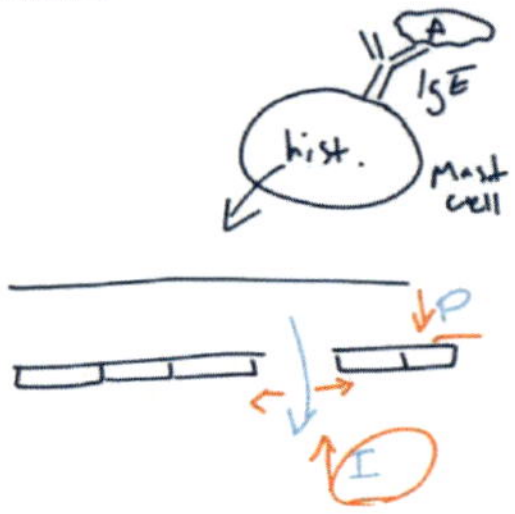

2. How would the redistribution of water be altered in the intracellular and extracellular fluid compartments in a patient who has been given an IV bolus of normal saline?

   - **↑ volume of the extracellular fluid compartment, but osmolarity is unchanged → no redistribution of water (isosmotic volume expansion)**

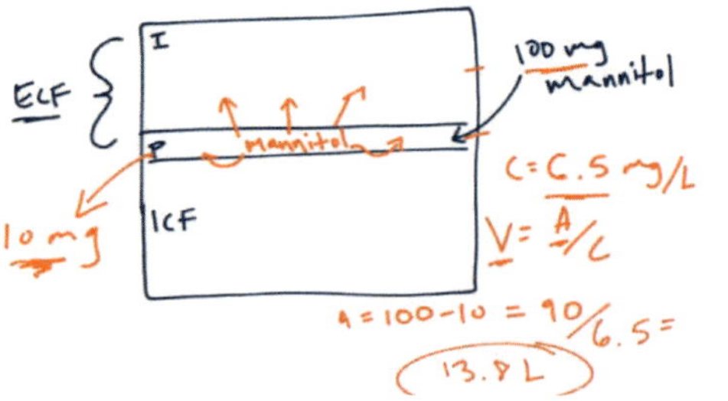

3. How would the redistribution of water be altered in the intracellular and extracellular fluid compartments in a patient who has been given an IV highly concentrated NaCl?

   - **↑ NaCl in the ECF → ↑ ECF osmolarity → water moves from the ICF to the ECF until the osmolarity has equilibrated → net ↓ ICF volume and ↑ ECF volume (hyperosmotic volume expansion)**

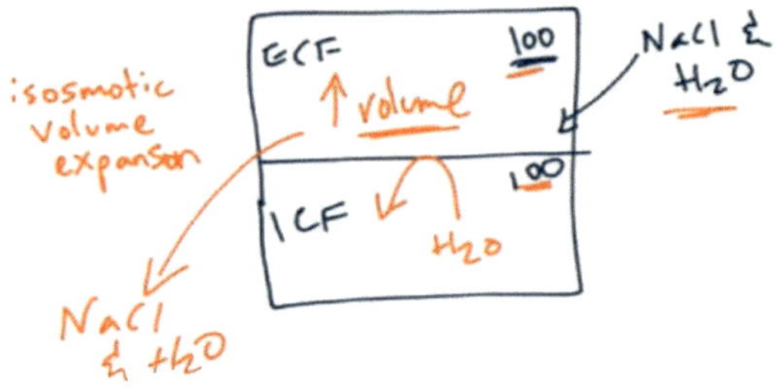

4. What neurological pathology is associated with hyperosmotic volume expansion?

   - **Central pontine myelinolysis**

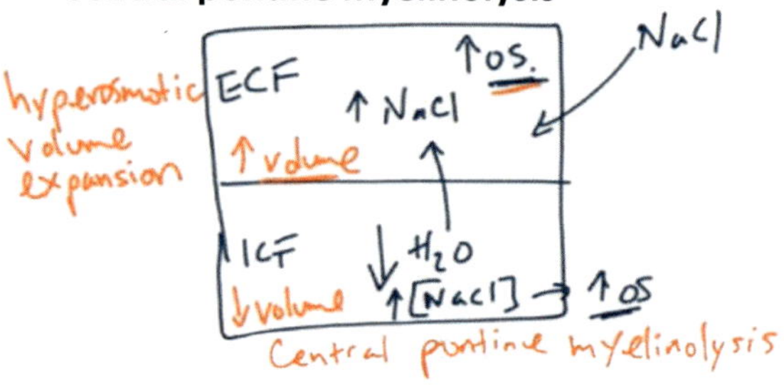

5. How would the redistribution of water be altered in the intracellular and extracellular fluid compartments in a patient who has been sweating during a long hike?

   - **In sweat, water loss is greater than NaCl loss → ↓ free water from ECF → ↑ ECF osmolarity → water moves from ICF to ECF → net ↓ ECF and ICF volume (hyperosmotic volume contraction)**

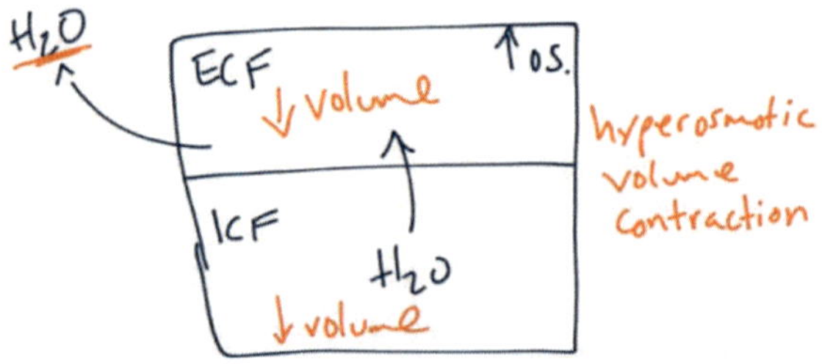

Section II - Nephrology Equations

I. Clearance

A. Clearance equation

$$C=UV/P$$

Where:
C = Clearance (mL/min)
U = Urine concentration (mg/mL)
V = Urine volume / time (mL/min)
P = Plasma concentration (mg/mL)

1. Clearance represents how much of a substance can be removed from a certain amount of plasma volume in a given amount of time.

II. Flow

A. Renal plasma flow (RPF)

$$RPF = MAP / RVR$$

Where:
RPF = renal plasma flow (mL/min)
MAP = mean arterial pressure (mmHg)
RVR = renal vascular resistance (mmHg/(mL/min))

1. MAP = cardiac output X total peripheral resistance
2. RVR refers to the total resistance within the kidney and is a function of the resistance of the afferent and efferent arterioles.
3. RPF is the volume of plasma that flows through the kidney into the afferent and efferent arterioles in a given amount of time.

B. RPF is measured clinically by using the clearance of para-aminohippuric acid (PAH).

$$RPF = C_{PAH} = [U]_{PAH}V / [P]_{PAH}$$

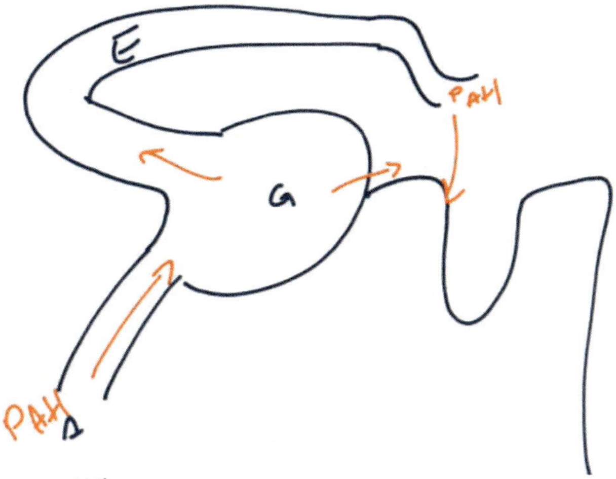

Where:
RPF = renal plasma flow (mL/min)
C_{PAH} = clearance of PAH (mL/min)
$[U]_{PAH}$ = urine concentration of PAH (mg/mL)
V = urine flow rate (mL/min)
$[P]_{PAH}$ = plasma concentration of PAH (mg/mL)

1. PAH is freely filtered by the glomerulus, actively secreted, and not reabsorbed. Nearly 100% of PAH is excreted as it enters the kidneys, making the clearance of PAH a good marker for RPF.
2. Filtration of PAH by the glomerulus is a process that cannot be saturated. Secretion of PAH in the PCT, however, is a transport-mediated process that can become saturated when plasma PAH levels rise.

C. Renal blood flow (RBF)

$$RBF = RPF / (1 - hematocrit)$$

Where:
RBF = renal blood flow (mL/min)
RPF = renal plasma flow (mL/min)

1. RBF is different from RPF because it includes red blood cells. Recall that plasma is what remains after the cells have been removed. In other words, RBF is the same thing as RPF after including the hematocrit and the plasma.

III. Filtration

A. Glomerular filtration rate (GFR)

$$\mathbf{GFR = [U]_{inulin}V/[P]_{inulin}}$$

Where:
GFR = glomerular filtration rate (mL/min)
$[U]_{inulin}$ = concentration of inulin in the urine (mg/mL)
V = urine flow rate (mL/min)
$[P]_{inulin}$ = concentration of inulin the plasma (mg/mL)

1. GFR is the flow rate of fluid that is filtered from the glomerulus into Bowman's space.
2. Inulin is freely filtered by the glomerulus but not reabsorbed or secreted which makes the clearance of inulin the most accurate measurement of GFR.
3. Creatinine clearance is more commonly used to measure GFR.
   a) Creatinine is a by-product of muscle metabolism and is produced at a relatively constant rate.
   b) It is freely filtered by the glomerulus and very little is reabsorbed or secreted.
   c) Due to these properties, creatinine clearance is commonly used as a surrogate for GFR and renal function.
   d) A rise in blood creatinine may indicate renal dysfunction.

B. Starling equation

$$\mathbf{GFR = K_f[(P_{GC} - P_{BS}) - (\pi_{GC} - \pi_{BS})]}$$

Where:
GFR = glomerular filtration rate
P_{GC} = hydrostatic pressure in the glomerular capillaries
P_{BS} = hydrostatic pressure in Bowman's space
π_{GC} = oncotic pressure in the glomerular capillaries
π_{BS} = oncotic pressure in Bowman's space
K_f = filtration coefficient

1. K_f is intrinsic to the glomerulus and is a function of the anatomy of each individual.

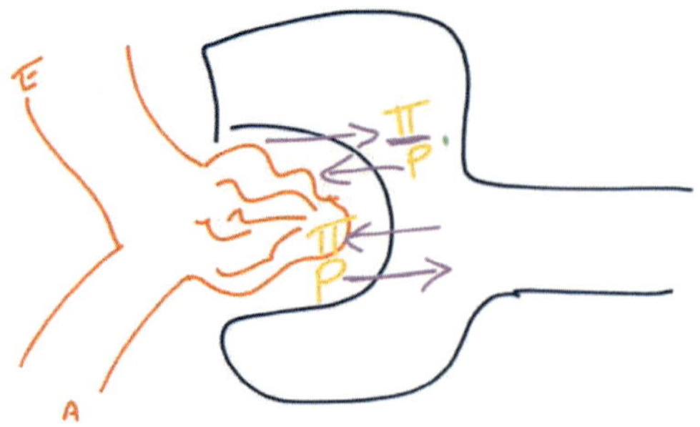

C. Filtration fraction

$$\mathbf{FF = GFR / RPF}$$

Where:
FF = filtration fraction
GFR = glomerular filtration rate (mL/min)
RPF = renal plasma flow (mL/min)

1. FF is the percentage of plasma that is filtered through the glomerulus compared to the total plasma that reaches the kidneys.

D. Filtered load (FL) or filtrate rate (FR)

$$\mathbf{FL = GFR\ X\ PC}$$

Where:
FL = filtered load (mg/min)
GFR = glomerular filtration rate (mL/min)
PC = plasma concentration (mg/mL)

E. Excretion rate (ER)

$$\mathbf{ER = FL - RR}$$

Where:
ER = excretion rate (mg/min)
FL = filtered load (mg/min)
RR = net reabsorption rate (mg/min)

1. ER is how much of a substance is filtered plus how much is secreted into the lumen of the nephron.

F. Reabsorption rate (RR)

$$\mathbf{RR = FL - ER}$$

Where:
RR = net reabsorption rate (mg/min)
FR = filtered load (mg/min)
ER = excretion rate (mg/min)

G. Fractional excretion (FE)

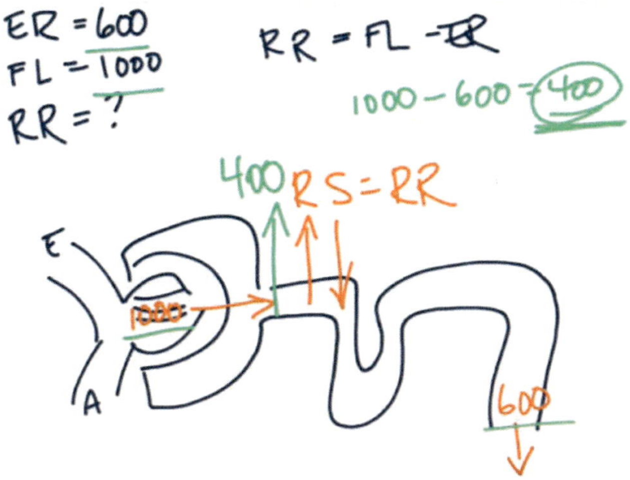

FE = amount excreted (mg) / amount filtered (mg)

Where:

FE = fractional excretion

1. Fractional excretion can be helpful in determining kidney function.

H. Henderson-Hasselbalch equation

$pH = 6.1 + \log [HCO_3^-] / (0.03 \times PCO_2)$

Where:

pH = the acidity of the blood

$[HCO_3^-]$ = the concentration of HCO_3^- in the blood

PCO_2 = the partial pressure of CO_2 in the arterial blood

1. Can be useful for determining the pH in a buffer system.

I. Anion-gap (AG)

$AG = Na^+ - (Cl^- + HCO_3^-)$

Where:

AG = anion gap

1. Used to diagnose a metabolic acidosis.

J. Winters formula

$PCO_2 = 1.5\,[HCO_3^-] + 8 \pm 2$

Where:

PCO_2 = the partial pressure of CO_2 in the arterial blood

HCO_3^- = the concentration of HCO_3^- in the blood

1. Used to diagnose a mixed acid-base disorder.

REVIEW QUESTIONS ?

1. A patient has a plasma glucose of concentration of 1.0 mg / mL, a urine glucose concentration of 0.01 mg / mL, and a flow rate of 1.5 mL/min. What is the clearance of glucose?

- **C = 0.015 mL/min**
- **This means the body is retaining most of the glucose and only excreting a small amount in the urine**

P = 1
U = 0.01
V = 1.5
(0.01 x 1.5) / 1 = 0.015 mL/min

2. How does the concentration of para-aminohippuric acid (PAH) change as it is filtered and passes through the nephron?

- **Some PAH is filtered by the glomerulus and the remaining PAH is actively secreted into the PCT until nearly 100% is excreted in the urine**
- **↓ PAH concentration in the glomerulus (some is lost as it is filtered)**
- **↑ PAH concentration in PCT (excess PAH is secreted into PCT)**

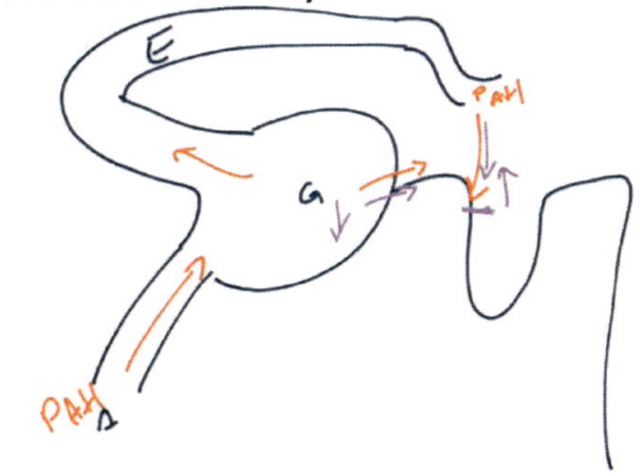

3. If the renal plasma flow is 10 mL/min and the hematocrit is 0.5, what is the renal blood flow (RBF)?

- **RBF = 20**

↑RBF = RPF/(1-hct)
RPF = 10 mL/min
hct = 0.5 → 0.7
RBF ?
10/(1 - 0.5) = 20
↑10/(1 - 0.7) = 33.3

REVIEW QUESTIONS

4. If the renal plasma flow is 10 mL/min and the hematocrit is 0.7, what is the renal blood flow (RBF)?

   - **RBF = 33**
   - **As the hematocrit ↑ → RBF ↑ (there is more blood reaching the kidneys)**

$RBF = RPF/(1-hct)$

$RPF = RBF \times (1-hct)$

RBF = 10 mL/min
hct = 0.5 → 0.7
RPF ?

$10 \times (1-0.5) = 5$

$10 \times (1-0.7) = 3$

5. What is renal plasma flow (RPF) if the RBF is 10 mL/min and the hematocrit is 0.5?

   - **RPF = 5**

6. What is renal plasma flow (RPF) if the RBF is 10 mL/min and the hematocrit is 0.7?

   - **RPF = 3**

7. ↑ hematocrit → ↓ RPF (↓ plasma reaches the kidneys because more RBCs occupy the volume of blood)

   - **RBF = 793.3 mL/min**
   - **The clearance of PAH can be used to estimate RPF**

8. The urine concentration of PAH is 110 mg/mL, the urine flow rate is 1.5 mL/min, the plasma concentration of PAH is 0.4 mg/mL and the hematocrit is 48%. What is the renal blood flow?

   - **V = 2 mL/min**
   - **The clearance of creatinine can be used to calculate GFR (GFR = UV/P). This equation can be rearranged to calculate urinary flow rate (V)**

$RBF = RPF/(1-hct)$

$C = \frac{UV}{P} = \frac{(110 \times 1.5)}{0.4} =$

412.5

$RBF = 412.5/(1-0.48) =$

793.3 mL/min

9. If the clearance of creatinine is 100 mL/min, the concentration of inulin in the urine is 50 mg/mL, and the concentration of inulin the plasma is 1.0 mg/mL, what is the urinary flow rate?

   - **Inulin can be used to estimate GFR (85 mL/min), because it is neither secreted or reabsorbed (only filtered)**
   - **If another compound (i.e. PAH indicated by purple drawing below) has a greater clearance than inulin, it is because it is filtered AND secreted**

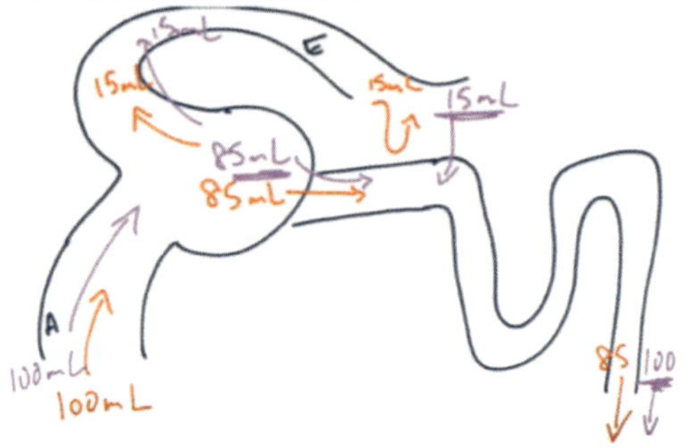

$C_{creatinine} = GFR = 100$ mL/min
$U_{inulin} = 50$ mg/mL
$P_{inulin} = 1.0$ mg/mL
V ?

$GFR = UV/P$

$V = (GFR \times P)/U$

$\frac{100 \times 1}{50} = 2$ mL/min

10. What is an example of a disease that would cause the oncotic pressure in Bowman's space to increase?

    - **Nephrotic and nephritic syndromes**

11. The GFR is measured to be 85 mL/min using inulin clearance, but 100 mL/min using the clearance of a newly discovered drug. What could explain why the GFR is higher when using the clearance of the new drug?

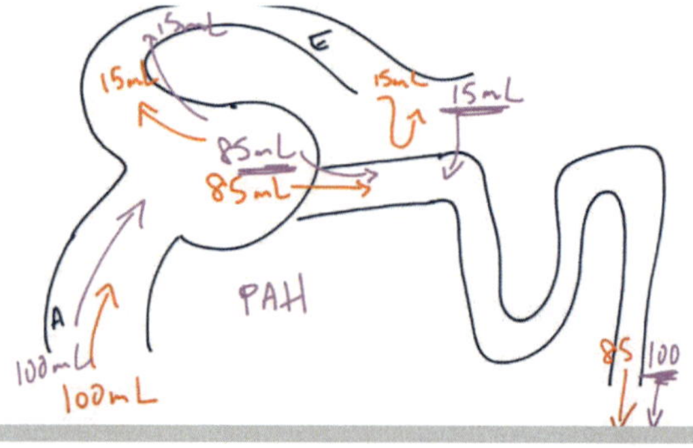

REVIEW QUESTIONS

12. How would the GFR be altered in a patient with one of these nephrotic or nephritic syndrome?

- **↑ filtration of protein → ↑ oncotic pressure in Bowman's space and ↓ oncotic pressure in glomerular capillaries→ ↑ water filtration due to change in oncotic forces → ↑ GFR**

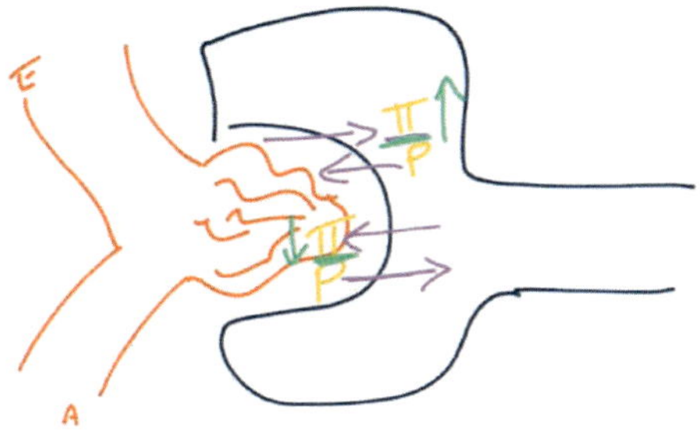

13. How would GFR be altered in a patient with severe benign prostatic hyperplasia (BPH)?

- **BPH → outflow obstruction → ↑ urine in Bowman's space → ↑ hydrostatic forces → ↓ GFR**

14. How would ANP impact GFR?

- **ANP dilates afferent arteriole → ↑ blood in glomerulus → ↑ hydrostatic forces → ↑ GFRHow would GFR be altered in a patient with severe benign prostatic hyperplasia (BPH)?**

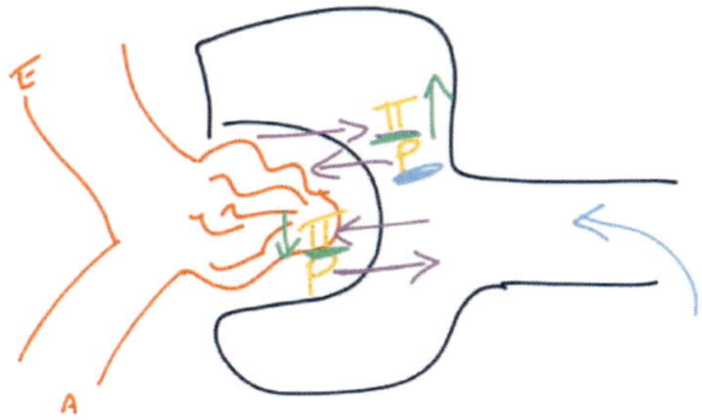

15. What would happen to GFR in a patient with polycythemia vera?

- **Polycythemia vera → ↓ renal plasma flow → ↓ volume of fluid that can be filtered through the glomerulus → ↓ GFR**

16. How would diabetes alter GFR?

- **Glucose reacts with efferent arteriole → ↓ efferent arteriole radius → ↑ hydrostatic forces in glomerulus → ↑ GFR**

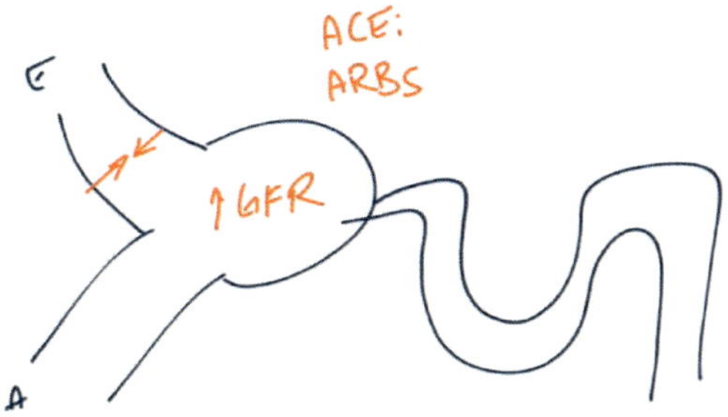

17. What drugs are useful in decreasing GFR and can be helpful in treating diabetics?

- **ACEi and ARBs**
- **These limit angiotensin II (normally constricts efferent arteriole) → dilation of efferent arteriole → ↓ GFR**

18. How does age alter GFR?

- **↑ Age → ↓ number of nephrons → ↓ GFR**

19. How would congestive heart failure alter GFR?

- **CHF → ↓ cardiac output → ↓ renal perfusion → ↓ GFR**
- **CHF → ↑ fluid accumulation in venous system → ↑ renal resistance → ↓ GFR**

20. What would the net filtration pressure be in a patient with a glomerular capillary hydrostatic pressure of 38 mmHg, a glomerular capillary oncotic pressure of 25 mmHg, a hydrostatic pressure in Bowman's space of 11 mmHg, and an oncotic pressure in Bowman's space of 3 mmHg?

- **GFR = 5**

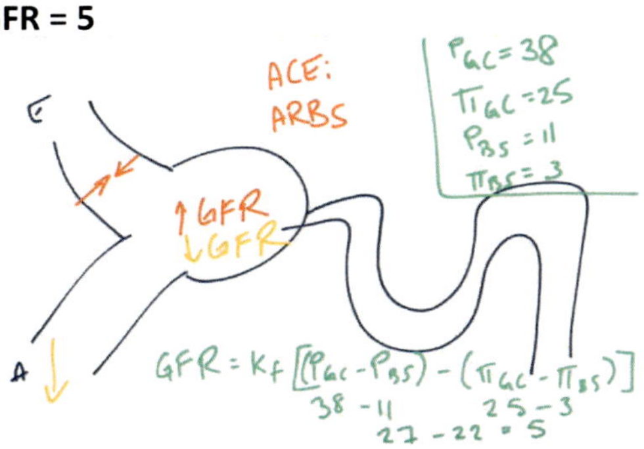

REVIEW QUESTIONS

21. What would happen to filtration fraction if the efferent arteriole is constricted?

- **Efferent arteriole constriction → ↑ volume in glomerular capillaries → ↑ hydrostatic forces → ↑ GFR → ↑ filtration fraction**

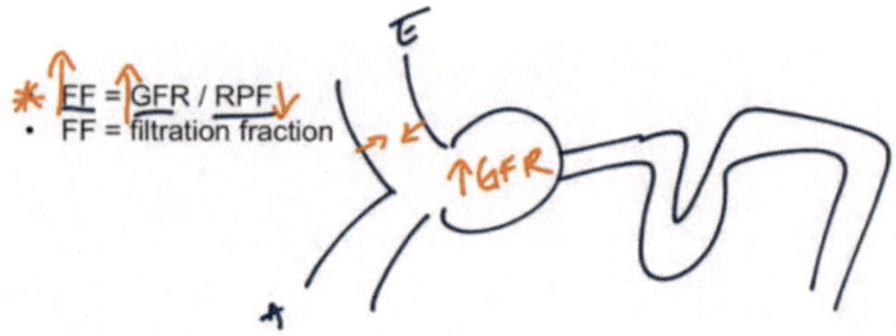

22. What would an increased filtration fraction indicate about glomerular oncotic pressure?

- **↑ FF → ↑ GFR relative to RPF (more fluid is being filtered and more protein is left behind) → ↑ glomerular oncotic pressure**

23. If the inulin clearance is 90 mL/min, the plasma concentration of substance X is 1 mg/mL, and the net reabsorption rate of substance X is 10 mg/min, what is the excretion rate (ER_x) of substance X?

- **Excretion rate = 80 mL/min**
- **Excretion rate = filtered load - net reabsorption rate**
- **Filtered load = GFR X plasma concentration**
- **The clearance of inulin = GFR**

$C_{inulin} = 90$ mL/min
$P_X = 1$ mg/mL
$RR_X = 10$ mg/min
$ER_X = ?$

FL = GFR × PC
C_{inulin} = GFR
FL = 90 × 1 = 90
ER = FL − RR
$ER_X = 90 - 10 = 80$ mg/min

24. If a patient is excreting 600 mg/min of a substance and filtering 1000 mg/min of the substance, what is the net reabsorption rate of the substance?

- **Reabsorption rate = filtered load - excretion rate**
- **RR = 1,000 - 600 = 400**
- **A positive value indicates reabsorption rather than secretion**

ER = 600
FL = 1000
RR = ?
RR = FL − ER
1000 − 600 = 400

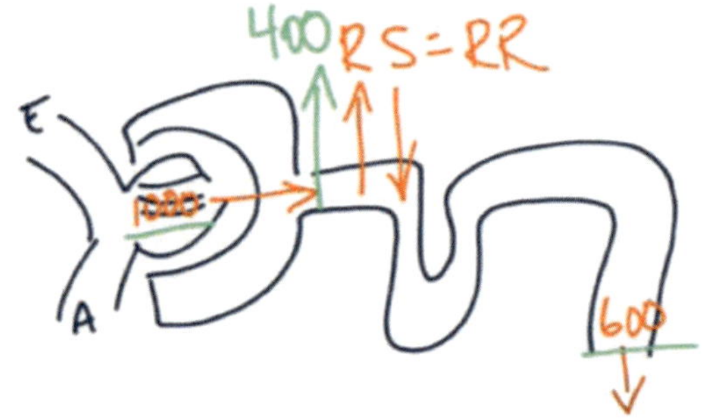

25. Drug X is freely filtered and actively secreted in the proximal convoluted tubule. The secretion process is transport-mediated. How would the excretion rate of drug X change as the plasma concentration of drug X increases?

- **Drug X is similar to PAH which is freely filtered and actively secreted**
- **The secretion of PAH is a transport-mediated process and can become saturated if plasma levels are too high. Filtration does not become saturated.**
- **Once the secretion process is saturated, the rate of excretion slows**

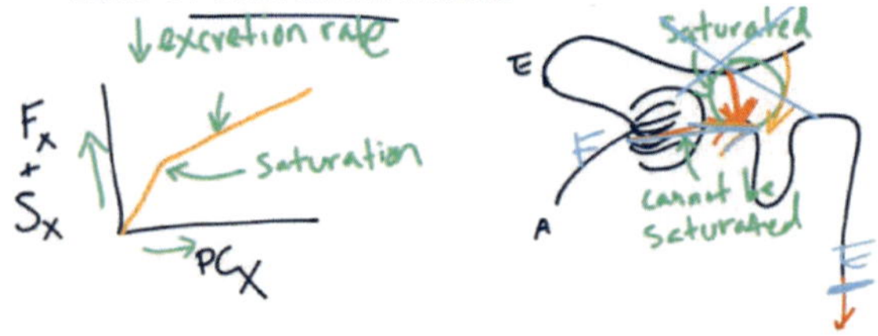

Section III - The Nephron

I. The Nephron (Figure 4.1)

A. Proximal convoluted tubule (PCT)

1. Bicarbonate

a) Within the cells of the PCT, CO_2 and H_2O react to form H^+ and HCO_3^-. The H^+ is secreted into the lumen of the nephron through the Na^+/H^+ antiporter and the HCO_3^- is reabsorbed into the blood.

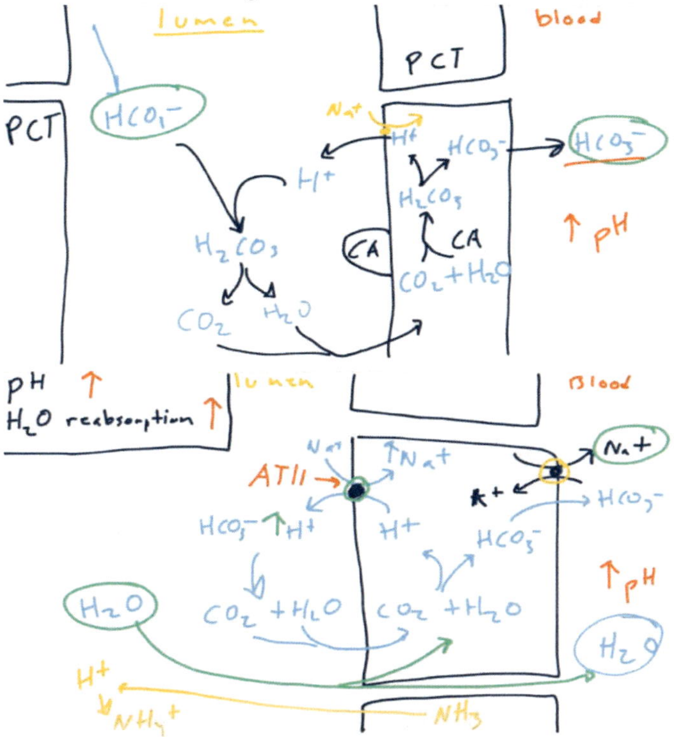

b) Within the lumen, the H^+ reacts with filtered HCO_3^- to form H_2O and CO_2. The CO_2 and H_2O diffuse across the cell membrane which can then react within the cell and start the cycle again.

c) The process results in a net reabsorption of HCO_3^- which was filtered through the glomerulus. The H^+ is continuously recycled, ultimately resulting in neither a net reabsorption or secretion.

d) Angiotensin II up-regulates the Na^+/H^+ antiporter resulting in reabsorption of Na^+ and loss of H^+.

2. Phosphate

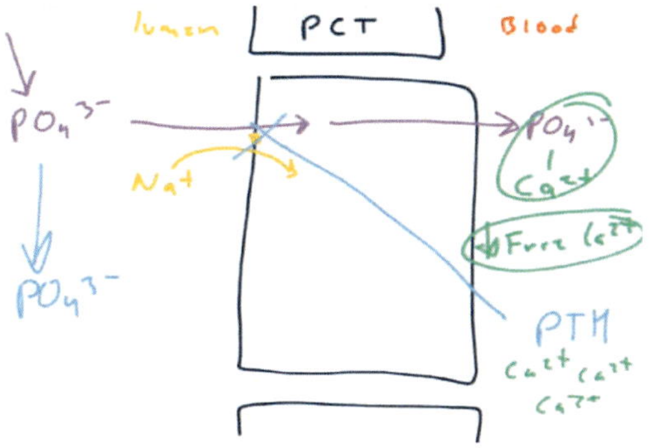

a) Reabsorbed via a Na^+/PO_4^{3-} cotransporter. Nearly 85% is reabsorbed by the PCT. The rest is excreted as urine.

b) PTH blocks the Na^+/PO_4^{3-} cotransporter, preventing Na^+ and PO_4^{3-} from moving from the lumen into the cell.

3. Amino acids

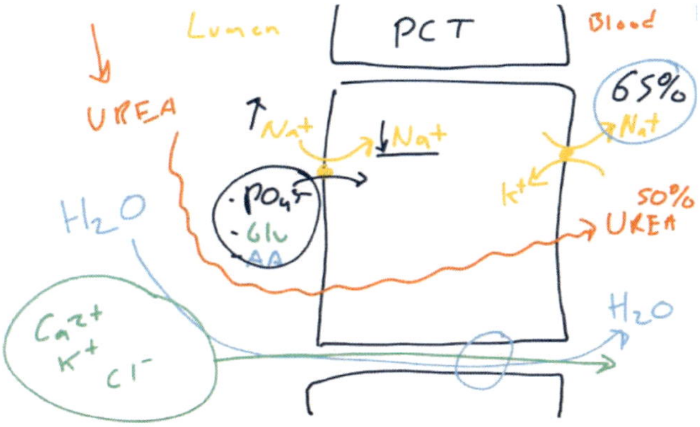

a) Reabsorbed via a Na^+/amino acid cotransporter. Nearly 100% is reabsorbed by the PCT.

4. Sodium (Na^+)

a) Sodium is filtered from the glomerulus into the lumen of the nephron.

b) The PCT reabsorbs ~65% of Na^+. Other parts of the nephron also reabsorb Na^+, allowing for less than 1% actually being excreted into the urine.

c) Water follows Na^+, so most (~65%) of the water filtered into the lumen is reabsorbed in the PCT.

5. Potassium (K^+)

a) K^+ is freely filtered by the glomerulus.

b) Approximately 65% of K^+ is reabsorbed in the proximal convoluted tubule (PCT).

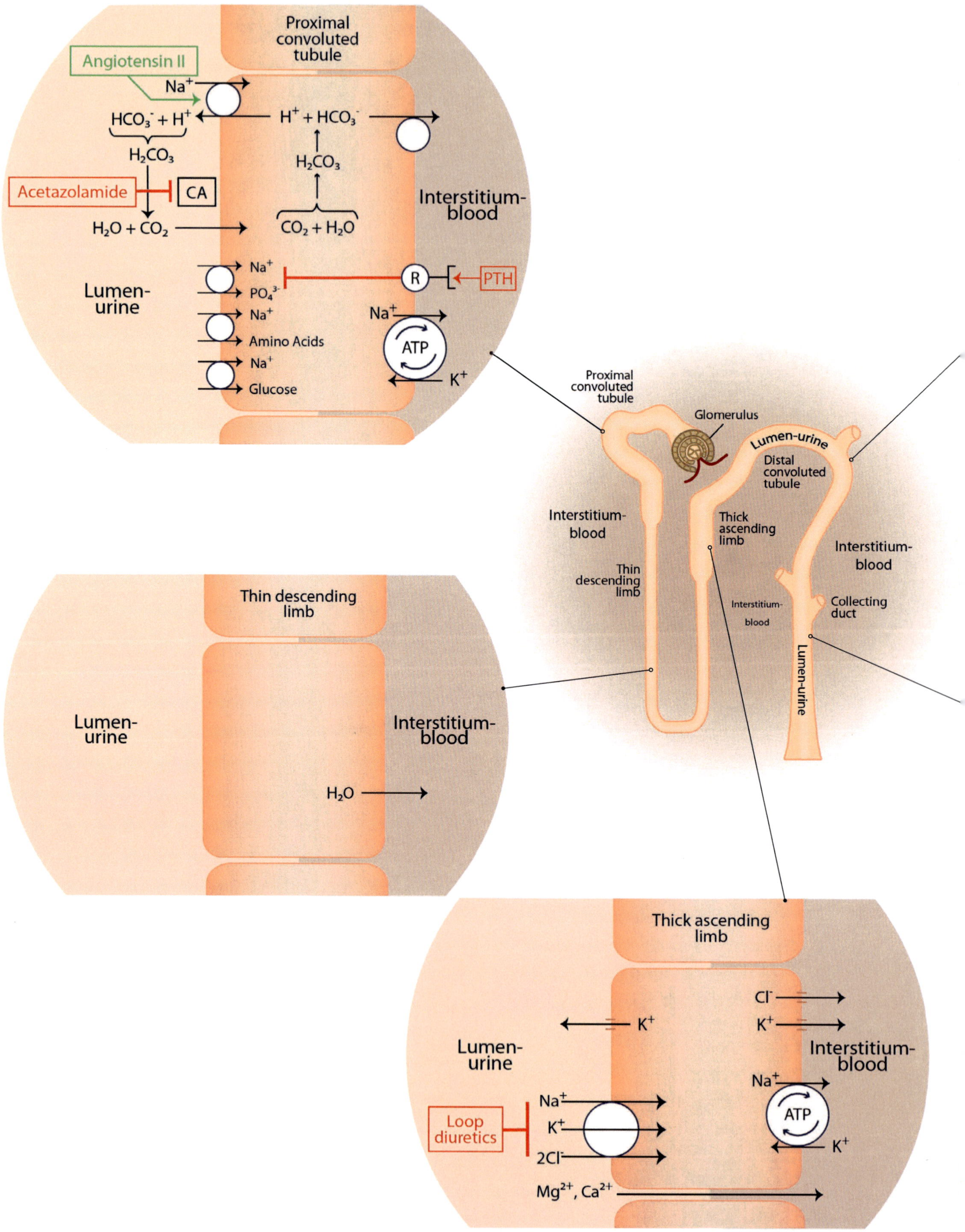

Figure 4.1 - Physiology of the nephron.

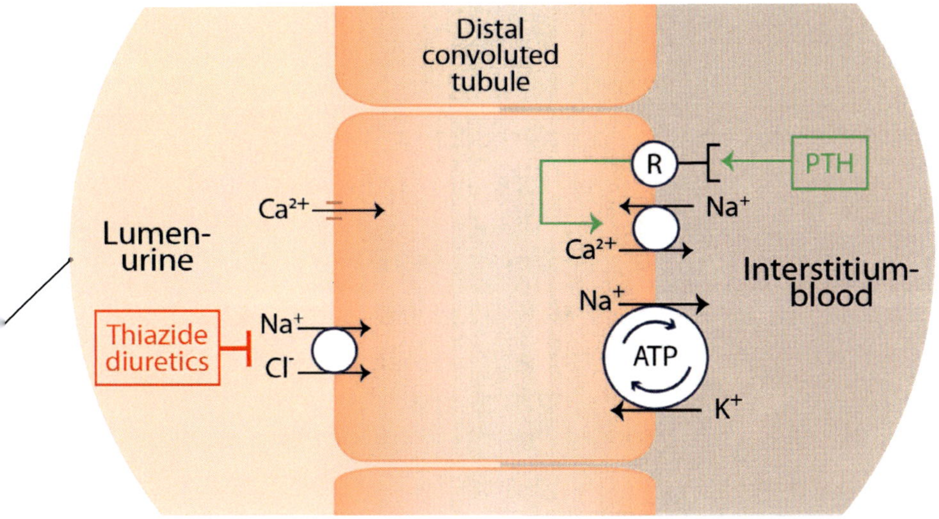
Distal convoluted tubule
Lumen-urine
Interstitium-blood
PTH
R
Na+
Ca2+
Ca2+
Na+
ATP
K+
Thiazide diuretics
Na+
Cl-

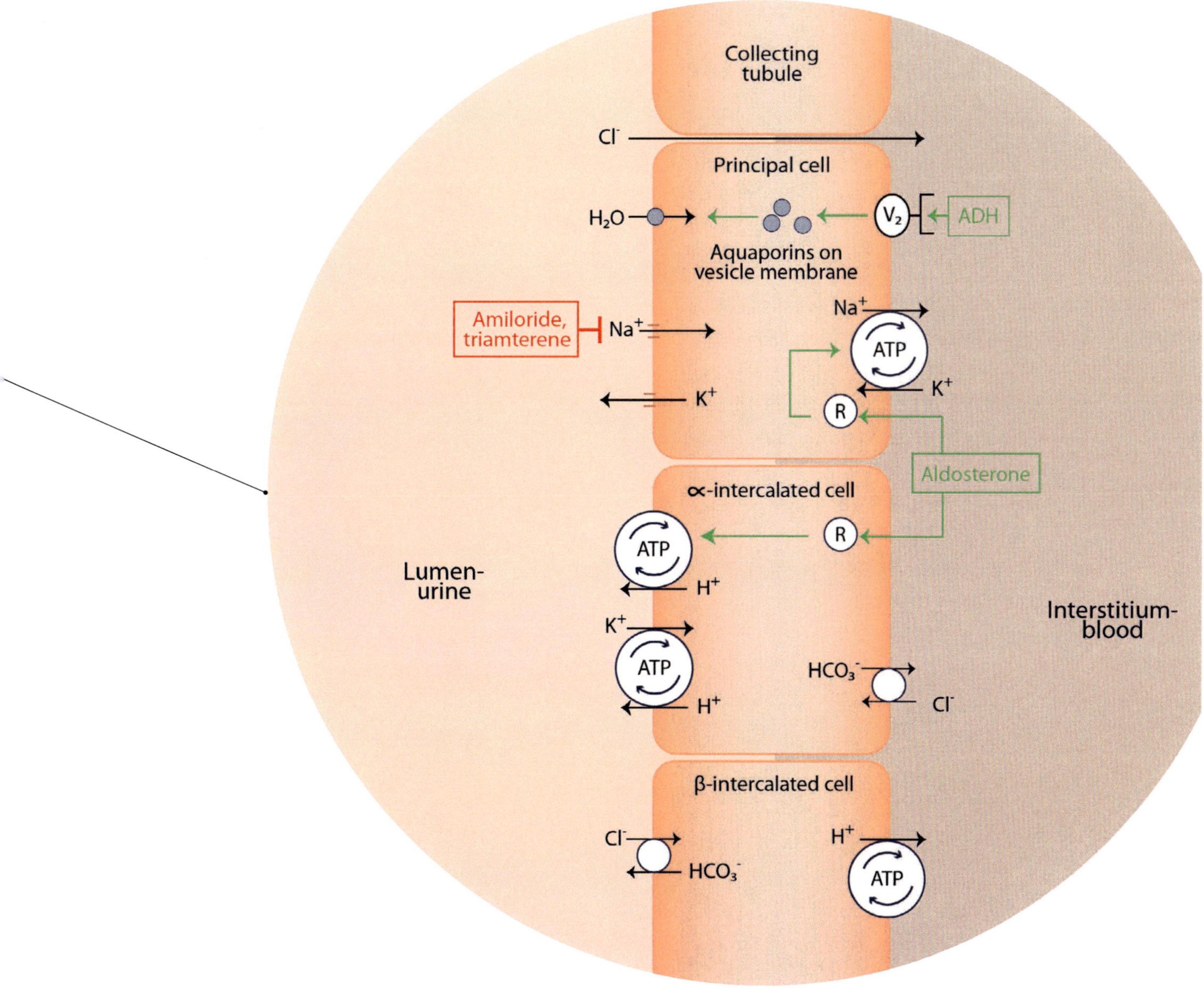
Collecting tubule
Cl-
Principal cell
H2O
V2
ADH
Aquaporins on vesicle membrane
Amiloride, triamterene
Na+
Na+
ATP
K+
K+
R
Aldosterone
∝-intercalated cell
R
ATP
H+
Lumen-urine
Interstitium-blood
K+
ATP
H+
HCO3-
Cl-
β-intercalated cell
Cl-
HCO3-
H+
ATP

c) Approximately 30% of K^+ is reabsorbed in the thick ascending limb of the loop of Henle by the NKCC channel.

d) The remaining 5% of K^+ is reabsorbed in the distal convoluted tubule (DCT).

e) K^+ regulation primarily occurs in the collecting ducts via principal and alpha intercalated cells.

(1) Principal cells secrete K^+

(2) Alpha cells reabsorb K^+

6. Glucose

a) Freely filtered and normally completely reabsorbed in the PCT

b) Glucose is reabsorbed on the luminal side of the PCT cells via an SGLT (sodium-glucose linked transporter). The glucose is then exported from the cell to the blood using GLUT transporters on the basolateral side.

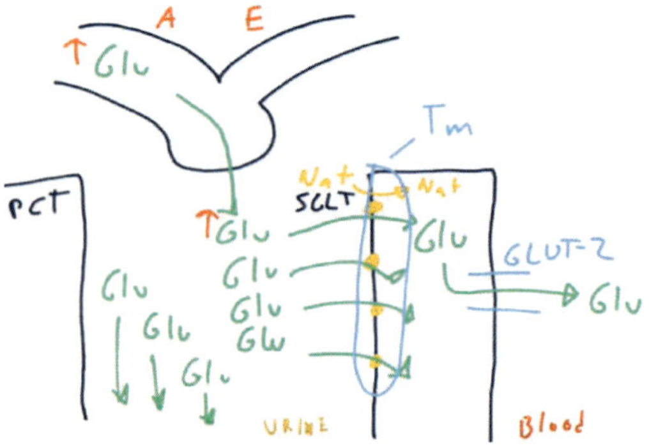

c) At 200 mg/dL glucose begins to appear in the urine due to partial saturation of SGLT transporters (all nephrons vary slightly so some become saturated at a lower concentration of glucose).

d) At 375 mg/dL all SGLT transporters are completely saturated.

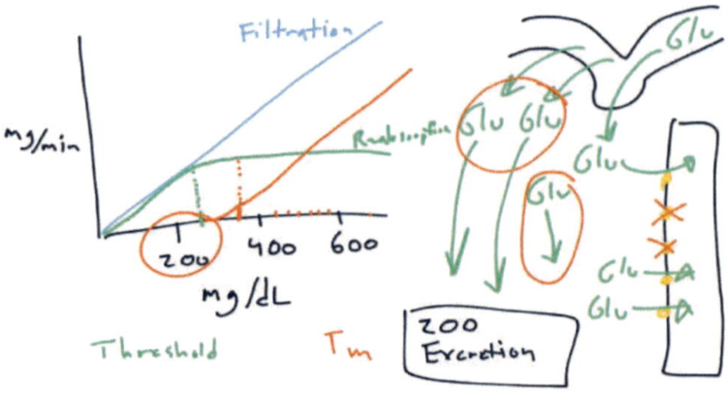

7. Urea

a) Urea is freely filtered by the glomerulus.

b) The PCT reabsorbs ~50% of the urea via simple diffusion.

8. Ammonia (NH_3)

a) Produced in the PCT

b) Secreted into the lumen to bind H^+ to form NH_4^+ → is the primary means of excreting acid in the kidney

B. Thin descending limb of the loop of Henle

1. Water is passively reabsorbed due to the hypertonic medulla, thereby increasing the osmolarity the tubular filtrate. This portion of the nephron is impermeable to Na^+.

2. Urea is secreted into the lumen by simple diffusion.

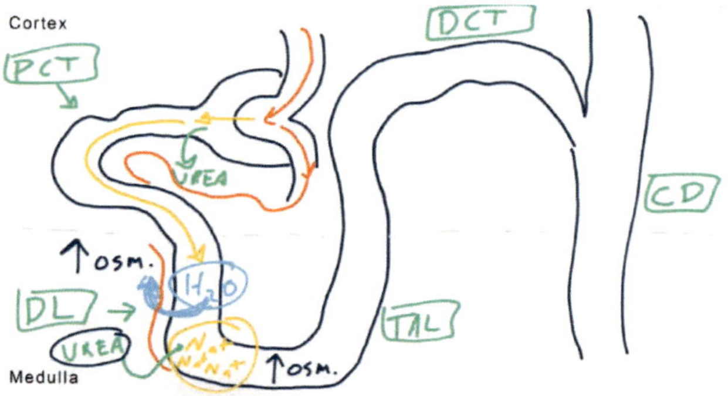

C. Thick ascending limb of the loop of Henle (TAL)

1. Electrolytes are actively pumped from the tubular lumen to the interstitium via the $Na^+/K^+/2Cl^-$ pump (NKCC). Because the TAL and early distal convoluted tubule (DCT) are impermeable to water the tubular fluid becomes hypotonic.

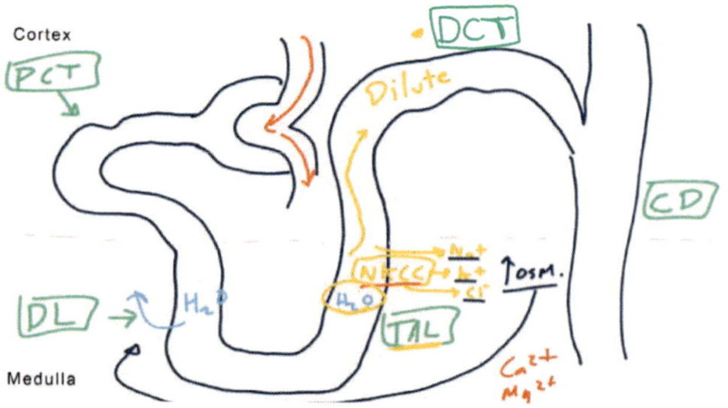

2. Magnesium and Calcium are reabsorbed paracellularly. This occurs as a result of the $Na^+/K^+/2Cl^-$ cotransporter (NKCC) which brings in K^+ that can then leak back through a luminal channel in the cell. This creates a net positive charge in the urine, stimulating the passive reabsorption of Ca^{2+} through

the paracellular space. Magnesium is also reabsorbed this way.

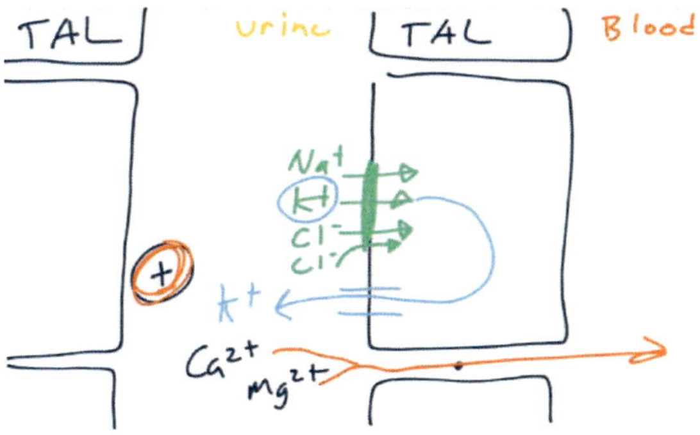

D. DCT

1. Na^+ and Cl^- are reabsorbed using a Na^+/Cl^- symporter on the luminal side of the cells. This further dilutes the tubular filtrate.

   a) Thiazide diuretics block the action of the Na^+/Cl^- symporter → increased excretion of Na^+ → increased excretion of H_2O → overall fluid loss.

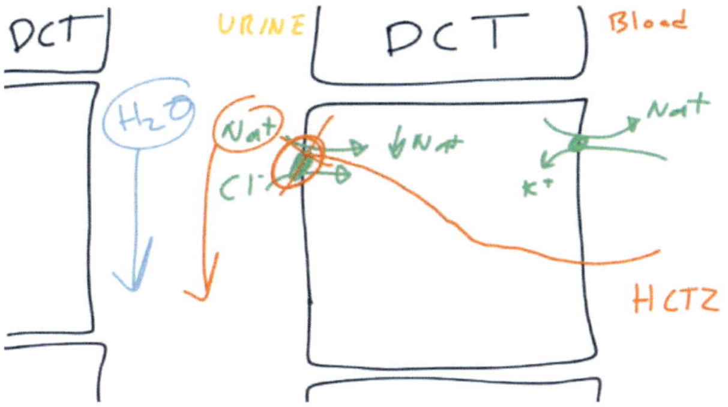

2. Ca^{2+} is reabsorbed using Ca^{2+} channels on the luminal surface and Na^+/Ca^{2+} antiporters (exchangers) on the basolateral surface.

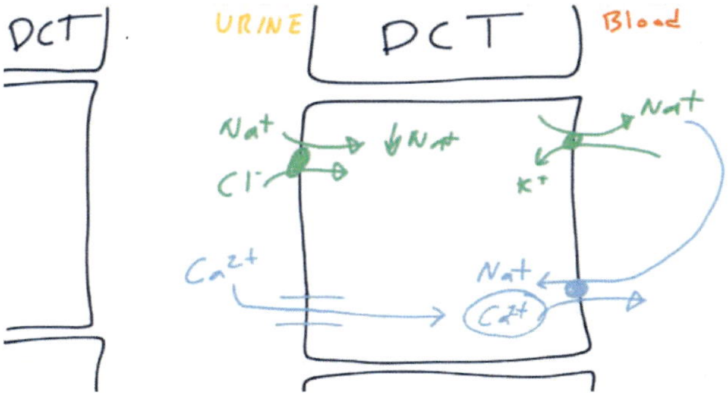

   a) PTH up-regulates the Ca^{2+}/Na^+ antiporter resulting in increased reabsorption of Ca^{2+}.

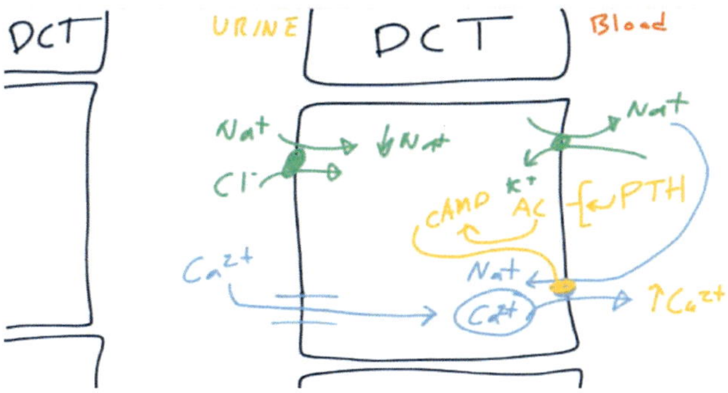

E. Collecting duct

1. Composed of principal cells, α cells, and β-intercalated cells

2. Principal cells

   a) Reabsorb Na^+ and H_2O, but secrete K^+

   b) When acted upon by ADH, principal cells will increase the number of aquaporins (water channels) on the luminal membrane → increased H_2O reabsorption.

   c) When acted upon by aldosterone, principal cells increase activity of Na^+/K^+ exchangers → increased Na^+ reabsorption and increased K^+ secretion.

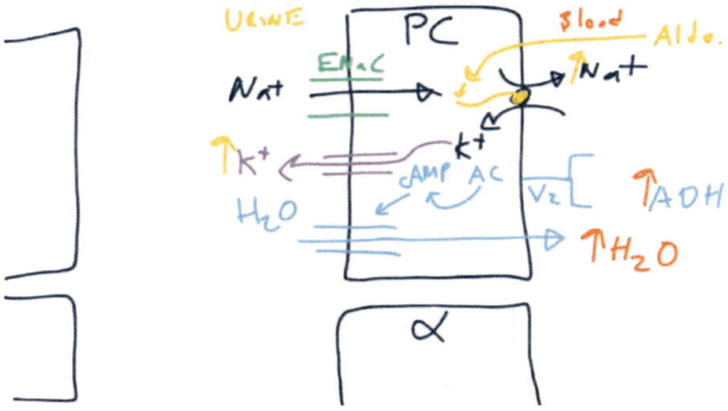

3. Alpha-intercalated cells

   a) Have a K^+/H^+ exchanger on the luminal surface to secrete H^+ and reabsorb K^+

   b) Have a H^+-ATPase which actively secretes H^+. On the basolateral surface, the cells have a HCO_3^-/Cl^- exchanger to reabsorb HCO_3^-.

      (1) Aldosterone upregulates H^+ secretion via H^+-ATPase. Increased H^+ secretion will lead to increased HCO_3^- reabsorption.

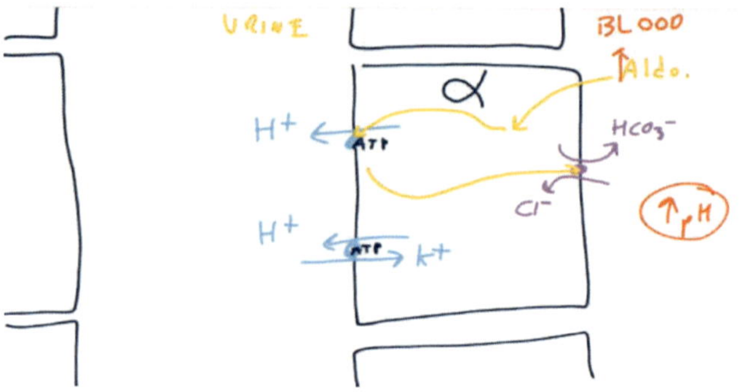

F. Renal tubular acidosis type I

1. α intercalated cell dysfunction → decreased secretion of H^+ → decreased reabsorption of HCO_3^- → metabolic acidosis
2. Decreased H^+ secretion → increased urinary pH (>5.5)→ increased risk for calcium phosphate kidney stones
3. Decreased H^+ secretion → decreased activity of H^+/K^+ antiporter → decreased reabsorption of K^+ → hypokalemia

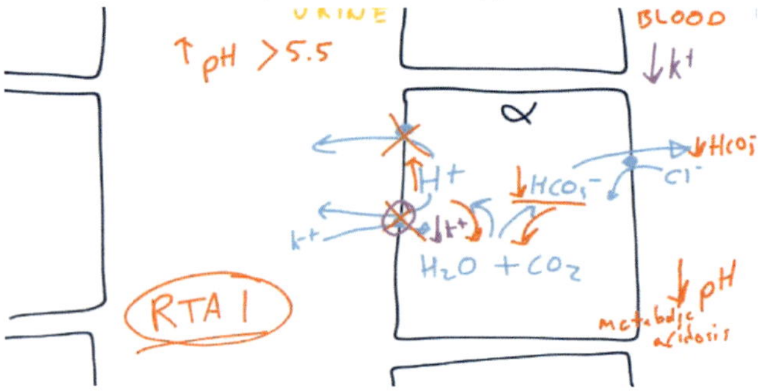

G. Renal tubular acidosis type II

1. Proximal convoluted tubule cell dysfunction → decreased HCO_3^- reabsorption and increased HCO_3^- excretion → temporary increase in urinary pH → eventual total body loss of HCO_3^- → metabolic acidosis and decreased excretion of HCO_3^- → decreased urinary pH (<5.5)
2. Acidic pH → decreased activity of H^+/K^+ antiporter → decreased reabsorption of K^+ → hypokalemia

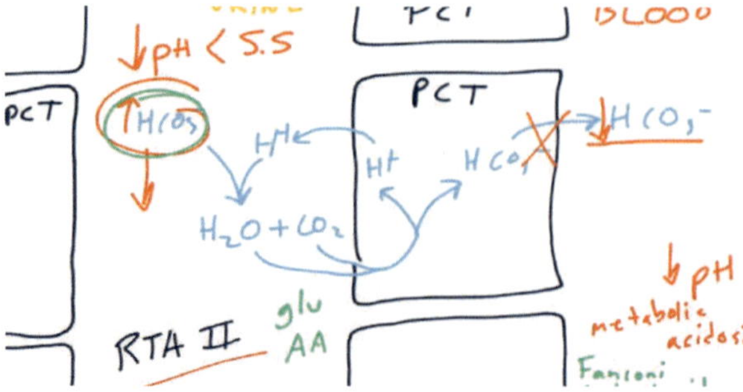

H. Renal tubular acidosis type IV

1. Hypoaldosteronism → hyperkalemia → decreased NH_3 synthesis in the PCT (mechanism not fully understood) → decreased NH_4^+ in urine → decreased urinary pH (<5.5)

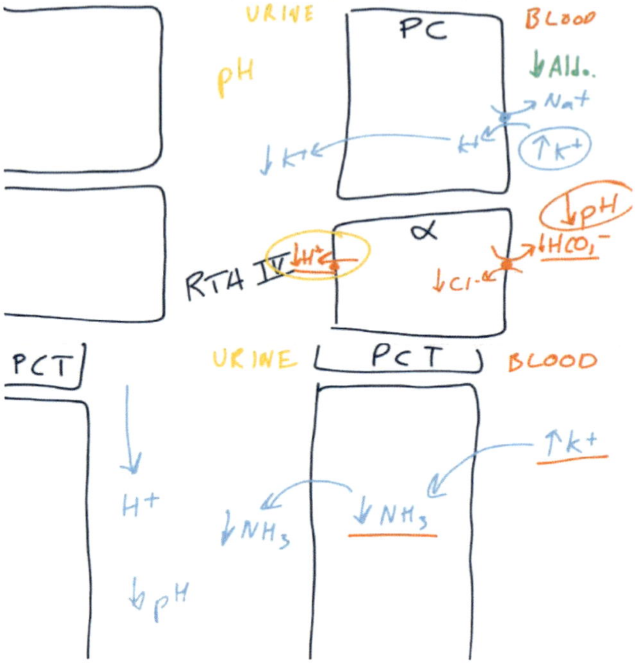

II. Secretion and Reabsorption

A. Tubular fluid (TF) to plasma (P) concentration ratio (Figure 4.2)

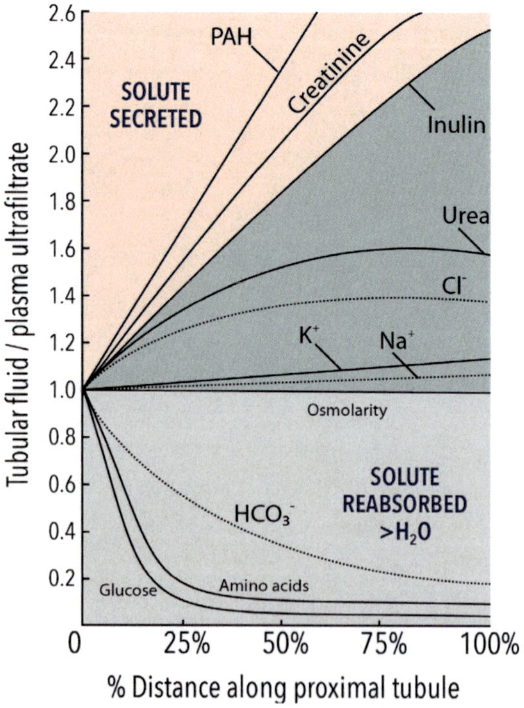

Figure 4.2 - Tubular fluid (TF) to plasma (P) concentration ratio

1. Used to determine the net reabsorption and secretion of a solute
2. Reabsorbed at a similar rate as H_2O
   a) TF/P = 1)
   b) Examples include Na^+ and K^+
3. Reabsorbed faster than H_2O
   a) TF/P < 1
   b) Glucose and amino acids
      (1) Highly reabsorbed → low TF concentration → very low TF/P ratio
   c) HCO_3^-
      (1) Highly reabsorbed → low TF concentration → very low TF/P ratio
4. Reabsorbed slower than H_2O
   a) TF/P > 1
   b) Urea and chloride reabsorbed, but at slower rate than K^+, Na^+, and H_2O → TF/P > 1

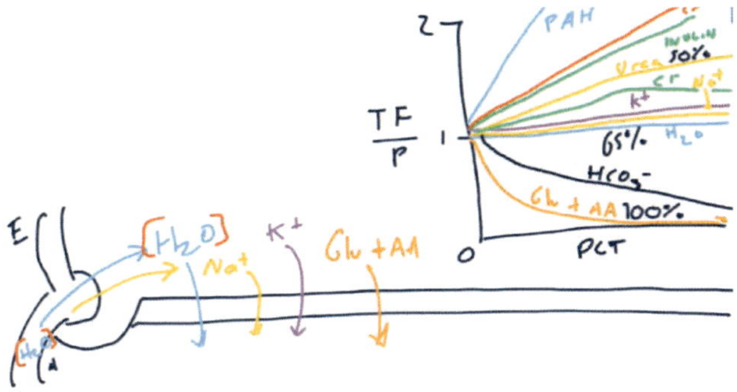

5. Secreted by PCT (TF/P > inulin)
   a) Inulin is not reabsorbed nor secreted → high TF concentration → high TF/P ratio
   b) Creatinine is slightly secreted → higher TF concentration → high TF/P ratio
   c) PAH is highly secreted → very high TF concentration → very high TF/P ratio

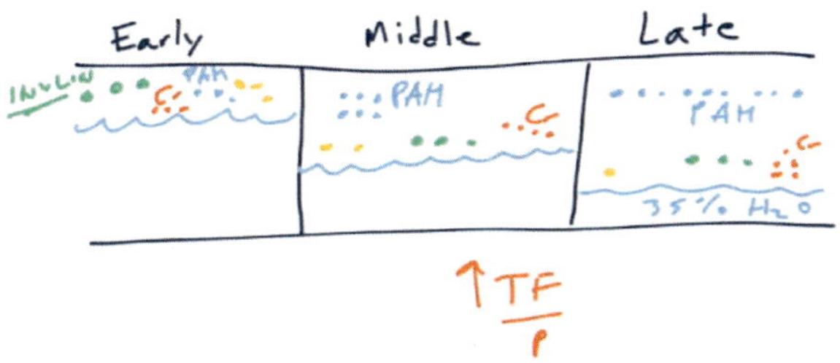

III. Electrolytes

Renal failure diminishes the kidneys ability to reabsorb secrete electrolytes appropriately.

A. Sodium (Na^+)

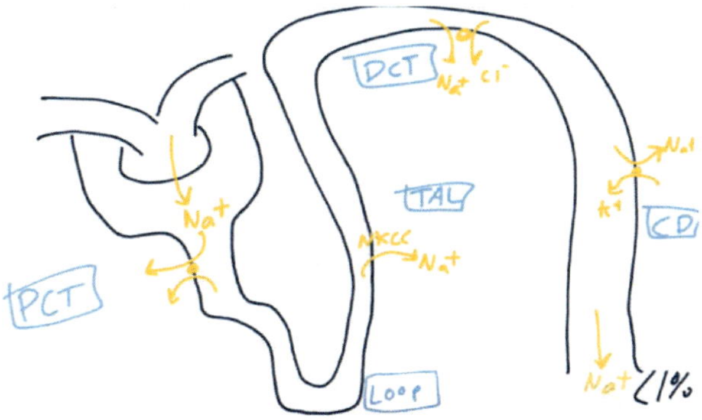

1. ~65% is reabsorbed in the proximal convoluted tubule via Na^+ symporters.
2. ~25% is reabsorbed in the loop of Henle via $Na^+/K^+/2Cl^-$ cotransporters.
3. ~10% is reabsorbed in the collecting duct and distal tubule via Na^+/Cl^- cotransporters (early distal tubule) and Na^+/K^+ exchangers and Na^+ channels (late distal tubule and collecting duct).
4. The amount that is actually excreted is typically discussed via the equation for the fractional excretion of sodium (FE_{Na}).
   a) Increases in FE_{Na} imply kidney dysfunction. Since most of it is to be reabsorbed, if FE_{Na} increases, then less is being reabsorbed and more is being excreted.
   b) Measured as excretion over filtered load.
      (1) As plasma levels rise, filtered load would increase to compensate.

B. Potassium (K^+)

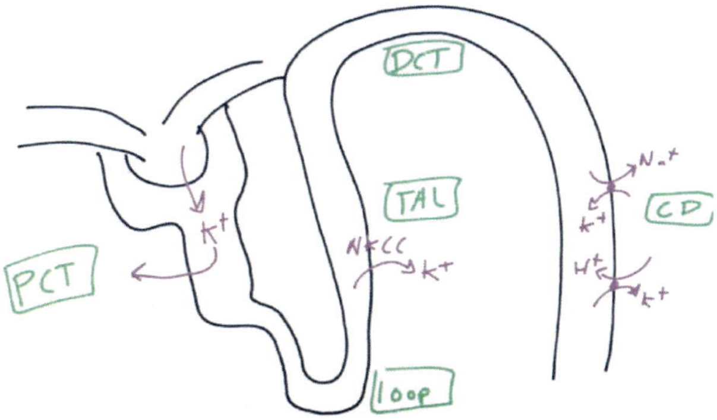

1. K^+ is freely filtered by the glomerulus.
2. Approximately 65% of K^+ is reabsorbed in the proximal convoluted tubule (PCT).
3. Approximately 30% of K^+ is reabsorbed in the thick ascending limb of the loop of

Henle by the $Na^+/K^+/2Cl^-$ cotransporters.

4. The remaining 5% of K^+ is reabsorbed in the distal convoluted tubule (DCT).
5. K^+ regulation primarily occurs in the collecting ducts via principal and alpha intercalated cells
    a) Principal cells secrete K^+.
    b) Alpha cells reabsorb K^+.

C. Chloride (Cl^-)

1. Reabsorbed in the proximal tubule, paracellularly with water, Ca^{2+}, K^{2+}.This is where the majority is reabsorbed.
2. The remainder is reabsorbed in the thick ascending limb via $Na^+/K^+/2Cl^-$ cotransporters, the distal tubule via Na^+/Cl^- symporters and the collecting duct via HCO_3^-/Cl^- exchangers.

D. Calcium (Ca^{2+})

1. ~90% reabsorbed in the proximal tubule and the loop of Henle via passive forces linked to Na^+ reabsorption.
    a) The reabsorption of Ca^{2+} that occurs in the proximal tubule is passive. As water is reabsorbed through the paracellular space, it drags Ca^{2+} ions with it.
    b) Passive reabsorption of Ca^{2+} in the ascending loop of Henle
    c) The $Na^+/K^+/2Cl^-$ cotransporter (NKCC) brings in K^+ that can then leak back through a luminal channel in the cell → net + charge in the urine → stimulates passive reabsorption of Ca^{2+} through paracellular space. Magnesium is also reabsorbed this way.
2. ~8% reabsorbed in the distal tubule via Na^+/Ca^{2+} exchange on the basolateral surface and a Ca^{2+} channel on the luminal surface.

E. Magnesium (Mg^{2+})

1. Reabsorbed in the proximal tubule paracellularly with water and Ca^{2+}.
2. Reabsorbed in the thick ascending limb, paracellularly with Ca^{2+}.
3. Reabsorbed in the distal tubule.

F. Urea

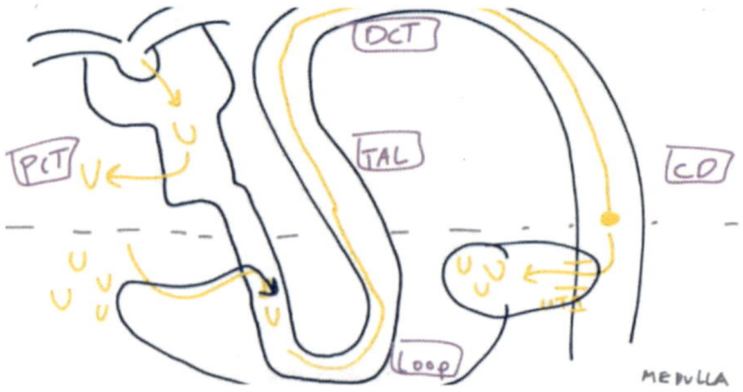

1. Urea is freely filtered by the glomerulus.
2. 50% of urea is reabsorbed in the PCT.
3. Urea passively diffuses from the interstitium into the loop of Henle, increasing the luminal concentration of urea.
4. ADH increases the permeability of urea channels in the medullary collecting ducts, allowing urea to move into the interstitium of the medulla. The increased interstitial urea increases the osmotic gradient of the medulla, allowing for increased reabsorption of water.

IV. Dilution and Concentration of Tubular Filtrate

A. Concentration of urine is compared to plasma to determine osmolarity.

1. Hyperosmolar urine is more concentrated than plasma.
2. Hypoosmolar urine is less concentrated than plasma.

B. The nephron concentrates urine by reabsorbing H_2O through the corticopapillary osmotic gradient of the interstitium.

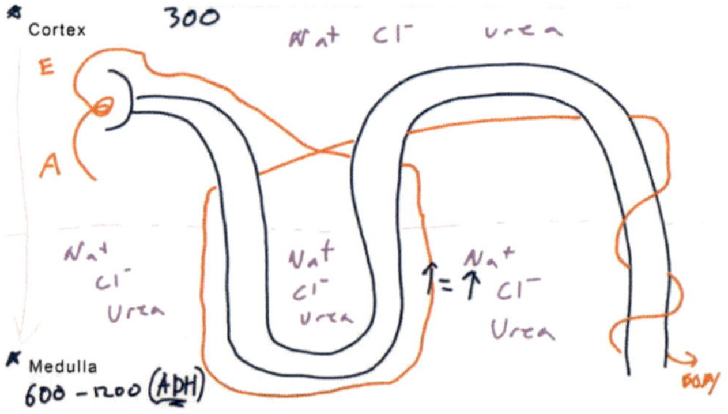

1. High concentration of Na^+, Cl^-, and urea in the interstitium creates a high osmolar gradient with which to reabsorb H_2O from the filtrate.

a) Urea can be recycled from the filtrate (urea recycling). Urea enters the loop of Henle through simple diffusion and exits the medullary collecting duct through UT1 channels.

b) Na^+ and Cl^- can be reabsorbed from the thick ascending limb (TAL) and the distal tubule, adding to the osmotic gradient of the interstitium.

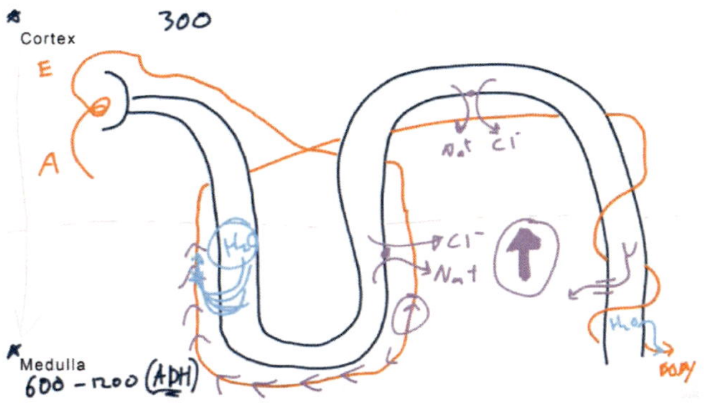

(1) Na^+ and Cl^- from the TAL can enter the vasa recta, creating a countercurrent multiplication which increases the osmolar gradient of the blood which travels to the loop of Henle. This allows greater reabsorption of H_2O in the thin descending limb.

c) ADH upregulates NaCl reabsorption in the TAL → increased Na^+ and Cl^- in the interstitium and increased countercurrent multiplication → increased corticopapillary gradient

d) ADH upregulates urea transporters (UT1) in the medullary collecting duct → increased urea in the interstitium → increased corticopapillary gradient

C. As the tubular filtrate passes through the different portions of the nephron the osmolarity ranges from 50-1200 mOsmol/L H_2O.

D. The osmolarity of tubular filtrate remains relatively constant in the PCT and the DCT, regardless of ADH concentration. It is considered isotonic compared to the osmolarity of the plasma.

E. High and low concentrations of ADH

1. The osmolarity of the tubular filtrate always increases as it approaches the bend in the **loop of Henle**, regardless of ADH status.

a) During conditions of low ADH, the osmolarity is approximately 600 mOsmol/L H_2O.

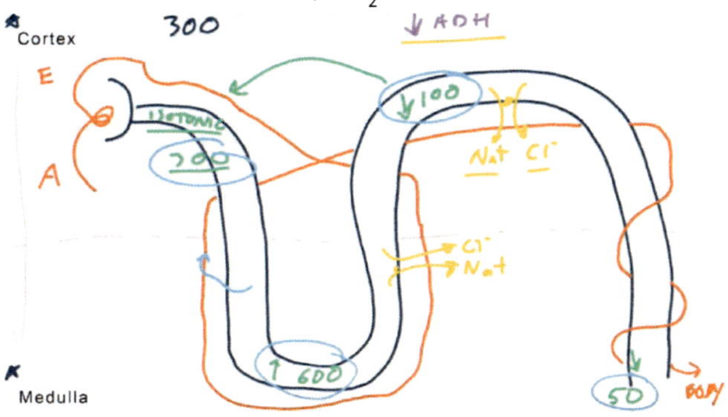

b) During conditions of high ADH, the osmolarity is approximately 1200 mOsmol/L H_2O.

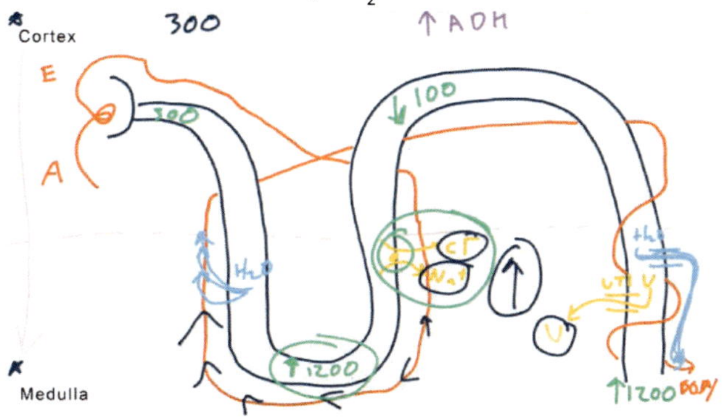

2. The osmolarity of the tubular filtrate in the **collecting tubules** varies widely depending on the concentration of ADH.

a) During conditions of low ADH, the osmolarity is approximately 50 mOsmol/L H_2O.

b) During conditions of high ADH, the osmolarity is approximately 1200 mOsmol/L H_2O.

F. ADH requires aquaporins as well as a high medullary osmolar gradient in order to reabsorb water in the collecting duct. Without the gradient, water will remain in the collecting duct, even in the presence of aquaporins.

REVIEW QUESTIONS

1. What would you expect the ammonium concentration to be in a patient with type 4 renal tubular acidosis (RTA)?

   - **RTA Type IV results from PCT dysfunction → decreased NH_3 production from PCT → decreased filtered H^+ binding to NH_3 (ammonia) → decreased urine NH_4 (ammonium)**

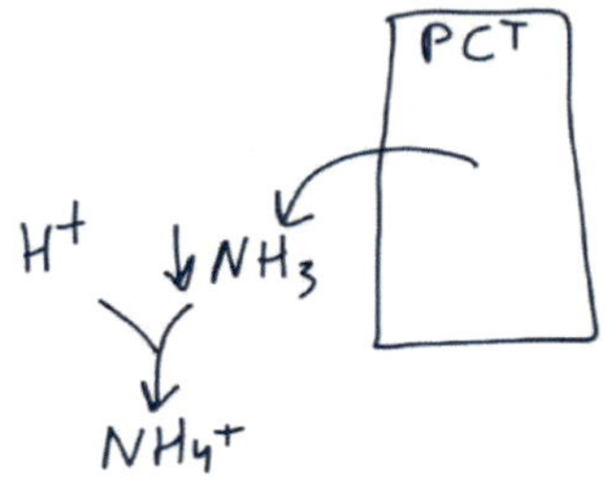

2. A patient has aminoaciduria and glucosuria, what would you expect the urinary pH to be and why?

   - **Amino acids and glucose are reabsorbed at the proximal convoluted tubule (PCT)**
   - **If amino acids and glucose appear in the urine, suspect PCT dysfunction → poor reabsorption of HCO_3^- → eventual loss of serum HCO_3^- → decreased HCO_3^- entering urine → decreased urine pH**

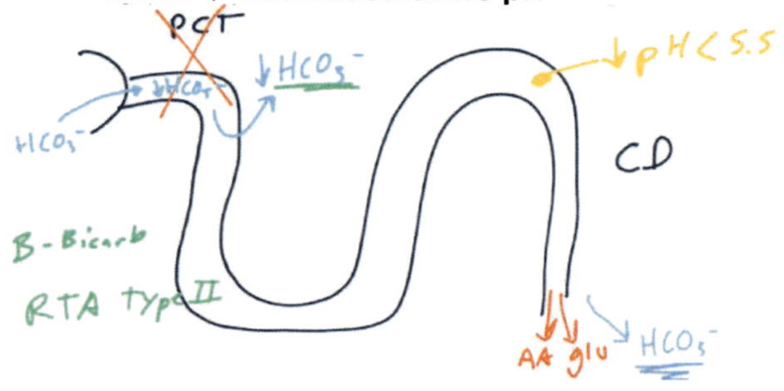

3. A patient with chronic respiratory acidosis, causing the proximal tubule to reabsorb bicarbonate at a faster rate. What then will happen to the line depicting bicarbonate in figure 4.6?

   - **Respiratory Acidosis (chronic): Prolonged respiratory acidosis → renal compensation → increased HCO_3^- reabsorption → decreased HCO_3^- in TF → decreased TF/P ratio for HCO_3^-**
   - **Fanconi Syndrome indicates dysfunction of PCT → decreased reabsorption of all solutes normally reabsorbed by PCT → increased solutes in TF → increased TF/P ratio for all of these solutes**
   - **Aminoaciduria indicates decreased amino acid reabsorption → increased amino acids in TF → increased TF/P ratio for amino acids**
   - **TF/P > 1 (in this case 1.7) indicates solute is reabsorbed slower than H_2O (or excreted in this case) → PAH must be the solute indicated**

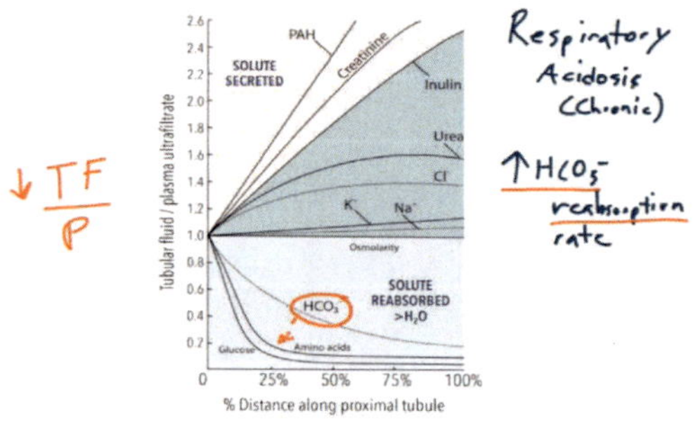

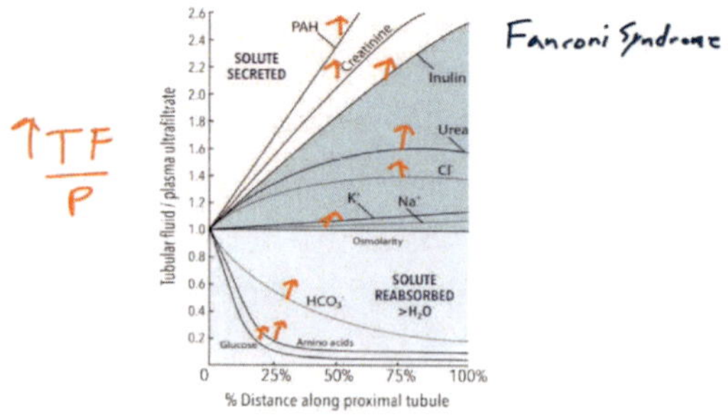

REVIEW QUESTIONS

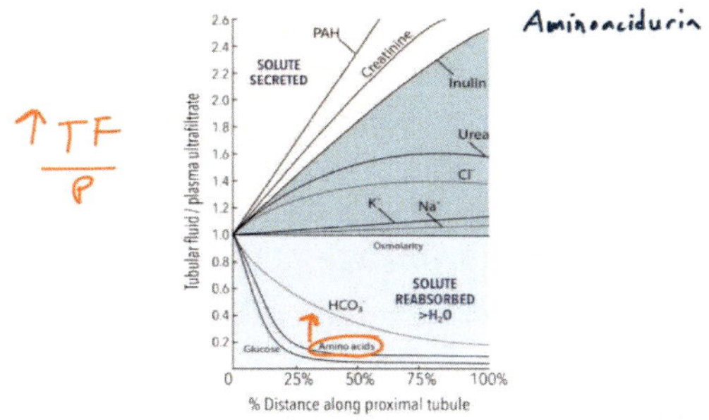

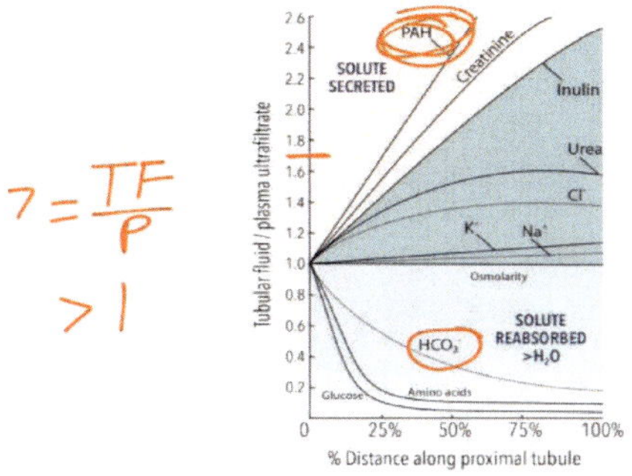

4. The FENa is 3% in a patient. What does this tell you about the function of the nephron?

- **FENa > 3% indicates excess excretion of Na^+**
- **The defect could be in any of the locations where Na^+ is normally reabsorbed (PCT, TAL, DCT, and collecting duct)**

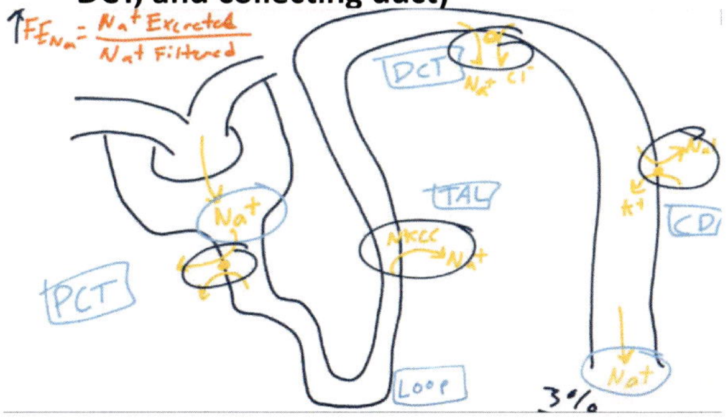

5. A patient has muscle cramps, heart arrhythmias and an EKG showing a flattened T wave. You suspect hypokalemia is present. If this patient has hypokalemia, what would you expect to happen to the concentration of potassium in the urine and why?

- **K^+ will be reabsorbed at the PCT and TAL, as usual**
- **There will be decreased secretion of K^+ at the collecting duct and decreased reabsorption as well**
- **Net effect would be decreased urinary K^+**

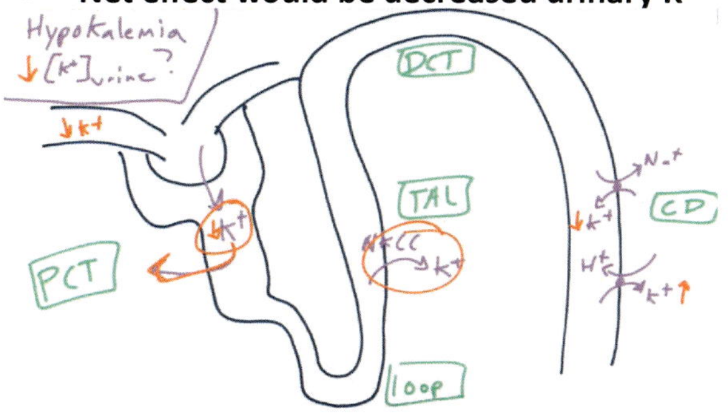

6. A patient is taking a thiazide diuretic. What will happen to the urinary excretion of potassium?

- **Thiazides block NaCl channel at DCT, leading to increased loss of Na^+ and H_2O**
- **RAAS will be stimulated, leading to greater K^+ excretion via aldosterone at collecting duct**

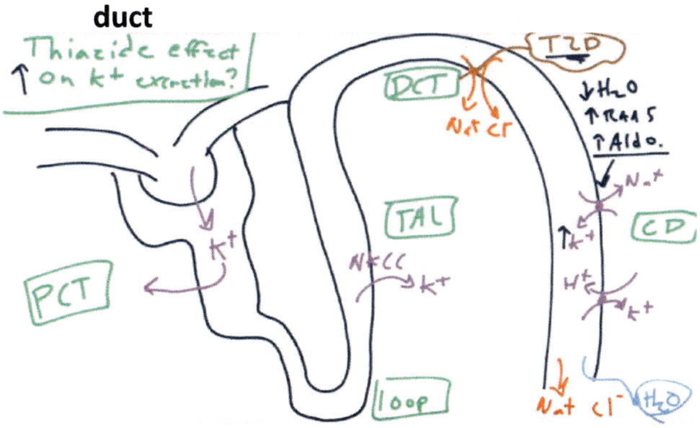

REVIEW QUESTIONS

7. How would a loop diuretic alter the osmolarity of the urine in the bottom of the loop of Henle, the distal tubule, the collecting duct, and the vasa recta?

   - **Loop diuretics block NKCC in TAL, causing excretion of Na^+, Cl^-, and H_2O**
   - **Blocking NKCC will also cause decrease Na^+ and Cl^- in the vasa recta (countercurrent), decreasing H_2O reabsorption at the descending loop of Henle (decreased hypertonicity)**
   - **Less osmotic power decreases H_2O reabsorption through aquaporins at collecting duct**
   - **DCT osmolarity cannot be determined**

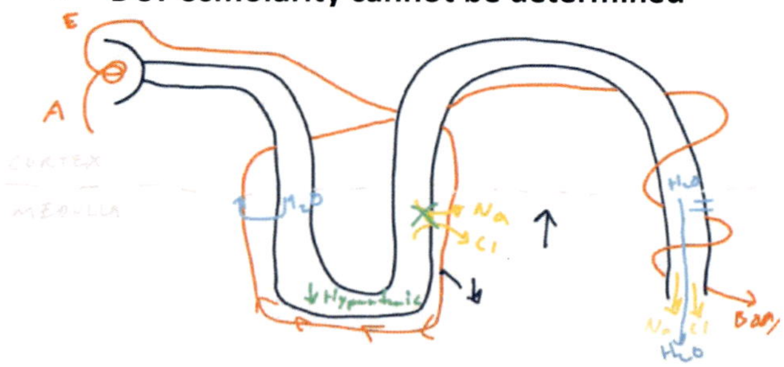

8. What would happen to the osmolarity at the bottom of the loop of Henle in a patient who is running a marathon?

   - **Running a marathon leads to water loss and increased serum osmolarity → ADH release from hypothalamus → increased Na^+ and Cl^- reabsorption from TAL → increased osmolarity of Vasa recta → increased water reabsorption from descending limb → increased tonicity at loop of henle**

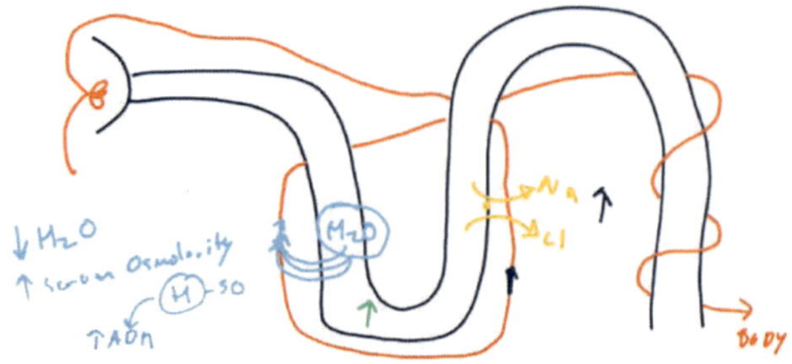

9. With very low levels of ADH, which segment of the nephron would have the lowest osmolarity and which would have the highest?

   - **Long distance running decreases H_2O and increases serum osmolarity, leading to increased ADH release**
   - **ADH increases NKCC activity at the TAL, leading to increased osmotic power of the vasa recta, leading to increased H_2O reabsorption at the descending loop (increased tonicity)**

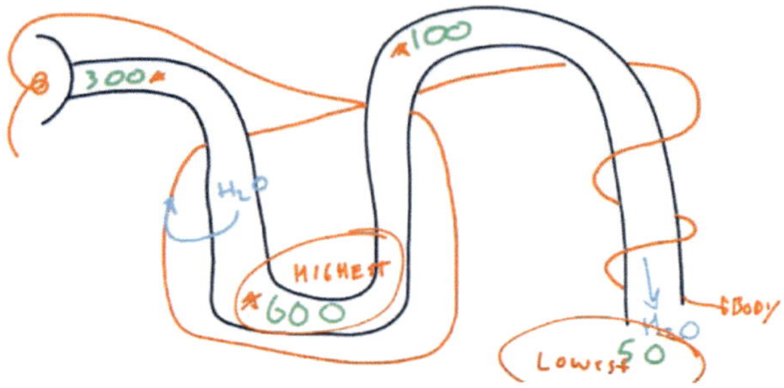

Section IV - Renin-Angiotensin-Aldosterone System

I. Prostaglandin

A. Dilate the afferent arteriole

II. Dopamine

A. At low doses → dilation of the afferent and efferent arterioles

B. At high doses → alpha-agonistic effect resulting in vasoconstriction

III. Bradykinin

A. Dilates arterioles

B. Broken down by ACE inhibitors

IV. Vitamin D and PTH are Discussed in Endocrinology

V. Atrial Natriuretic Peptide

A. Released from atria in response to increased volume

B. Dilates afferent arteriole

VI. Renin-Angiotensin-Aldosterone System (RAAS)

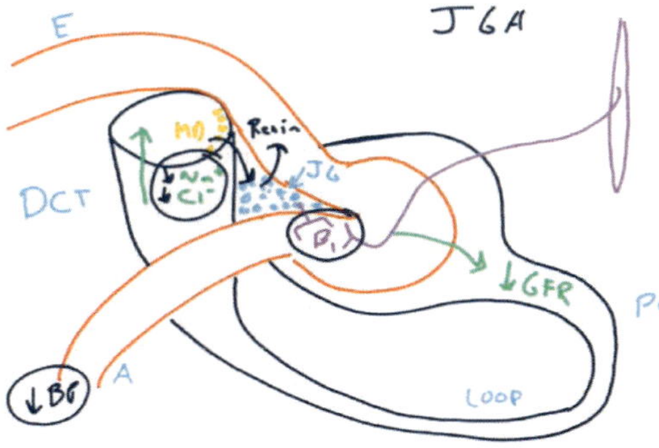

A. The juxtaglomerular apparatus (JGA) release renin in response to certain stimuli.

1. The JGA consists of macula densa cells, juxtaglomerular cells, and extraglomerular mesangial cells.

a) Macula densa cells are present in the distal tubule of the nephron and monitor flow rate and salt content. These cells then transmit the signal to the juxtaglomerular cells.

(1) Decreased Na^+ delivery to the macula densa → increased renin

b) Juxtaglomerular cells are modified smooth muscle cells located in the afferent arteriole. These cells regulate the release of renin in response to signals from the macula densa.

c) Extraglomerular mesangial cells are wedged between the afferent and efferent arterioles and contain renin, but their role is not well understood.

d) Beta receptors on the JG cells of the kidneys respond to the sympathetic nervous system by releasing renin. Increased sympathetic tone → increased renin release

e) Decreased blood flow / blood pressure to the macula densa → increased renin

B. Renin is released into the blood and converts serum angiotensinogen from the liver to angiotensin I (ATI).

C. Angiotensin converting enzyme (ACE) which is produced in the pulmonary vasculature converts angiotensin I to angiotensin II.

D. Angiotensin II upregulates the hypothalamic pituitary axis, thereby increasing production of aldosterone.

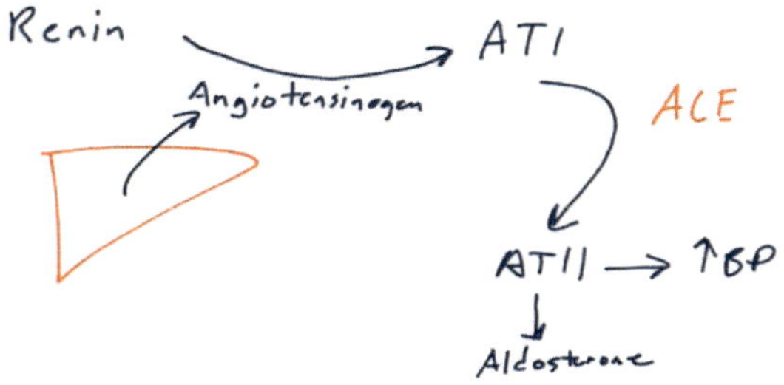

E. Aldosterone Functions

1. Constricts the efferent arteriole.

2. Up-regulates the Na^+/H^+ pump in the PCT → Increased H^+ secretion → increased HCO_3 reabsorption → increased serum pH

F. Angiotensin II functions

1. ATII also increases Na^+ and H_2O reabsorption to increase fluid levels.
2. ATII, which will then increase serum pH. The fluid loss, or contraction, will not be entirely overcome by ATII, so the patient will remain in a state of "contraction," but nevertheless be alkalotic. Therefore, ATII causes the alkalotic part of contraction alkalosis and seeks to reverse the contraction part.
3. ATII is a potent vasoconstrictor.

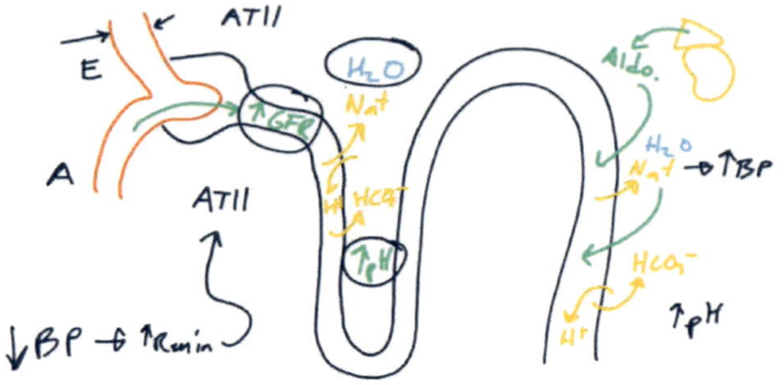

VII. ADH

A. Osmoreceptors are present in the supraoptic nucleus of the hypothalamus which produce ADH in response to increased blood osmolarity and decreased blood pressure.

Situations to think about:

1. Shock (low BP), →↑ renin
2. Chronic kidney disease →↓ renin
3. Adrenal tumor overproducing aldosterone →↑ BP →↓ renin

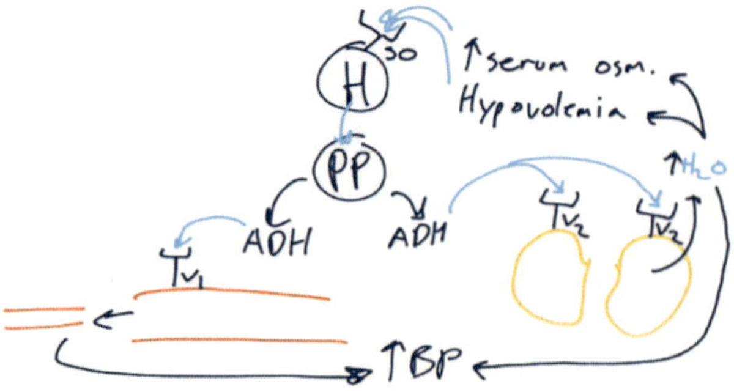

VIII. Autoregulation

A. This is how the kidneys maintain a normal level of blood flow (RBF) and GFR.

B. Dilation of the afferent arteriole and constriction of the efferent arteriole both result in increased GFR.

C. Increased blood pressure would stimulate the afferent arterioles to constrict via a reflexive myogenic response.

D. Decreased blood pressure would cause the afferent arterioles to produce more metabolic waste products such as K^+, adenosine, and lactate → dilation of the afferent arteriole.

REVIEW QUESTIONS ?

1. What would meloxicam do to the GFR?

- **Meloxicam inhibits COX activity**
- **COX enzymes increase prostaglandins which would dilate the afferent arteriole and increase GFR**
- **With decreased COX activity and decreased prostaglandins, GFR would be decreased**

2. If the diameter of the afferent and efferent arterioles are changing equally, what would happen to GFR?

- **GFR would remain unchanged**

3. A patient has hypertension, what would happen to the sodium chloride delivery to the macula densa?

- **HTN increases GFR, increasing Na^+ and Cl^- that reaches the macula densa, decreasing its stimulation of the JG cells, thereby decreasing renin**

4. What would happen to the GFR and potassium level in a patient taking an ACE inhibitor?

- **ACEi will decrease ATII, which normally constricts the efferent arteriole**
- **With decreased ATII, there will be a relative dilation of the efferent arteriole and decreased GFR**
- **Low aldosterone leads to low K^+ secretion and high serum K^+**

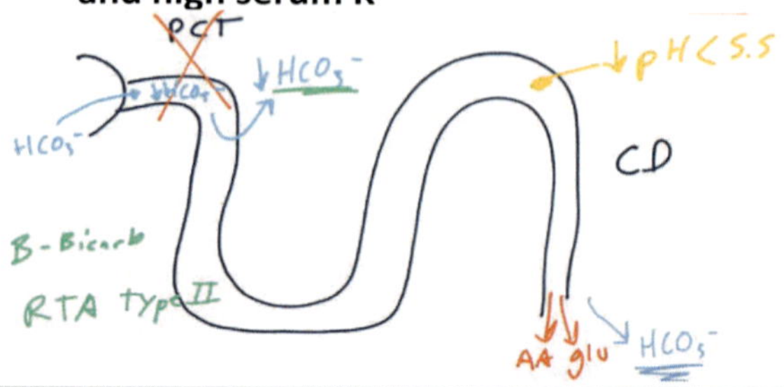

REVIEW QUESTIONS

5. A patient has chronic anxiety, what would happen to his or her aldosterone level?
   - **Sympathetic activity will stimulate β_1 stimulation on the JG cells, triggering RAAS**
6. What would happen the RAAS in a patient with HF?
   - **CHF decreases blood flow to the JGA, triggering RAAS**

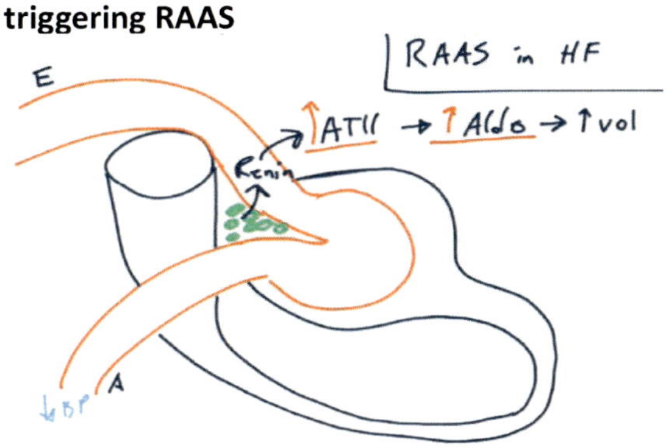

7. What would happen to the receptors of the supraoptic nucleus in a patient with psychogenic polydipsia?
   - **Psychogenic polydipsia leads to increased H_2O and decreased serum osmolarity, decreasing activity of the supraoptic nucleus**

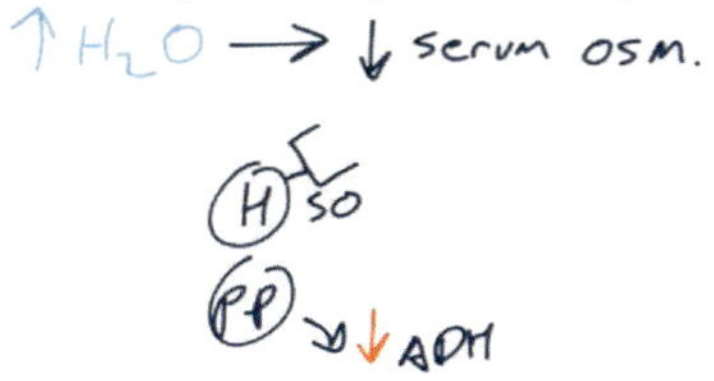

8. In a patient with new hyperaldosteronism, what would happen to tubuloglomerular feedback?
   - **High blood pressure (from increased aldosterone) increases Na^+ and Cl^- reaching the macula densa, inhibiting release of renin from the JG cells**

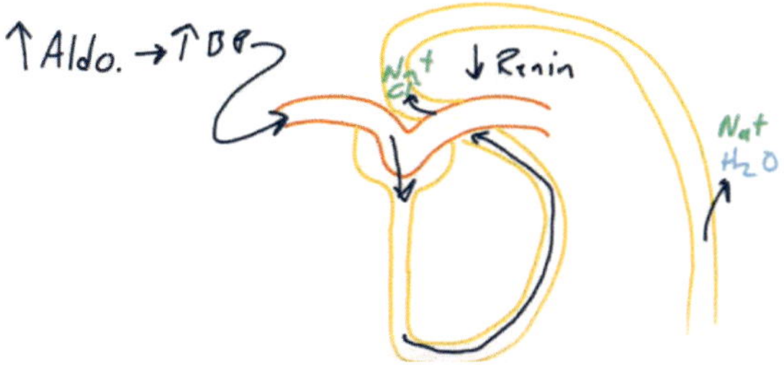

9. What would loop diuretics do to the RAAS?
   - **Loop diuretics block NKCC, initially increasing Na^+ and Cl^- reaching the macula densa, thereby decreasing release of renin from the JG cells**
   - **However, once enough H_2O is diuresed, GFR will decrease enough to decrease Na^+ and Cl^- reaching the macula densa and RAAS will be stimulated**

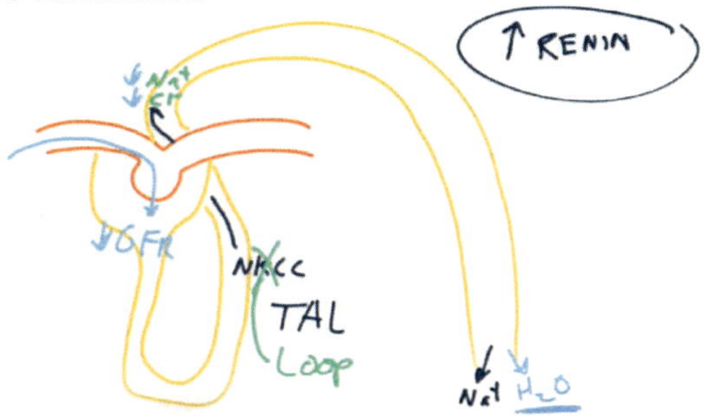

10. What would happen to the GFR in a patient with renal artery stenosis?
    - **GFR would decrease, leading to increased stimulation of the macula densa, JG cells, and increased release of renin**
    - **Note: This same mechanism would be seen in anything that decreases blood flow to the kidneys (e.g. severe dehydration, hypotension, etc)**

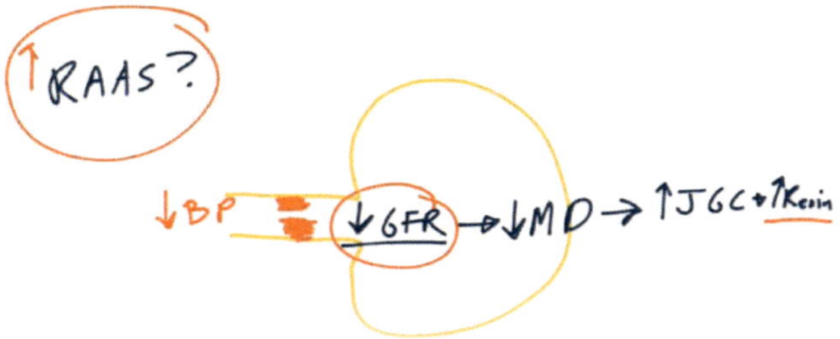

11. What would happen to renin secretion in a severely dehydrated patient?
    - **Decreased blood flow/volume triggers increased release of renin**

Section V - Acid-Base

I. Acid-base

A. Acid production

1. Volatile acid

a) CO_2 is the major physiologic volatile acid.

2. Nonvolatile acid

a) Includes several molecules such as phosphoric acid, sulfuric acid, and lactic acid.

B. Buffers

1. A buffer is comprised of an acid and conjugate base that work to prevent significant changes in pH when H^+ ion concentrations change.

2. Henderson-Hasselbalch equation

$pH = 6.1 + \log [HCO_3^-] / (0.03 \times PCO_2)$

Where:

pH = the acidity of the blood

$[HCO_3^-]$ = the concentration of HCO_3^- in the blood

PCO_2 = the partial pressure of CO_2 in the arterial blood

a) Can be useful for determining the pH in a buffer system.

b) When the concentrations of HCO_3^- and CO_2 are equal the buffer system is most effective.

3. Extracellular buffers

a) The major extracellular buffers include HCO_3^- and inorganic phosphate (PO_4^{3-}).

4. Intracellular buffers

a) The major intracellular buffers include organic phosphates (ATP, ADP, and AMP), hemoglobin, and deoxyhemoglobin.

5. Urinary buffers

a) NH_3^+

(1) The amino acid glutamine can be converted to NH_3 throughout the nephron.

(2) NH_3 is secreted into the lumen of the nephron which can then act as a buffer by binding H^+ to form NH_4^+.

(3) NH_3 synthesis is greatly enhanced during states of acidosis.

b) HPO_4^{2-}

(1) HPO_4^{2-} is a product of metabolism and is freely filtered by the glomerulus.

(2) HPO_4^{2-} can act as a buffer by binding H^+ to form $H_2PO_4^-$.

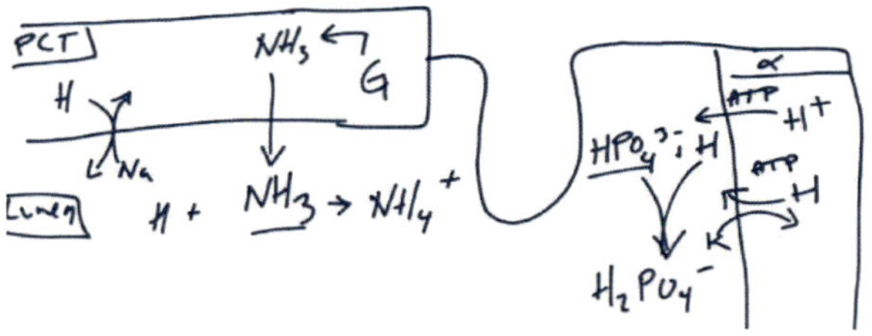

II. Making a diagnosis (Figures 4.3 and 4.4)

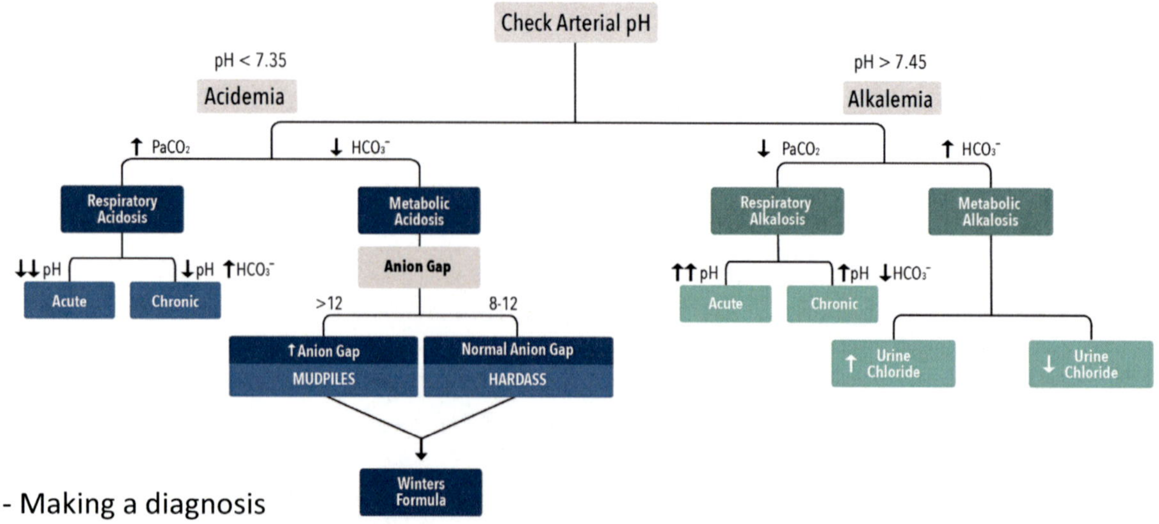

Figure 4.3 - Making a diagnosis

Steps to acid-base

Step 1: Check pH

If >7.45 → alkalosis
If < 7.35 → acidosis

Step 2: Measure CO_2 and HCO_3^-

Elevated concentrations of CO_2 is the primary disturbance in respiratory acidosis.

1. Decreased concentrations of CO_2 is the primary disturbance in respiratory alkalosis.
2. Decreased concentrations of HCO_3^- is the primary disturbance in metabolic acidosis.
3. Elevated concentrations of HCO_3^- is the primary disturbance in metabolic alkalosis.

Step 3: Measure the anion gap to distinguish different causes of a metabolic acidosis.

Step 4: Use the Winters formula to diagnosis a mixed metabolic acidosis and concomitant respiratory disturbance.

Step 5: Measure the concentrations HCO_3^- in conjunction with the pH to determine a chronic versus an acute respiratory disturbance.

A. Disorders

III. Respiratory acidosis

A. Caused by hypoventilation and subsequent retention of CO_2.

B. Excess CO_2 in the arterial blood gets converted to H^+ via carbonic anhydrase.

C. Can be acute (<8 hours) or chronic (>24 hours).

D. Renal compensation is present in chronic respiratory acidosis.

1. Excess H^+ can be excreted in the form of NH_4^+ and $H_2PO_4^-$.
2. Excess H^+ also increases intracellularly within the PCT.
3. The H^+ can enter the lumen of the nephron via the Na^+/H^+ pump in the PCT which can

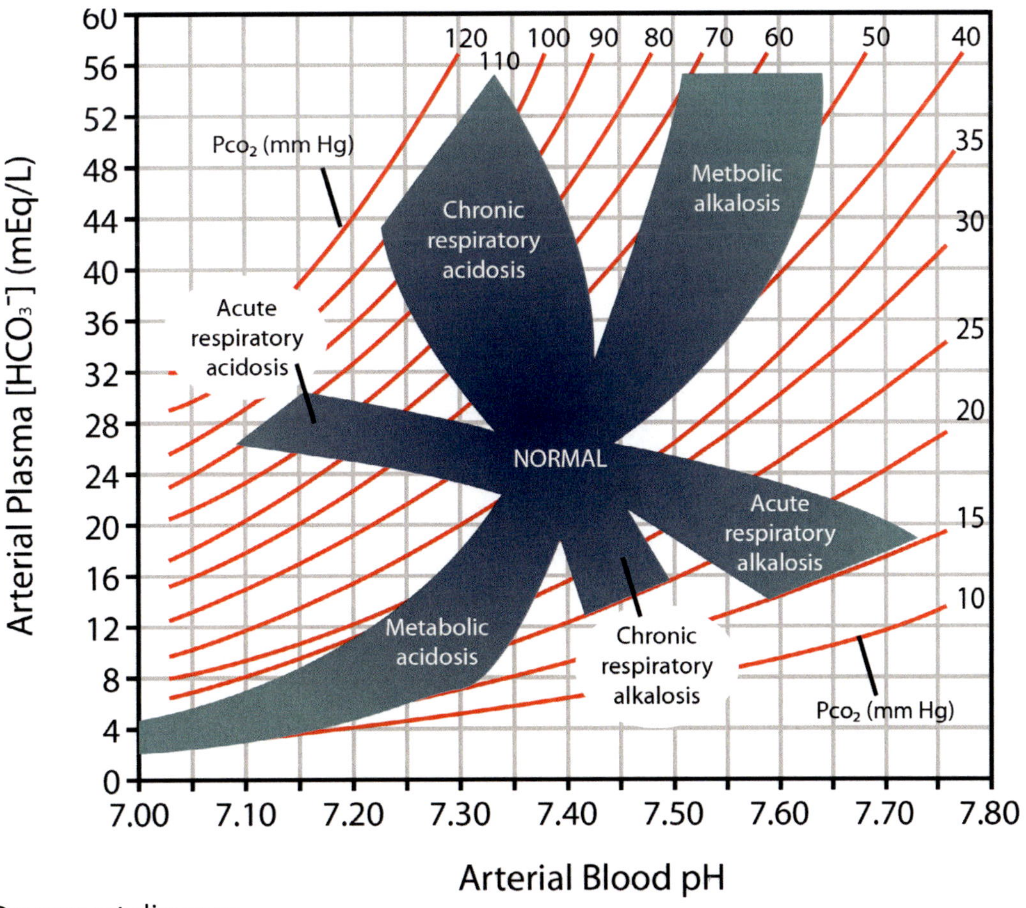

Figure 4.4 - Davenport diagram

then react with filtered HCO_3^- to form CO_2 and H_2O.

4. This mechanism results in increased bicarbonate reabsorption and is the basis for renal compensation during respiratory acidosis.

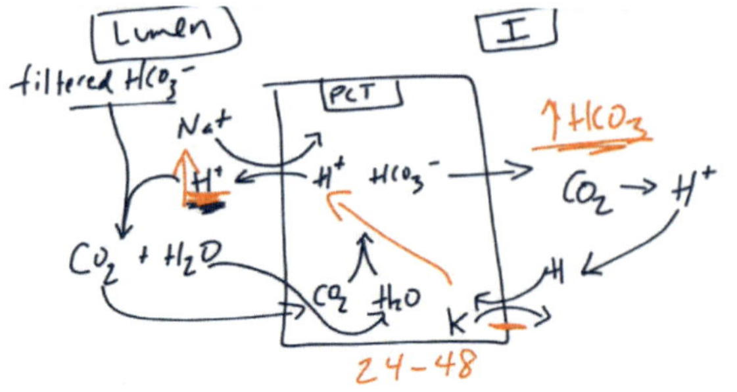

IV. Respiratory Alkalosis

A. Caused by hyperventilation and a subsequent drop in CO_2.

B. Decreased CO_2 in the arterial blood results in decreased H^+ due to mass action.

C. Can be acute (<8 hours) or chronic (>24 hours).

D. Renal compensation is present in chronic respiratory alkalosis.

1. Decreased H^+ results in decreased intracellular H^+ within the PCT.

2. The decreased intracellular H^+ results in decreased H^+ within the lumen of the nephron and a subsequent decrease in the formation of CO_2 and H_2O from filtered HCO_3^-.

3. This mechanism results in decreased bicarbonate reabsorption and is the basis for renal compensation during respiratory alkalosis.

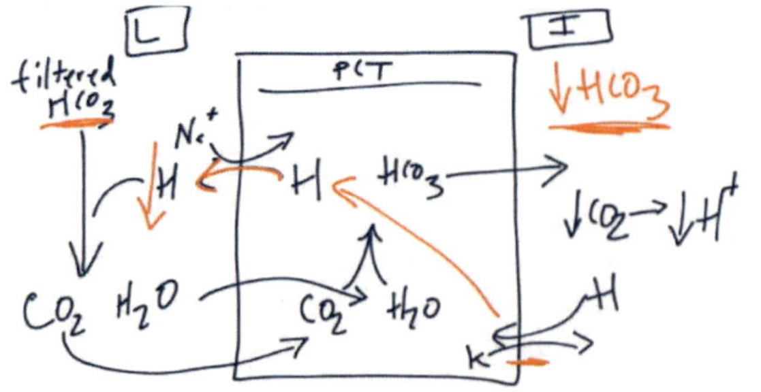

V. Metabolic Acidosis

A. Excess accumulation of acid or loss of base results in decreased concentrations of HCO_3^- in the blood.

B. The drop in HCO_3^- results in increased free H^+.

C. H^+ can be decreased in the form of CO_2 which is the basis for respiratory compensation and resultant hyperventilation.

D. The pH can be further corrected as the kidneys secrete additional NH_4^+ and $H_2PO_4^-$ and reabsorb additional HCO_3^-.

VI. Anion-gap

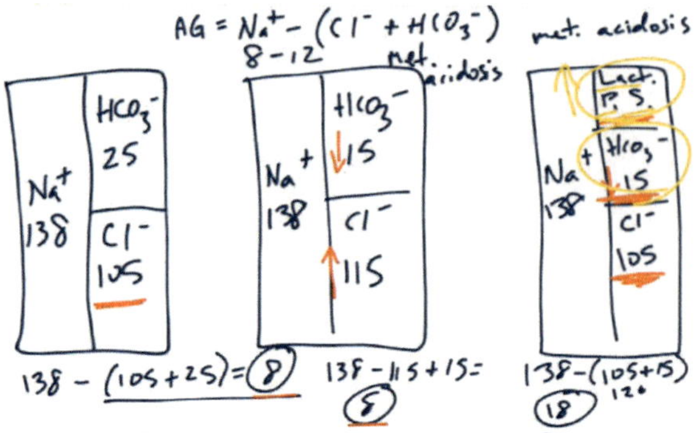

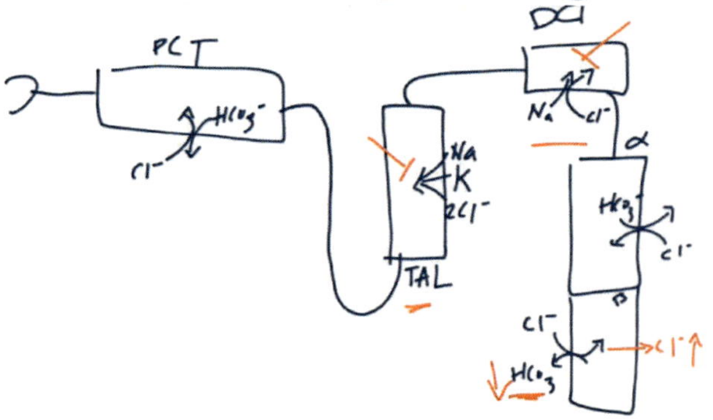

$$AG = Na^+ - (Cl^- + HCO_3^-)$$

Where:
AG = anion gap

A. A normal anion-gap is approximately 8-12 mEq/L.

B. An anion-gap is representative of unmeasured anions in the blood.

C. During a state of metabolic acidosis the HCO_3^- is decreased.

D. The loss of negatively charged HCO_3^- can disrupt the physiologic electroneutrality if the concentration of other anions does not increase.

E. If Cl^- increases in response to the loss of HCO_3^- then the anion-gap is normal.

F. If other unmeasured anions increase in response to the loss of HCO_3^- then the anion-gap is increased.

VII. Mixed Acid-base Disorders

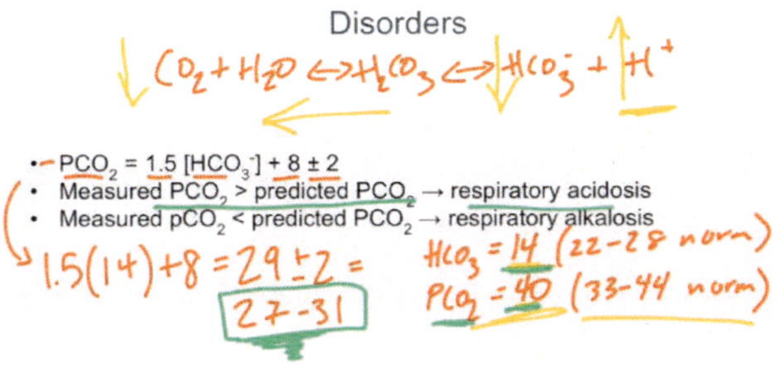

A. A mixed acid-base disorder occurs when there is not an adequate compensatory response from the kidneys or lungs to a primary acid-base disturbance.

B. A mixed metabolic acidosis and respiratory acid-base disturbance can be determined using the Winters formula.

$$PCO_2 = 1.5\ [HCO_3^-] + 8 \pm 2$$

Where:

PCO_2 = the partial pressure of carbon dioxide in the blood

HCO_3^- = the concentration of bicarbonate in the blood

VIII. Metabolic Alkalosis

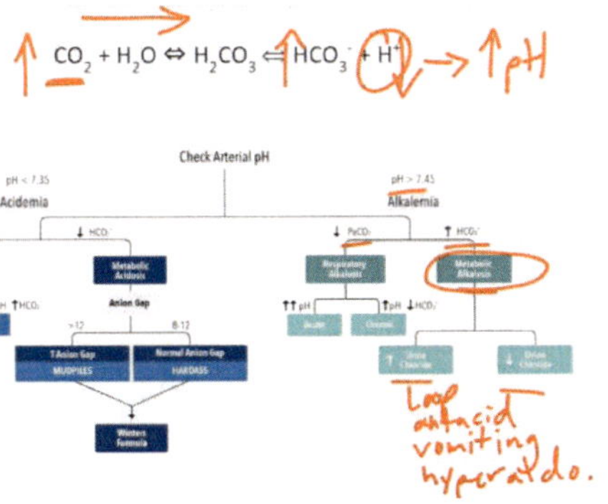

A. Elevated concentrations of HCO_3^- is due to a loss of H^+ or a gain of base.

B. The rise in HCO_3^- results in decreased free H^+.

C. Hypoventilation ensues as a means of retaining CO_2 which can then be converted to H^+ and is the basis for respiratory compensation.

D. The decreased H^+ results in decreased intracellular H^+ within the PCT.

E. The decreased intracellular H^+ results in decreased H^+ within the lumen of the nephron and a subsequent decrease in the formation of CO_2 and H_2O from filtered HCO_3^-.

F. This mechanism results in decreased bicarbonate reabsorption and is the basis for renal compensation during respiratory alkalosis.

G. Common causes

1. Loop diuretics and antacids

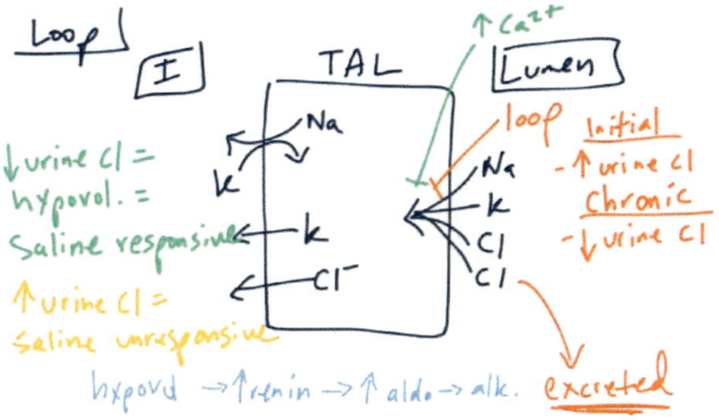

2. Vomiting

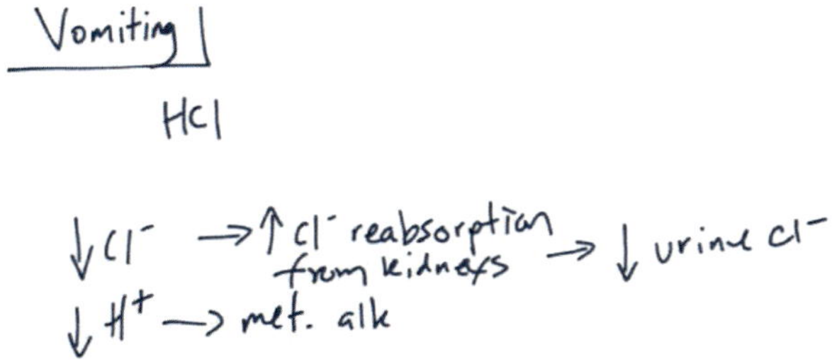

3. Hyperaldosteronism

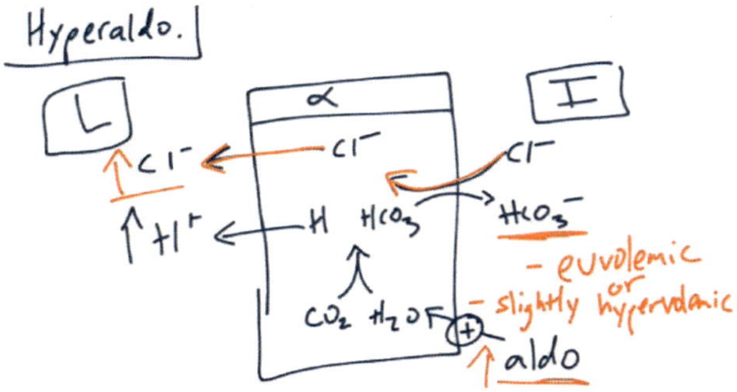

REVIEW QUESTIONS

1. How would the concentration of ammonium in the urine change in a patient with diabetic ketoacidosis, or DKA?

   - **DKA → ↓ insulin → ↑ lipolysis → ketoacids**
   - **As ketoacids accumulate in the nephron $NH_3 \rightarrow NH_4^+$**

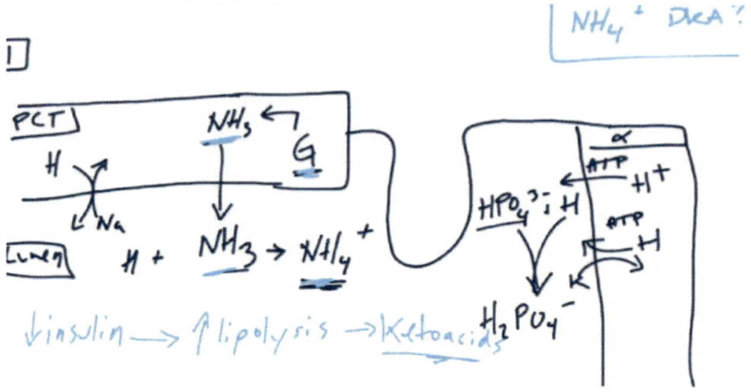

2. How would the pH, pCO_2, HCO_3^-, and urinary pH change in a patient with a 2 year history of asthma?

   - **Asthma → ↑ bronchoconstriction → ↑ PCO_2 → ↑ H^+ → ↓ pH**
   - **↑ H^+ stimulates the reabsorption of HCO_3^- → ↑ HCO_3^-**
   - **↑ acid excretion in the form of NH4+ and dihydrogen phosphate → ↓ urinary pH**

pH | PCO_2 | HCO_3^- | PaO_2

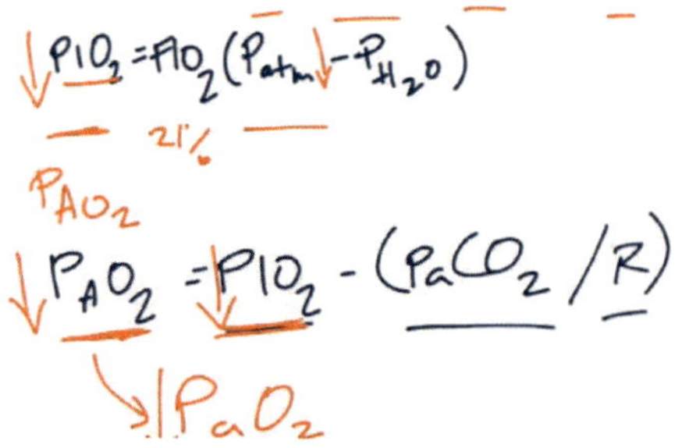

3. What drugs are commonly associated with an acute respiratory acidosis?

   - **Opioids (i.e. heroin)**

4. How would the pH, pCO_2, HCO_3^-, and the partial pressure of oxygen within the arterial system change in a patient who is climbing Mount Everest for the first time?

   - **↑ altitude → ↓ Patm → ↓ PIO_2 → ↓ PAO_2 → ↓ PaO_2**
   - **↓ PaO_2 → stimulation of chemoreceptors → hyperventilation → ↓ PCO_2**
   - **A left shift occurs → ↓ H^+ → ↑ pH**
   - **As ↓ H^+ → HCO_3^- excretion in the nephron increases → ↓ HCO_3^-**

5. A middle aged man with a history of depression has attempted suicide by ingesting an unknown substance. His pH is 7.2 (normal: 7.35-7.45), PCO_2 is 21 (normal: 33-44 mmHg), HCO_3^- is 10 (normal: 22-28 mEq/L), sodium is 140 (normal: 136-145 mEq/L), and chloride is 100 (normal: 95-105 mEq/L). What is the likely diagnosis?

   - **pH 7.2 = acidosis**
   - **↓ PCO_2 = metabolic acidosis**
   - **Anion gap = 30**
   - **Winters formula = PCO_2 = 1.5 [HCO_3^-] + 8 +/- 2 = 21-25**
   - **Predicted PCO_2 ~ actual PCO_2 = adequate respiratory compensation**
   - **Ddx includes MUD PILES**

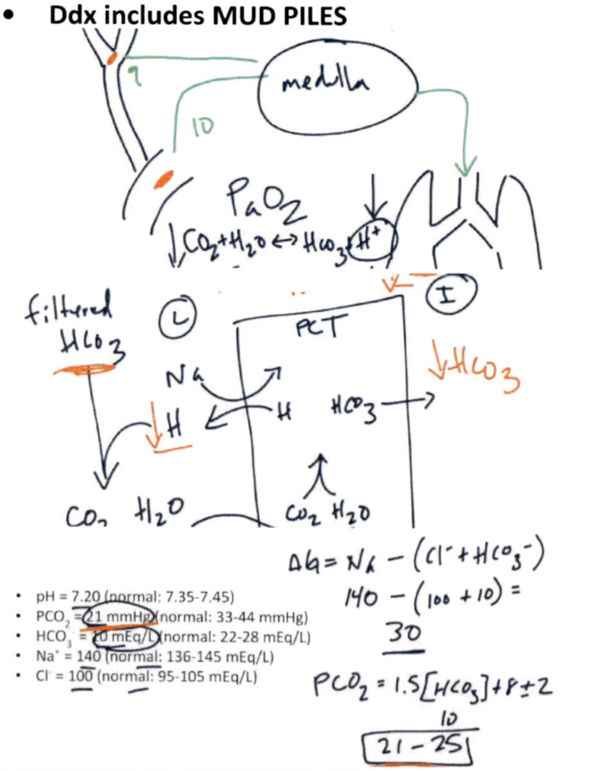

REVIEW QUESTIONS

6. There is a 21-year-old female who presents to the ED. She is sweating profusely, she is tachycardic and says her symptoms came on spontaneously several hours ago. Her pH is high, her PCO_2 is low, and her HCO_3^- is low-normal. What is the likely diagnosis?

- **Panic attack (she has an alkalosis with a ↓ PCO_2 likely due to hyperventilation)**
- **An acute change in respiratory status would not provide sufficient time for renal compensation (normal bicarbonate)**

↑pH | ↓PCO_2 | ↓/↔ HCO_3^-

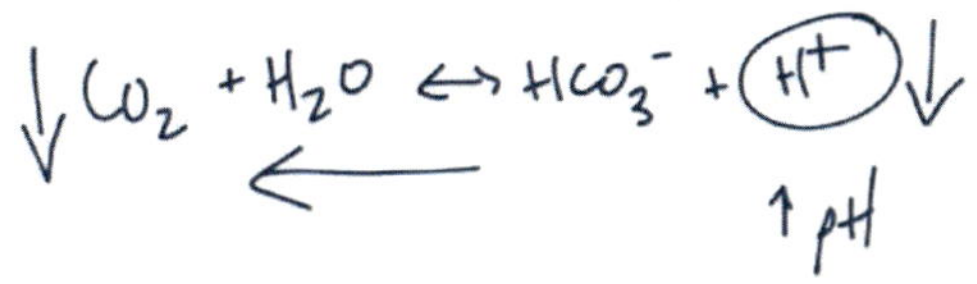

7. How would the bicarbonate concentration be altered in a patient with lactic acidosis?

- **From MUD PILES → "L" = lactic acidosis → must have an anion gap metabolic acidosis**
- **Lactic acid reacts with and consumes HCO_3^- → ↓ HCO_3^-**

↓ HCO_3^-

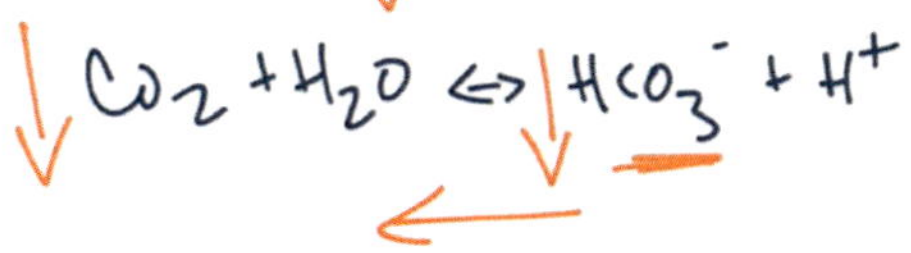

8. How would renal failure alter the pH of the serum?

- **Renal failure → kidneys are unable to reabsorb bicarbonate as effectively + unable to secrete acid as effectively → ↓ serum pH**

Renal failure | pH

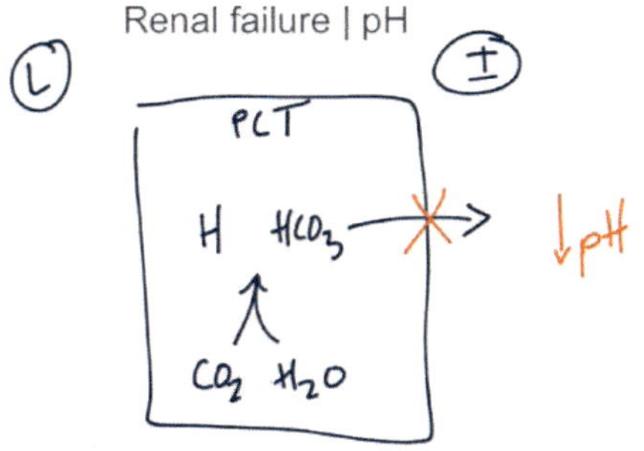

9. An 8-year-old girl presents to the ED because she is hyperventilating. Her pH is 7.33 (normal: 7.35-7.45), PCO_2 is 24 (normal: 33-44 mmHg), HCO_3^- is 19 (normal: 22-28 mEq/L), sodium is 145 (normal: 136-145 mEq/L), and chloride is 105 (normal: 95-105 mEq/L). What is the likely diagnosis?

- **↓ pH = acidosis**
- **↓ PCO_2 & ↓ HCO_3^- = metabolic acidosis**
- **Anion gap = 21**
- **Winters formula = PCO_2 = 1.5 [HCO_3^-] + 8 +/- 2 = 34.5-38.5**
- **Predicted PCO_2 < actual PCO_2 = inadequate respiratory compensation (the patient is breathing too fast than what is expected → concomitant respiratory alkalosis)**
- **Ddx includes MUD PILES (likely salicylate poisoning given metabolic acidosis and concomitant respiratory alkalosis)**

↓pH | ↓PCO_2 | ↓HCO_3^-

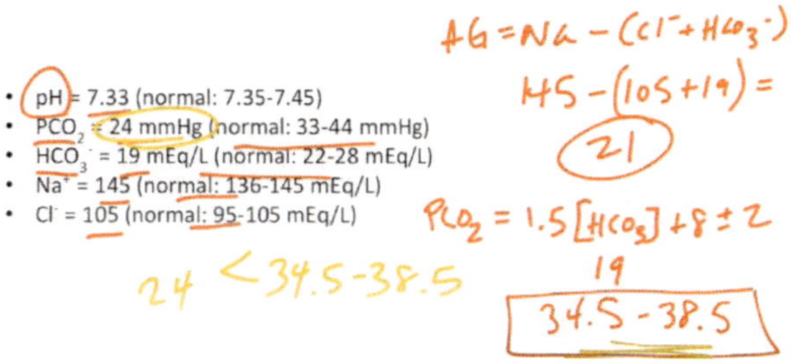
- pH = 7.33 (normal: 7.35-7.45)
- PCO_2 = 24 mmHg (normal: 33-44 mmHg)
- HCO_3^- = 19 mEq/L (normal: 22-28 mEq/L)
- Na^+ = 145 (normal: 136-145 mEq/L)
- Cl^- = 105 (normal: 95-105 mEq/L)

10. How would acetazolamide alter the concentration of ammonium and dihydrogen phosphate in the lumen of the nephron?

- **Acetazolamide blocks luminal and intracellular carbonic anhydrase → ↓ luminal H^+ → ↓ $H_2PO_4^-$ and NH_4^+ formation**

Acetazolamide | NH_4^+ | $H_2PO_4^-$

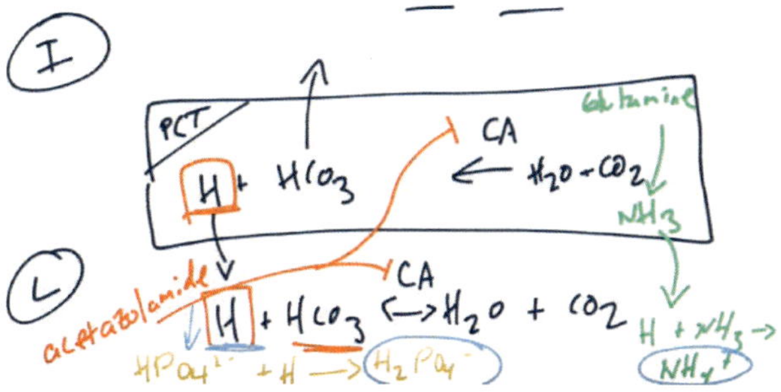

REVIEW QUESTIONS

11. What would the pH, PCO_2, bicarb, and anion gap be in a patient with severe diarrhea from a viral infection?

- **"HARD ASS" = Non-anion gap metabolic acidosis**
- **"D" = diarrhea → bicarbonate loss in stool → ↑ H^+ → ↓ pH**
- **Respiratory compensation → ↓ PCO_2**

pH | PCO_2 | HCO_3^- | AG

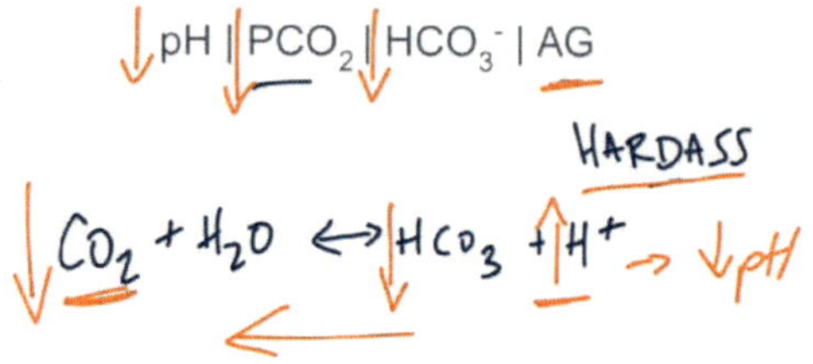

12. A 52-year-old woman presents to the ED with decompensated congestive heart failure. After her condition is stabilized and her volume status is controlled with bumetanide, she is told to follow up with her primary care physician. After several weeks she sees the primary care physician who is now concerned about an acid-base abnormality. What would the blood pH, urine chloride, and blood bicarbonate concentration likely be in this patient?

- **Loop diuretics (i.e. bumetanide) block the NKCC channel → ↑ H_2O loss → ↑ RAAS → ↑ H^+ excretion → ↑ blood HCO_3^-**
- **Loop diuretics also ↑ chloride excretion by blocking the NKCC channel → ↑ urine chloride**
- **Chronic blockage of the NKCC → ↓ urine chloride**

pH | urine Cl^- | HCO_3^-

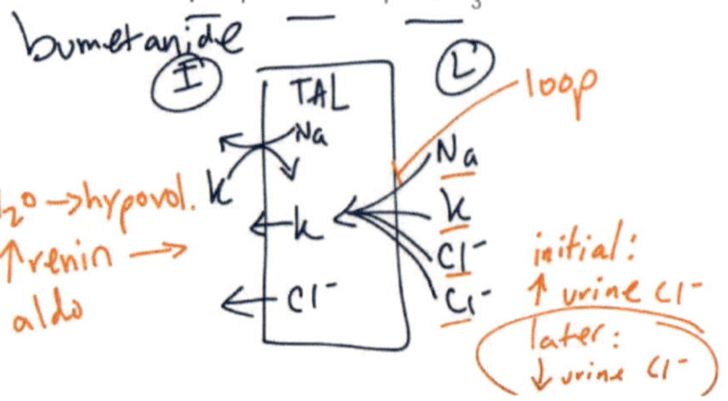

GASTROENTEROLOGY

Section I - Gastrointestinal Overview

I. Oral Cavity (Figure 5.1)

A. α-Amylase is an enzyme secreted by the salivary glands and begins the of starch.

B. R protein from the salivary glands promotes the absorption of vitamin B_{12}.

II. Esophagus

A. Contraction of the muscles of the pharynx initiates swallowing by moving a bolus of food into the esophagus.

B. Peristalsis assists in moving the bolus from the superior aspect of the esophagus to the lower esophageal sphincter (LES).

C. The LES must relax in order for food to move from the esophagus into the stomach.

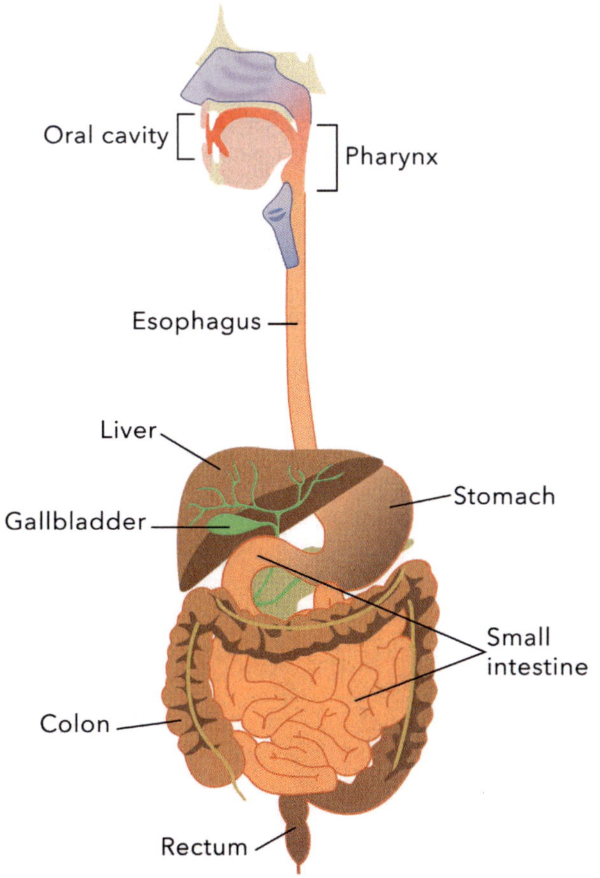

Figure 5.1 - GI Anatomical overview

III. Stomach

A. Gastric cells (Figure 5.2)

1. Parietal cells located in the body of the stomach secrete HCl and intrinsic factor.
2. Chief cells located in the body of the stomach secrete pepsinogen which gets cleaved into pepsin in the acidic environment of the stomach. Pepsinogen begins the process of protein metabolism.
3. Mucous cells located in the antrum of the stomach secrete the mucus responsible for the protective barrier near the gastric epithelium.
4. G cells located in the antrum of the stomach secrete gastrin which stimulates the parietal cells to secrete acid.
5. D cells located in the antrum of the stomach secrete somatostatin.
6. Stem cells are present in the isthmus of the gastric pits and are responsible for replenishing the gastric epithelium.

B. The stomach has three primary functions:

1. Intrinsic factor secretion by parietal cells facilitates vitamin B_{12} absorption which is ultimately absorbed in the terminal ileum (Figure 5.3).
2. A reservoir which regulates how frequently boluses of food can enter the duodenum.
3. Acid secretion which facilitates protein digestion.
   a) Parietal cells found in the gastric mucosa produce HCl. The H^+ is secreted into the lumen of the stomach in exchange for K^+. This is achieved via primary active transport (i.e. requires ATP).
   b) Acid secretion occurs in three phases (Figures 5.4 and 5.5):

(1) The cephalic phase of acid secretion is mediated by the vagus nerve and is triggered by the taste, sight, smell, and thought of food.

(2) The gastric phase of acid secretion occurs as a result of food entering the stomach which causes the release of gastrin and subsequent stimulation of histamine and acid secretion.

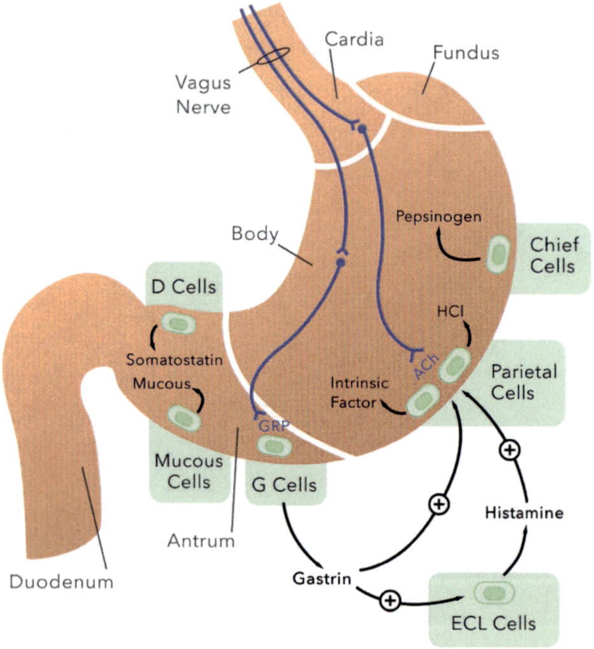

Figure 5.2 - Gastrointestinal hormones

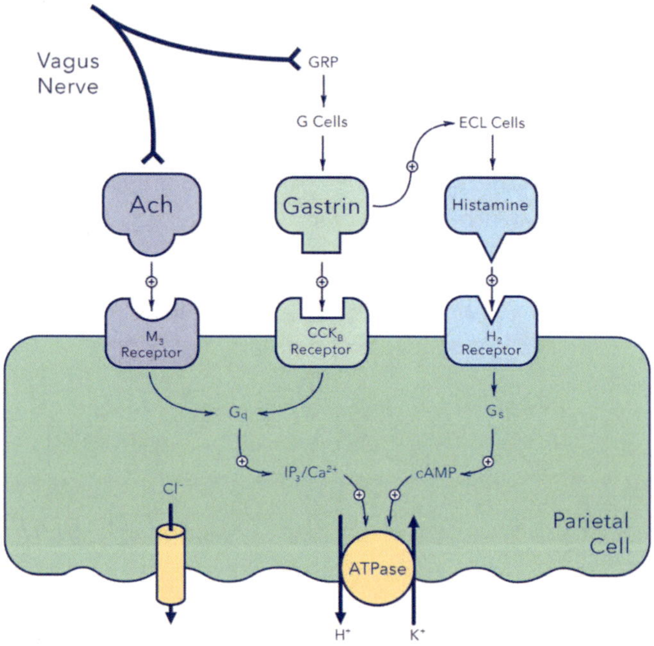

Figure 5.4 - Acid production

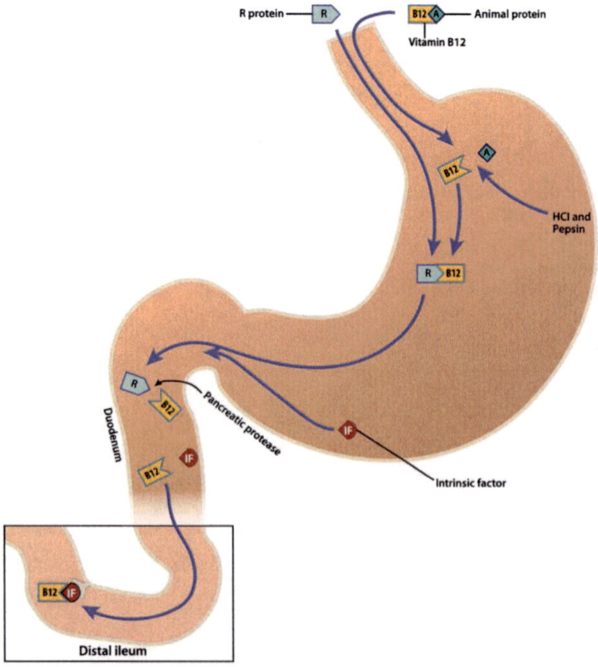

Figure 5.3 - Vitamin B12 absorption

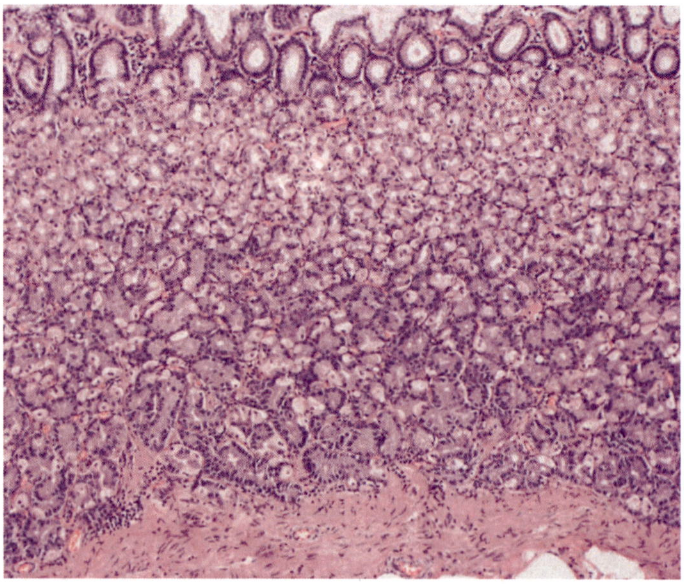

Figure 5.5 - Histological image of the stomach

(3) The intestinal phase of acid secretion occurs when protein enters the duodenum. Although the initial part of this phase stimulates acid secretion, the overall effect is to reduce acid secretion. This occurs as the ileum and colon release peptide YY which acts on the enterochromaffin-like cells (ECLs) and inhibits the release of histamine.

Figure 5.4 - Acid production

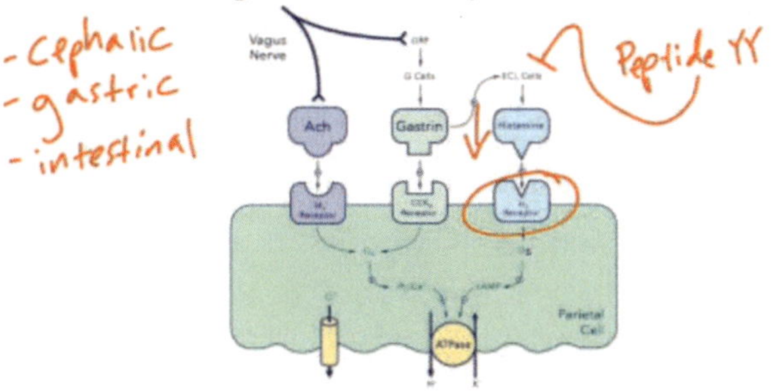

C. Factors that protect the stomach against the acidic environment:

1. Highly vascularized epithelium allowing the blood to sweep away excess acid.
2. Mucus barrier that prevents acid from eroding the tissue.
3. Bicarbonate secretion from the gastric epithelium into the mucus layer, thus neutralizing acid that reaches the barrier.
4. Prostaglandin E (PGE) which facilitates bicarbonate and mucus production.

IV. The small intestine consists of the duodenum, jejunum, and ileum.

V. Large Intestine

A. The normal flora in the colon produce folate and vitamin K from undigested sugars and also protect the mucosa from pathogenic bacteria.

B. The large intestine is especially prone to developing diverticula when intraluminal colonic pressure increases.

REVIEW QUESTIONS ?

1. What is the underlying cause associated with formation of a Zenker diverticulum?

- **Pharyngeal muscle dysmotility → ↑ pressure → mucosal herniation**

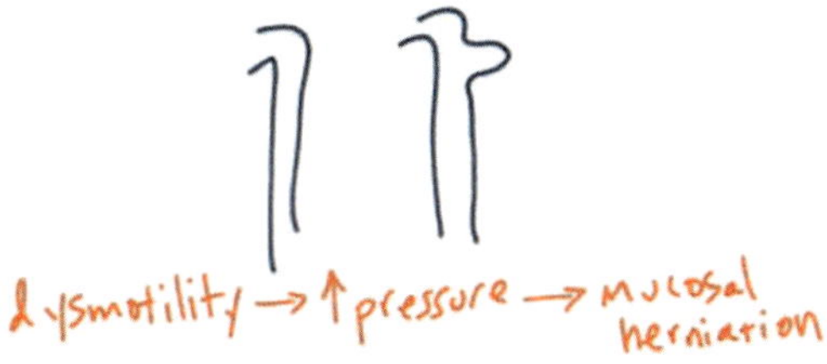

2. What disorder results in a decreased ability of the lower esophageal sphincter (LES) to relax?

- **Achalasia**
- **Loss of the inhibitory ganglion cells → ↑ contraction of the lower esophageal sphincter**

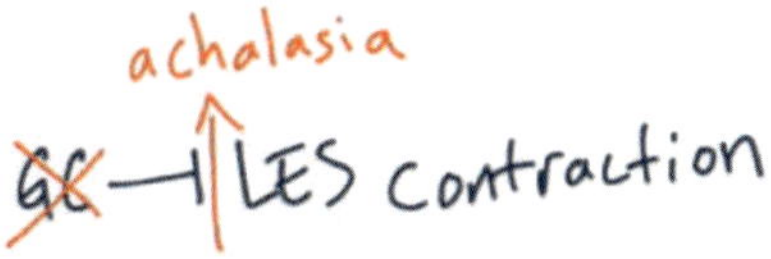

3. What is a disorder associated with a transient decrease in tone of the LES?

- **Gastroesophageal reflux disease (GERD)**
- **↑ laxity of the lower esophageal sphincter → reflux of acid into the esophagus**

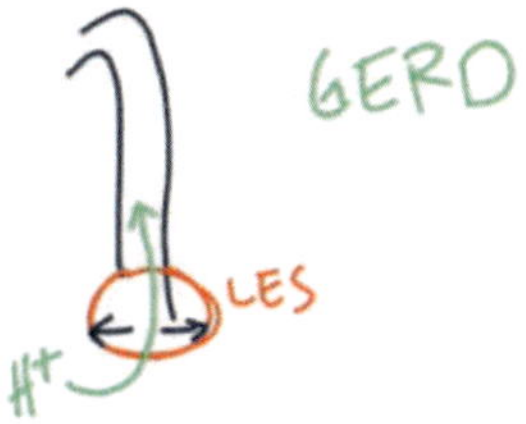

4. Which cell is inhibited by omeprazole (see figure 5.5)?

- **Parietal cells**
- **Proton pump inhibitors (omeprazole) block the hydrogen-potassium-ATPase channel**

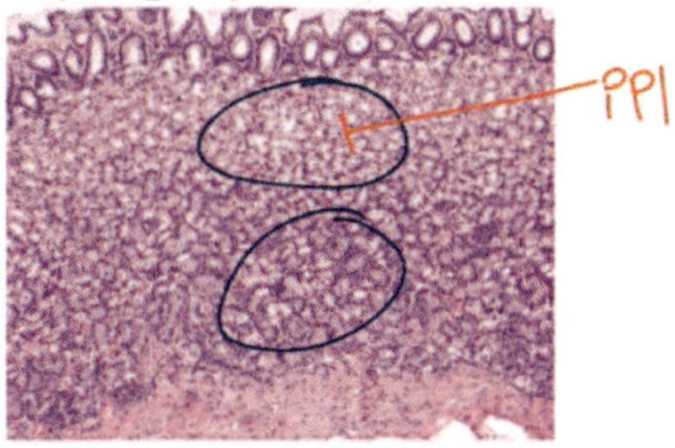

REVIEW QUESTIONS

5. A 36-year-old female presents with a 6 month history of fatigue. Her MCV is 124. The physician believes her symptoms are due to an autoimmune disorder. What is the most likely diagnosis?

   - **MVC>100 → macrocytic anemia**
   - **Pernicious anemia**

6. How would pernicious anemia alter gastrin levels?

   - **Autoimmune destruction of parietal cells → ↓ acid → ↑ G cell production of gastrin**

7. What is the only essential function of the stomach?

   - **Intrinsic factor production**

8. A patient has a gastrectomy due to gastric cancer and the esophagus is directly sutured to the duodenum. The patient is prophylactically given high doses of vitamin B12 to prevent anemia. What other symptom is the patient likely to have?

   - **Gastrectomy → ↑ osmotic load in the small intestine → ↑ intraluminal H_2O → diarrhea**

   ↑ osmotic load → ↑ H_2O lumen → diarrhea

9. A 4 week old boy presents with nonbilious projectile vomiting. How will this disorder alter his electrolyte concentration?

   - **Pyloric stenosis → vomiting → loss of HCl → hypochloremic metabolic alkalosis**

   Pyloric stenosis

   HCl

   ↓H^+ → alkalosis

   ↓Cl → hypochloremia

10. How can H. pylori cause damage to the gastric mucosa?

    - **H. Pylori produces urease (converts urea → NH3 → NH4+ → gastric epithelial damage)**

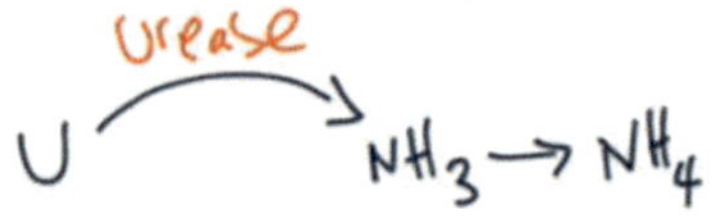

11. A patient is prescribed antibiotics for suspected strep throat. The patient also takes warfarin due to a history of blood clots. How will the warfarin dose likely need to be altered due to the new prescription of antibiotics?

    - **Warfarin inhibits epoxide reductase (converts oxidized vitamin K to reduced vitamin K) → ↓ function of coagulation factors → anticoagulation**
    - **Antibiotics → colonic bacteria death → ↓ vitamin K**
    - **Less warfarin is needed to have the same anticoagulative effect**

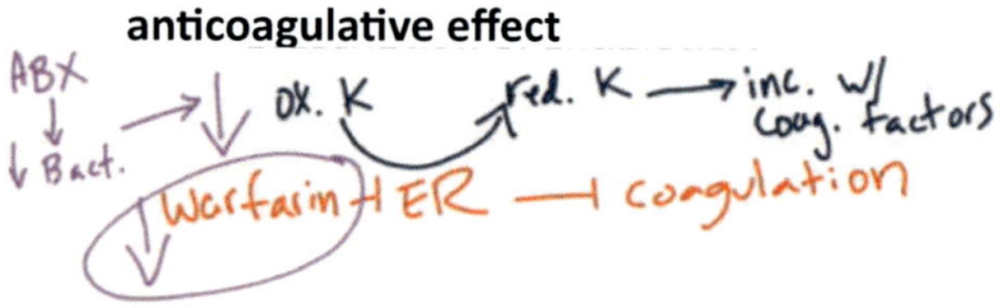

12. How can age increase the risk for developing diverticulitis?

    - **Age ↓ type III collagen (provides structural support to the colon) → ↑ rate of diverticula formation → ↑ risk of diverticulitis**

Section II - Exocrine Pancreas and Metabolism

I. Pancreas (Figure 5.6)

A. Endocrine pancreas

1. The endocrine pancreas secretes several hormones including insulin, glucagon, and somatostatin.

B. Exocrine pancreas

1. The exocrine pancreas secretes electrolytes and inactive enzymes called zymogens which become activated upon entering the duodenum.

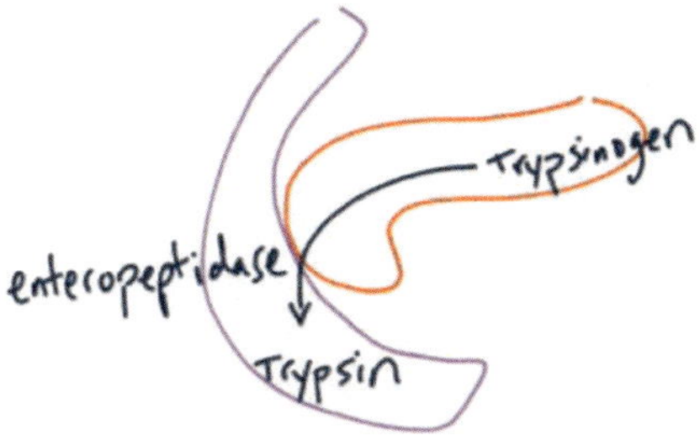

a) The pancreas also secretes colipase, a cofactor necessary for optimal activity of the enzyme lipase.

2. Pancreatic secretions are normally isotonic with the plasma (Na^+ & K^+ concentrations in pancreatic juice and the plasma are equal).

a) Pancreatic ductal cells exchange luminal chloride for intracellular bicarbonate, thereby increasing the amount of bicarbonate that reaches the duodenum.

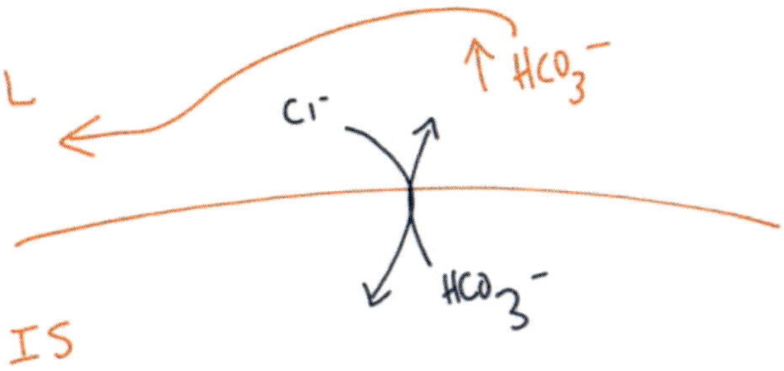

3. Pancreatic enzymes are involved in the digestion of fat, carbohydrates, and protein.

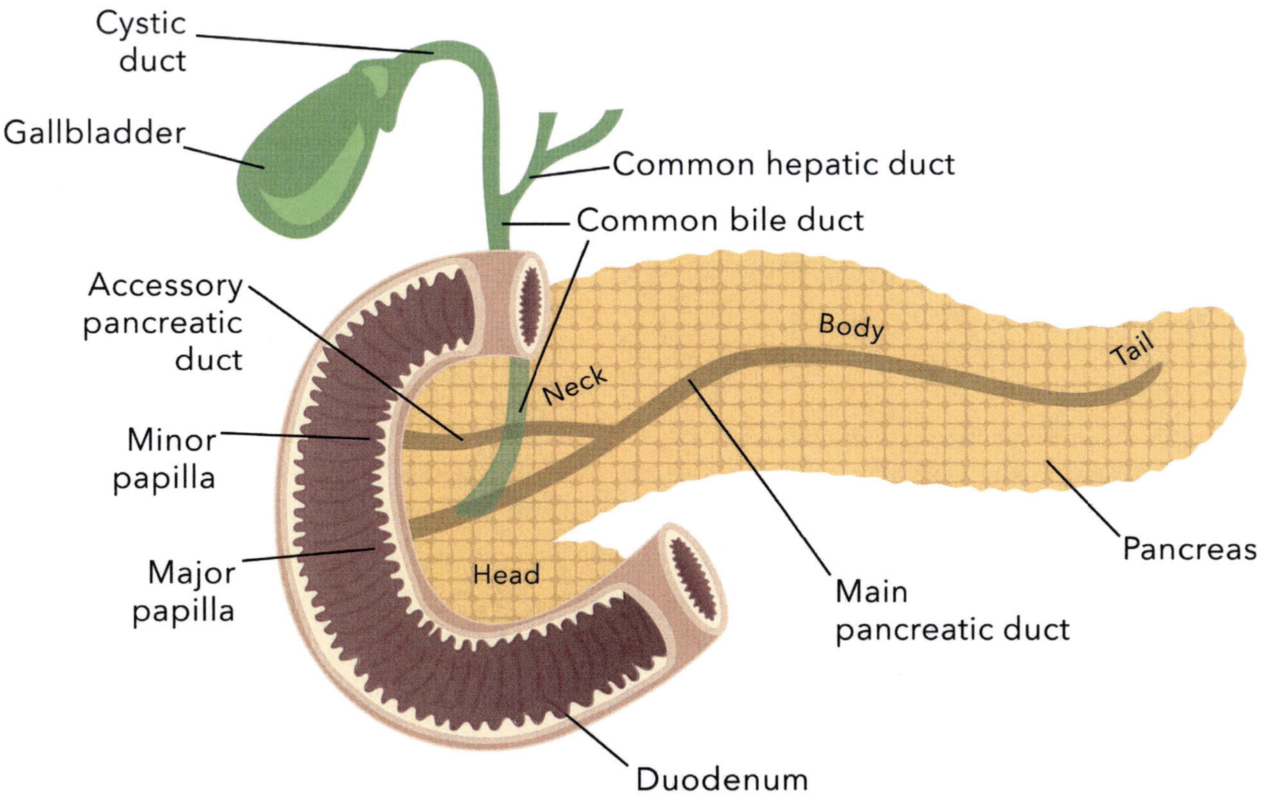

Figure 5.6 - The pancreas

II. Digestion and Absorption (Table 5.1)

Table 5.1 - Enzyme synthesis and functions

Active enzyme	Site of synthesis	Function
Trypsin	Pancreas	Proteolysis
Chymotrypsin	Pancreas	Proteolysis
Carboxypeptidase	Pancreas	Proteolysis
Elastase	Pancreas	Proteolysis
Pepsin	Stomach	Proteolysis
Brush border enzymes (enteropeptidase/ enterokinase, aminopeptidase, carboxypeptidase, etc.)	Brush border	Proteolysis
Lipase	Pancreas	Lipolysis
Amylase	Salivary glands & pancreas	Carbohydrate catabolism
Brush border enzymes (lactase, glucoamylase, sucrase, etc.)	Brush border	Carbohydrate catabolism

A. Lipids (Figure 5.7)

1. Large dietary lipids are primarily digested in the duodenum by pancreatic enzymes including cholesterol esterase, lipase, and phospholipase A2.
2. Bile salts assist with lipid metabolism by emulsifying the fatty acids and monoglycerides into micelles.
3. The micelles are further metabolized into fatty acids by pancreatic lipase.
4. The fatty acids can diffuse into the enterocytes where the fat is then packaged into chylomicrons.
5. The chylomicrons pass into the lacteals which then merge to form the larger lymphatic vessels.
6. Lipid absorption occurs primarily in the jejunum.

B. Carbohydrates (Figure 5.8)

1. Large carbohydrates are digested into smaller oligosaccharides via salivary and pancreatic amylase.
2. The intestinal brush border contains additional enzymes such as lactase, glucoamylase, and sucrase which digest the oligosaccharides into monomers (fructose, galactose, and glucose) which can the be absorbed by the enterocyte.
    a) Lactase is normally expressed in the small bowel and hydrolyzes lactose into glucose and galactose.
3. Carbohydrate monomers are absorbed by the enterocytes and then transferred into the blood.

C. Protein (Figure 5.9)

1. Protein metabolism begins in the stomach with pepsin.
2. Enteropeptidase (enterokinase) in the brush border is a protease that cleaves the inactive trypsinogen to trypsin.
3. Trypsin activates other inactive proteases which results in cleavage of dietary proteins into oligopeptides and amino acids.
4. Additional brush border proteases (aminopeptidase, carboxypeptidase, etc.) also facilitate the digestion of small peptides.

5. Amino acids enter the enterocyte by a sodium ion co-transporter.
6. Dipeptides and tripeptides enter the enterocyte by a hydrogen ion co-transporter.
7. Larger peptides may also enter the enterocyte via transcytosis.
8. Amino acids, peptides, and larger peptides are then transferred into the blood.

D. Micronutrients

1. Iron is absorbed in the duodenum as Fe^{2+}.
   a) In an alkaline environment iron is in the Fe^{3+} state.
   b) The acidic environment of the stomach maintains iron in the Fe^{2+} state and thus promotes iron absorption.
2. Copper
   a) Copper is normally absorbed in the stomach and duodenum and then transported into the blood.
   b) Once in the blood, copper binds to albumin and is transported to the liver where it is incorporated into other protein to form ceruloplasmin.
   c) Ceruloplasmin can be reabsorbed into the blood or secreted into the bile which then be excreted with stool.

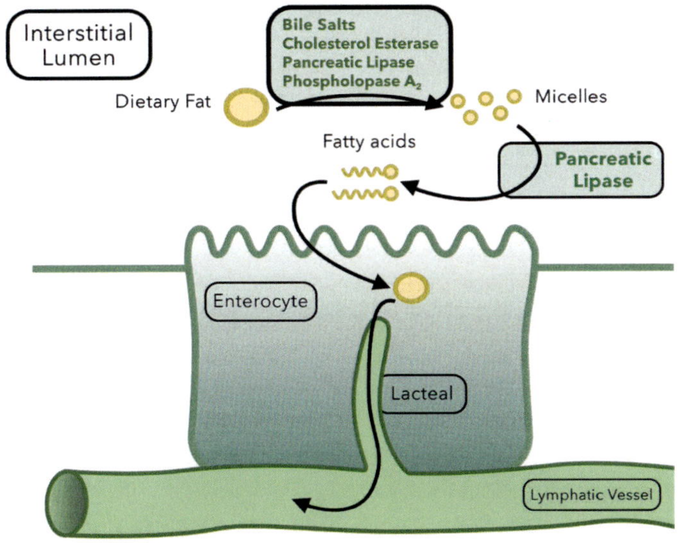

Figure 5.7 - Fat metabolism

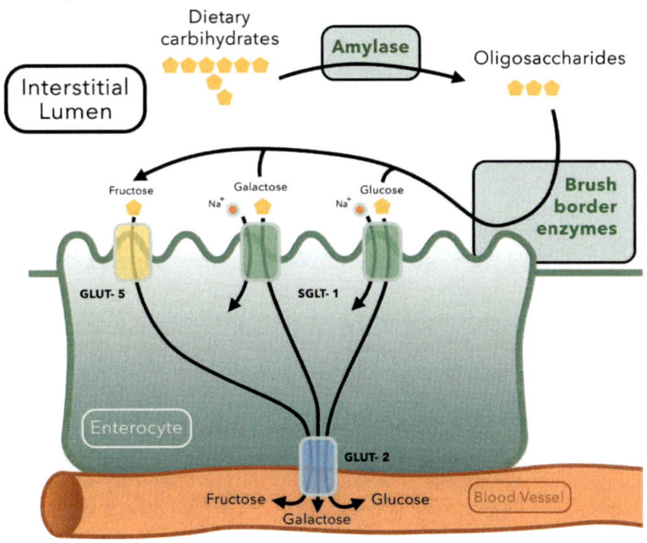

Figure 5.8 - Carbohydrate metabolism

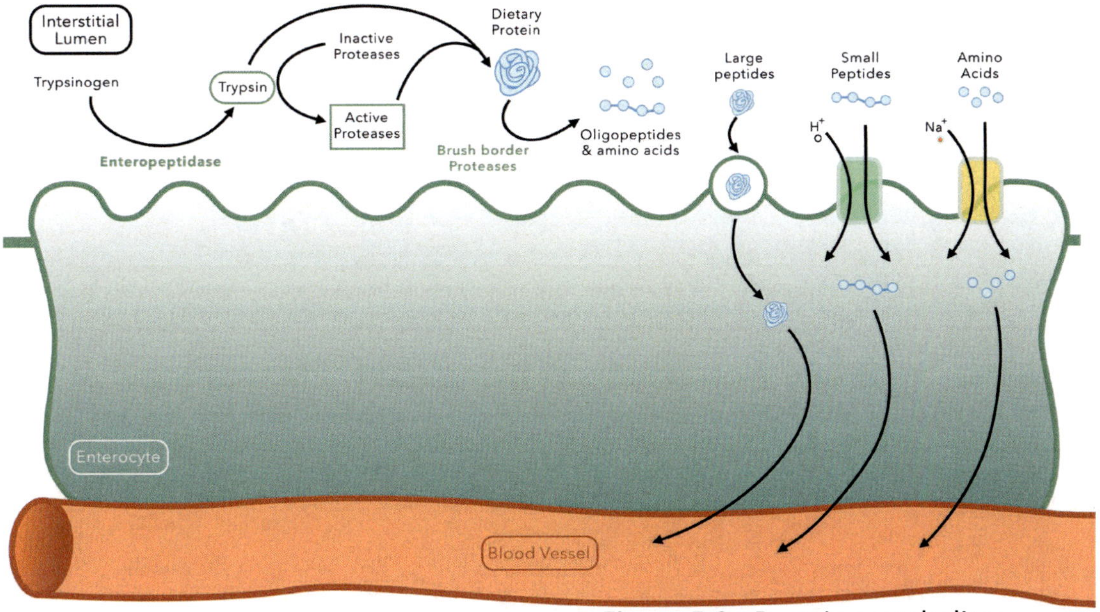

Figure 5.9 - Protein metabolism

REVIEW QUESTIONS

1. A 24-year-old female with a known past medical history of cystic fibrosis presents with abdominal pain and foul-smelling, greasy stools. What supplement would likely alleviate these symptoms?

    - **Pancreatic enzymes (i.e. lipase)**

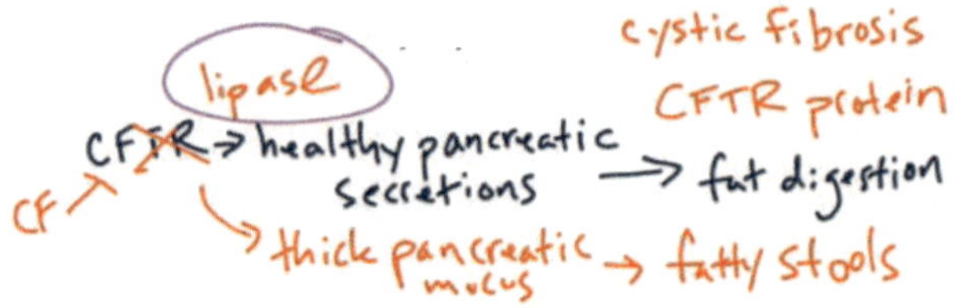

2. A 19-year-old female is in an automobile accident resulting in trauma to the abdomen. Labs show an elevated lipase and the physician suspects organ failure of the associated structure. How would the pH in the duodenum be altered as a result?

    - **↓ duodenal pH (pancreas cannot produce HCO3-)**

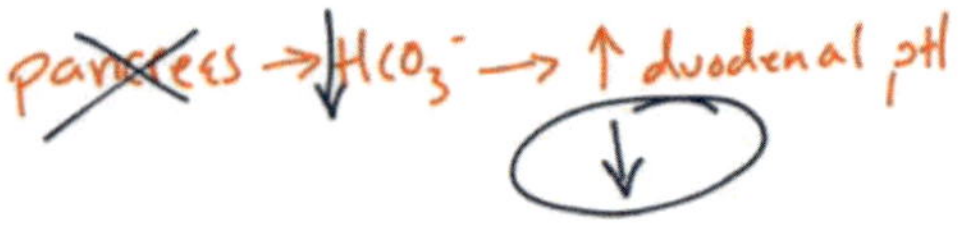

3. A 4-year-old boy presents with fatty stools. The physician suspects that the underlying cause of the patient's symptoms may be due to a defective coenzyme. What coenzyme does the physician likely have in mind?

    - **Colipase**
    - **The pancreas normally secretes colipase (a coenzyme necessary for optimal lipase function)**

4. A 4-year-old boy presents with night vision loss and swollen testicles. What is most likely responsible for the night vision loss?

    - **↓ vitamin A**
    - **Pancreatitis → pancreatic failure → ↓ ability of the body to absorb fat soluble vitamins**

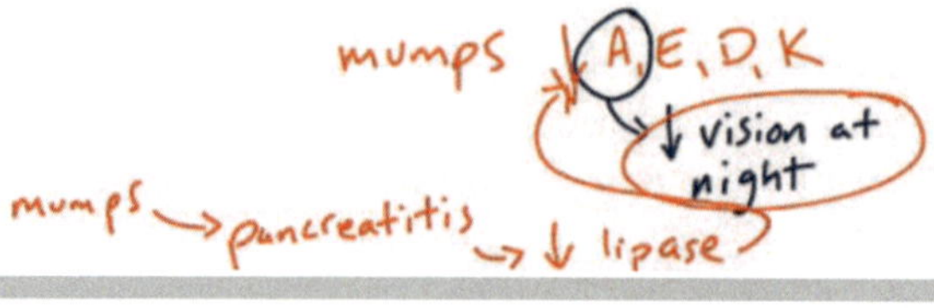

5. Where is the primary site for fat digestion? Absorption?

    - **Most fat digestion occurs in duodenum**
    - **Most fat absorption occurs in the jejunum**

6. What is a d-xylose test?

    - **Administered orally and measured in the urine**
    - **If mucosa is intact (even in the absence of digestive enzymes), D-xylose will be absorbed and found in the urine**
    - **If mucosa is damaged (e.g. celiac disease), D-xylose will not be fully absorbed in the intestines and minimal amount will appear in the urine**

7. A 47-year-old with type II diabetes and hypertriglyceridemia presents with epigastric pain. The physician suspects pancreatic involvement. What enzyme was most likely inappropriately activated resulting in the patient's epigastric pain?

    - **Trypsinogen**
    - **Hypertriglyceridemia → activation of trypsinogen → pancreatitis**

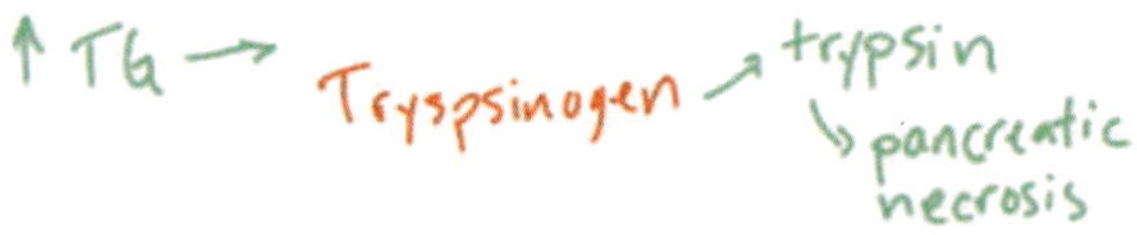

REVIEW QUESTIONS

8. A 32-year-old female presents with a 2 month history of bloody diarrhea. A colonoscopy is performed and a biopsy shows noncaseating granulomas. She is treated appropriately but 2 months later she returns with complaints of watery diarrhea that occurs after eating ice cream. How will the patient's hydrogen content in the breath compare to that of a healthy individual?

- **↑ breath hydrogen content**
- **This patient has Crohn's disease with secondary lactose intolerance (occurs due to damage to intestinal mucosa)**
- **Bacteria fermentation of undigested lactose → ↑ hydrogen**

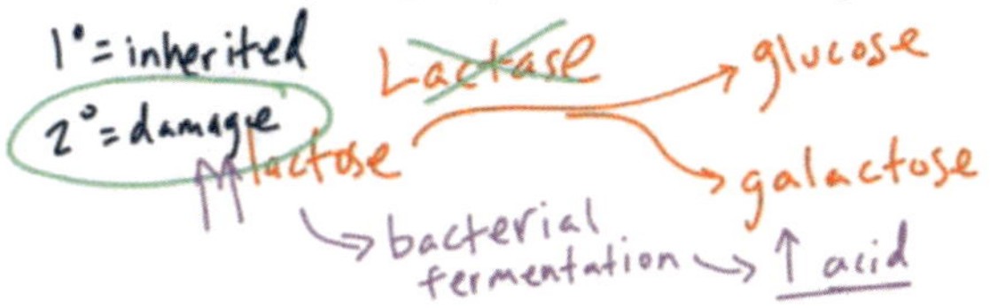

9. How would a gastrectomy alter iron absorption?

- **Gastrectomy → ↓ acid → ↓ Fe absorption**

10. Where is copper absorbed and excreted?

- **Absorbed: stomach and duodenum**
- **Excreted: duodenum (from the common bile duct)**

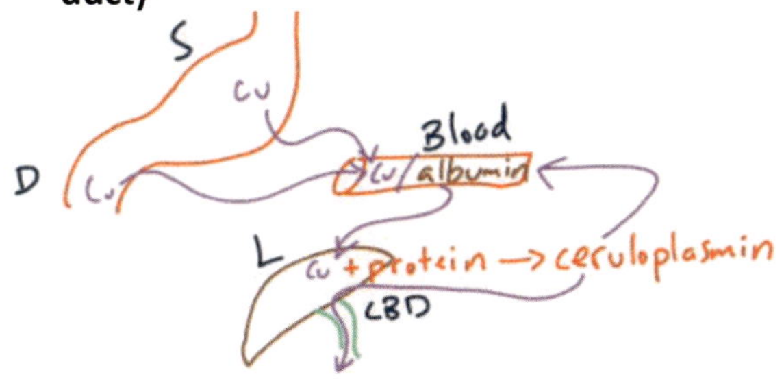

Section III - Liver and Bilirubin Metabolism

I. Anatomy Overview (Figure 5.10)

A. The hepatic artery proper, portal vein, and the common bile duct comprise the portal triad.

B. Branches of the portal triad surround liver lobules.

C. Arterial blood passes through zones I, II, and III of the lobule → exits through the central vein → returns venous blood to vena cava.

D. Substances absorbed from intestines enter the portal vein → travel through liver in the same manner as arterial blood.

E. Bile flows opposite of portal vein and arterial blood → exits liver through common bile duct.

II. Detoxification

A. Substances (drugs, toxins, etc) absorbed by digestive tract enter portal vein before entering into systemic circulation (first pass metabolism)

1. Ammonia (NH_3) is formed within intestines from nitrogenous substances (proteins) → sent to liver via portal vein → converted to urea → enters systemic circulation → excreted in urine.

a) Cirrhosis → excess ammonia → hepatic encephalopathy

Figure 5.10

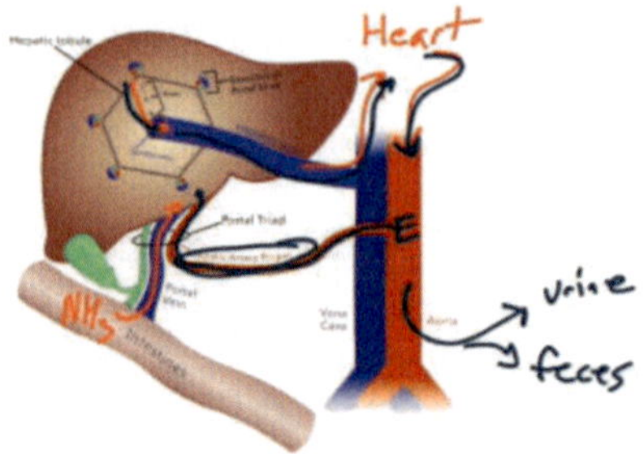

2. Estrogen is formed in tissues throughout body → sent to liver via hepatic artery proper → broken down into metabolites → excreted in urine, feces and bile.

a) Cirrhosis → excess estrogen

(1) Localized arteriole dilation → spider angiomas

(2) Gynecomastia

(3) Negative feedback on hypothalamus → decreased GnRH, FSH, and LH release → testicular atrophy (males) or amenorrhea (females)

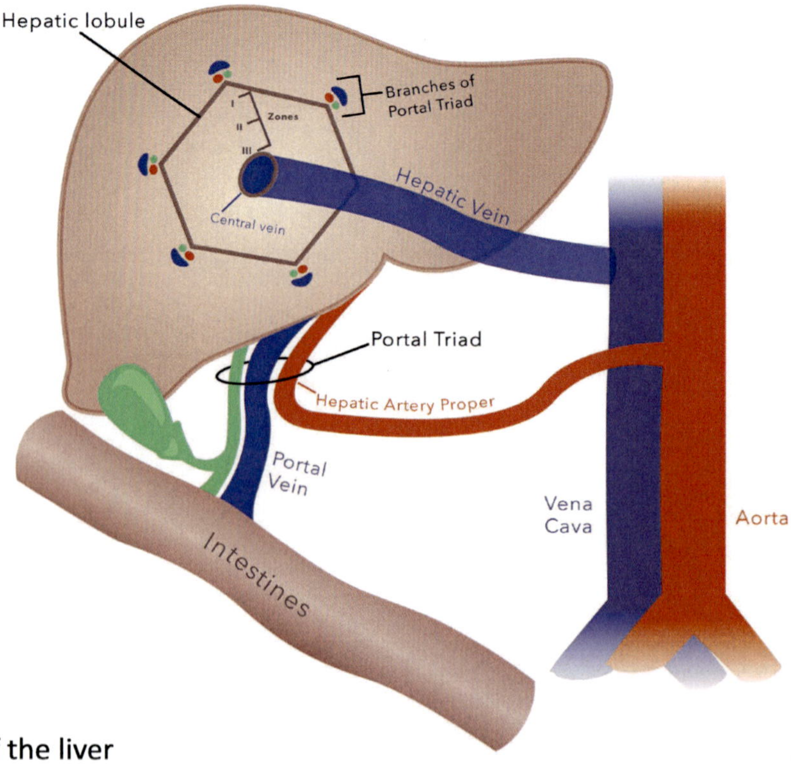

Figure 5.10 - Overview of the liver

III. Phase I and II Metabolism

A. Phase I metabolism occurs in zone III

1. Mediated primarily by cytochrome P-450 enzymes
2. Redox reactions and hydrolysis → creates slightly polar metabolites (and potentially metabolic toxins → zone III damage)

B. Phase II metabolism occurs in zone I

1. Mediated by transferases
2. Conjugation reactions → creates very polar metabolites → renal excretion

Figure 5.10

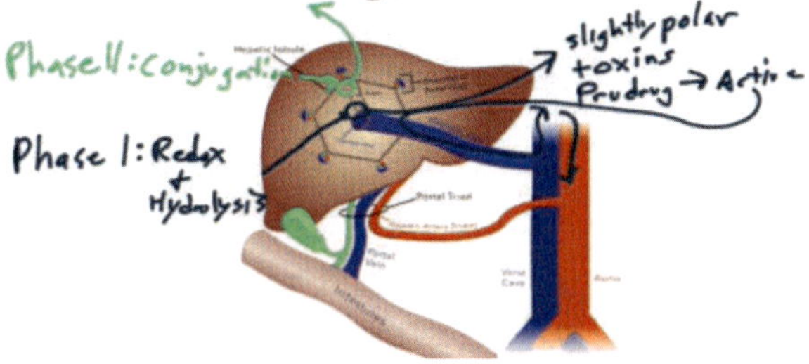

IV. Protein Production

Table 5.2 - Protein functions

Protein	Function
Carrier proteins	Albumin (fat soluble substances) Transferrin (iron) Ceruloplasmin (copper) Sex hormone-binding globulin (testosterone)
Hemostasis proteins	Procoagulation: Factors I-XII, fibrinogen and fibronectin Anticoagulation: Antithrombin III, proteins S and C
Immunity and inflammation	Complement proteins C1-C9 C-reactive protein Ferritin (sequesters iron from microbes)
Hormones	Insulin-like growth factor 1 (anabolic growth) Thrombopoietin (platelet production) Angiotensinogen (RAAS)

A. The liver is responsible for producing and releasing many important proteins, including hormones, carrier proteins, and other proteins involved in hemostasis.

B. Cirrhosis and loss of proteins

1. Loss of albumin → decreased oncotic pressure → edema
2. Loss of hemostasis proteins → coagulation disorders
3. Loss of thrombopoietin → thrombocytopenia

V. Carbohydrate Metabolism

A. Gluconeogenesis

B. Glycogen storage

C. Glycogenolysis → glucose released into bloodstream

VI. Lipid Metabolism

A. Production of cholesterol and lipoproteins

B. Cholesterol metabolism

1. HMG-CoA reductase is the rate limiting enzyme in cholesterol synthesis.
2. Normally converted into bile acid which can then be excreted in the bowels.

VII. Bilirubin Metabolism (Figure 5.11)

A. Macrophages break down RBCs → heme is broken down into iron and protoporphyrin → iron is recycled, protoporphyrin is converted to unconjugated bilirubin (UCB)

B. UCB is not water soluble and must be transported to the liver by albumin.

C. Uridine glucuronyl transferase (UGT) converts UCB to conjugated bilirubin (CB).

D. Conjugated bilirubin (CB)

1. CB in hepatocytes enter bile canaliculi → stored in gallbladder → released into duodenum with bile → intestinal flora break down CB into urobilinogen
2. Urobilinogen can:
    a) Remain in intestines → degraded to stercobilin and secreted in stool, making it brown
    b) Be reabsorbed by intestines → enter blood → converted to urobilin → portal vein → converted to CB (enterohepatic circulation) or filtered by kidney and excreted in urine, making it yellow

E. Additional notes on conjugated bilirubin and unconjugated bilirubin

1. UCB → CB → stercobilin enters feces, urobilin enters urine
2. CB failing to enter duodenum → clay-colored stool (loss of brownness of stercobilin)
3. CB can be filtered by kidney → dark urine in cases of excess CB
4. UCB cannot be filtered by the kidney → no dark urine in cases of excess UCB
5. UCB does not get excreted in feces → no clay-colored stool in cases of bile obstruction

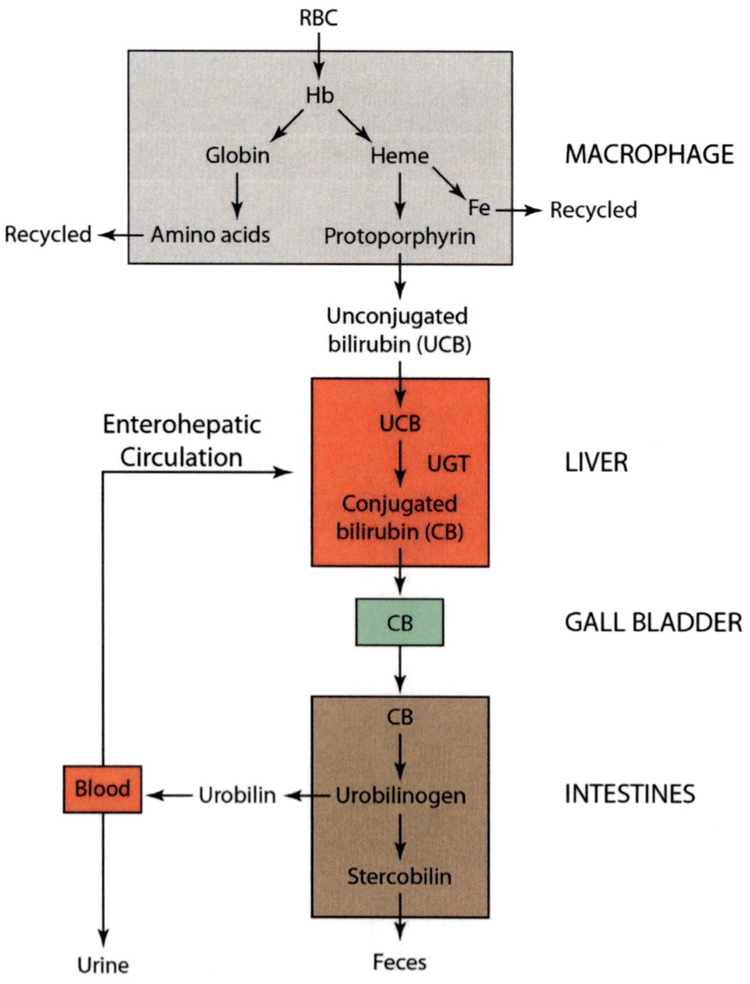

Figure 5.11 - Bilirubin metabolism pathway

REVIEW QUESTIONS

1. A male patient with known hepatic cirrhosis develops gynecomastia. Why?

Liver breaks down E + NH_3

2. A patient with chronic liver failure demonstrates purpura and petechiae. Why?

- **Chronic liver failure can cause decreased TPO, leading to decreased platelets.**
- **Note: recall that purpura are large and petechiae are small**

3. A patient with Wilson's Disease has low ceruloplasmin. How did the copper get to the liver?

- **Once absorbed by the small intestine, copper is bound to albumin and is transported to the liver via the portal vein**
- **Once in the liver, ceruloplasmin is created, which is how it is transported throughout the body**

copper carried by ceruloplasmin (from liver)

copper carried by albumin (from intestines to liver)

4. A statin drug inhibits an enzyme to decrease cholesterol synthesis. Where in the body does it directly act?

- **Statins inhibit HMG-CoA reductase which resides in liver hepatocytes**

5. A female patient with type II diabetes injects insulin. What would happen to glycogenolysis and gluconeogenesis?

- **The liver is responsible for glycogenolysis and gluconeogenesis**
- **Insulin acts to inhibit these actions of the liver, decreasing circulating blood sugar**

6. An infant is jaundiced at birth. Serum analysis shows elevated unconjugated bilirubin. Will the urine of the infant appear dark?

- **UCB is not water soluble and will not enter the urine to make it dark**
- **Note: Conjugated bilirubin (CB), if high, will enter the urine and make it dark**

Figure 5.11

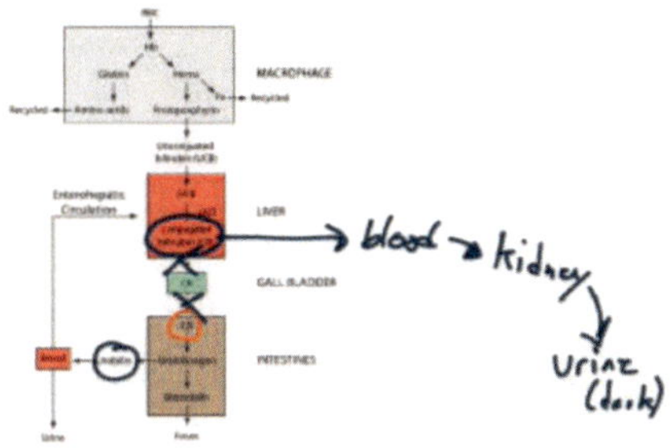

7. It is determined that this infant has normal physiological jaundice. Will this patient have clay-colored stool?

- **Unlike in Criglar-Nijaar in which UGT is completely dysfunctional, normal physiologic jaundice has some UGT function, causing the creation of some conjugated bilirubin (CB)**
- **The presence CB will allow the creation of stercobilin in the stool, making it brown**

Figure 5.11

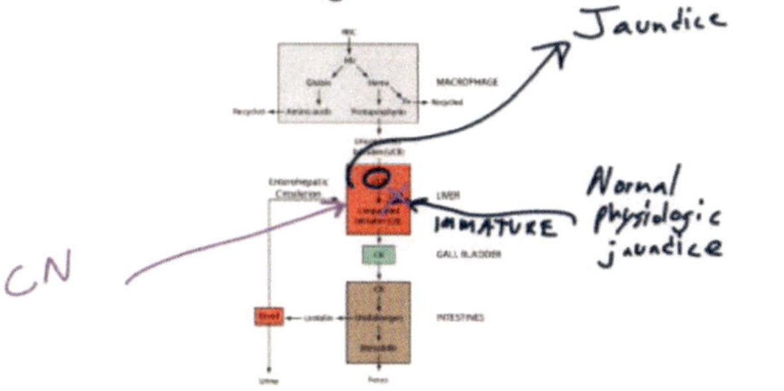

UCB
UGT
CB → Gallbladder → Intestines
brown ← Stercobilin

REVIEW QUESTIONS

8. A 60-year-old male with a history of alcoholism and pancreatitis presents with painless jaundice and epigastric pain. What is the most likely diagnosis?

- **If chronic pancreatitis suddenly presents with jaundice, suspect pancreatic mass compressing the common bile duct (obstructive jaundice)**
- **Obstructive jaundice prevents stercobilin in the stool, leading to clay-colored stools**

Chronic pancreatitis → Jaundice (compression of CBD)
↗ Pancreatic cancer

Figure 5.10

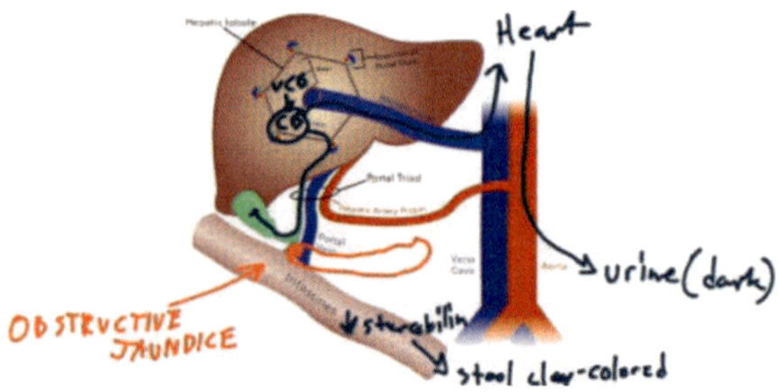

Section IV - Gallbladder

I. Anatomy Overview

A. Right and left hepatic ducts combine to form common hepatic duct

B. Cystic duct exits the gallbladder and combines with the hepatic duct to form the common bile duct.

C. Common bile duct places bile into the duodenum via the ampulla of Vater.

II. Bile Composition

A. Emulsifies fat → improved breakdown and absorption of fats

B. Composed of:

1. Bile salts (deoxycholic acid and lithocholic acid) → addition of glycine and taurine → bile acids
2. Cholesterol
3. Phospholipids
4. Bilirubin (CB)
5. Electrolytes
6. H_2O

III. Gallstone Overview

Figure 5.10

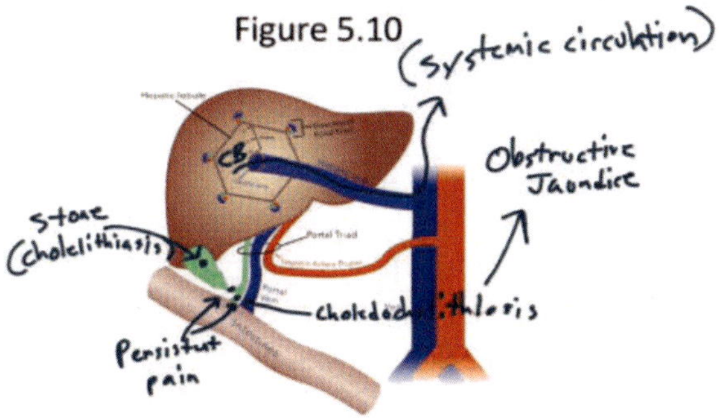

A. Caused by components of bile precipitating out

B. Cholesterol → cholesterol stones (radiolucent from low calcium)

1. Estrogen upregulates HMG-CoA Reductase → increased cholesterol
2. Estrogen, hypercholesterolemia, loss of bile acids (e.g. Crohn's disease), stasis (e.g. parenteral nutrition)

C. Bilirubin (CB) → black stones (radiopaque from high calcium)

1. Although bile is mostly CB, what precipitates with calcium is UCB.
2. Extravascular hemolysis or biliary infection

IV. Gallstone Symptoms

A. RUQ pain is caused by stone being lodged in cystic duct or common bile duct (choledocholithiasis)

B. Pain subsides within hours → gallstone has moved back into gallbladder → biliary colic

C. Persistent pain → gallstone is stuck

D. Jaundice → gallstone is lodged in common bile duct → cessation of bile outflow → conjugated bilirubin spills into bloodstream (obstructive jaundice)

V. Hepatobiliary (HIDA) Scan

A. Radioactive tracer injected into venous system (arm) → travels to liver and biliary system → hepatobiliary system visualized

B. Gallbladder not visualized → acute cholecystitis

C. Common bile duct not visualized → choledocholithiasis

VI. Bile Acid Recycling

A. Bile is released into duodenum via ampulla of Vater → bile emulsifies fat to aid in digestion.

B. Some bile is excreted in the feces.

1. Excretion of cholesterol
2. Conjugated bilirubin causes feces to be brown

C. Bile acids are reabsorbed in the terminal ileum → portal vein → liver hepatocytes for recycling into bile

D. Failure to recycle bile acids → gallstones (mostly cholesterol)

REVIEW QUESTIONS

1. A pregnant woman develops gallstones. She reports that she has never had gallstones before. Why might she be getting gallstones for the first time while she is pregnant?

   - **Pregnancy increases estrogen, which upregulates HMG-CoA Reductase**
   - **Increased cholesterol increases precipitation of cholesterol gallstones**

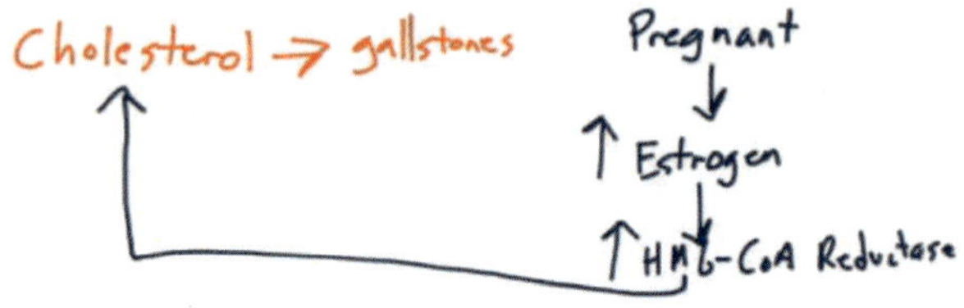

2. A 32-year-old female presents with abdominal pain in the right upper quadrant after eating fried chicken. The pain persists through the next day when she shows signs of jaundice. Where must the gallstone be lodged?

   - **Persistent pain indicates stone is in the cystic duct (no jaundice) or the common bile duct (jaundice)**

Figure 5.10

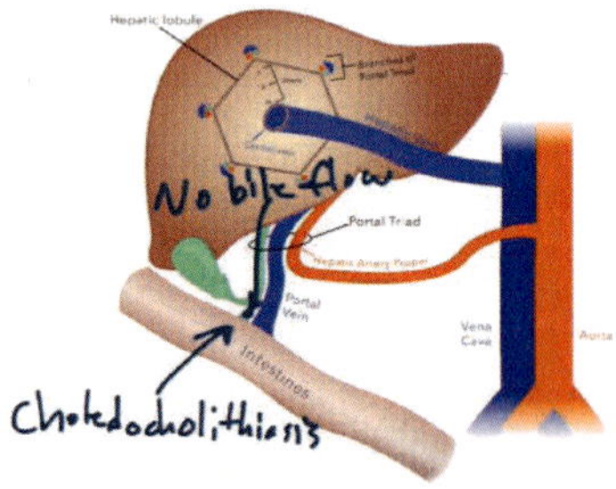

3. In a certain patient, the enteroendocrine cells responsible for releasing CCK are dysfunctional. What impact would decreased CCK have on the hepatobiliary system?

   - **Decreased CCK causes decreased gallbladder contraction**
   - **With decreased contraction, there will be stasis of bile, leading to precipitation of gallstones**

4. A 32-year-old female patient has persistent abdominal pain in the RUQ and vomiting for the last 2 days. Her current temperature is 103 F. A HIDA scan is performed and the gallbladder is not visualized but the common bile duct is. What is the likely pathology?

   - **Lack of visualization of gallbladder following a HIDA scan is pathognomonic for acute cholecystitis**

5. A patient with Crohn's disease frequently develops gallstones. Why?

   - **Bile acids are normally reabsorbed in the terminal ileum**
   - **In Crohn's disease, the terminal ileum is often involved/dysfunctional, leading to decreased bile acid reuptake**
   - **HIgh cholesterol to bile acid ratio leads to the precipitation of gallstones**

Section V - GI Hormones

I. Cholecystokinin (CCK) (Figure 5.12)

A. Produced by I cells in duodenum

B. Stimulated by fats and lipids

C. Aids in fat digestion

1. Gallbladder contraction and sphincter Oddi relaxation → release of bile → emulsification of fat

2. Pancreatic secretions → pancreatic enzymes → breakdown of fat

Figure 5.12

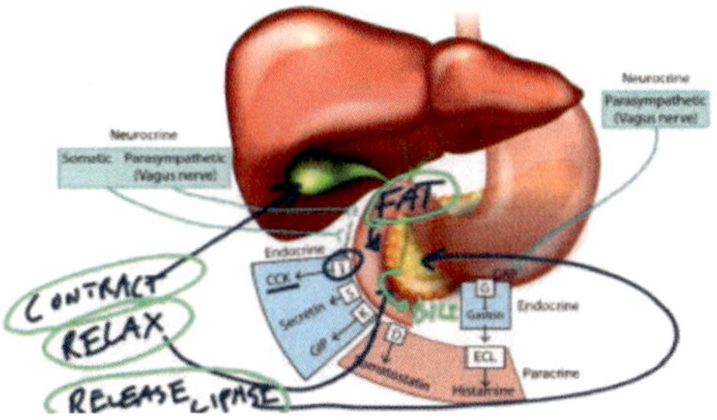

D. Decreased gastric emptying (increased satiety)

E. Cholecystokinin (CCK) is released from duodenal I cells in response to fat entering the duodenum.

II. Secretin

A. Produced by S cells in duodenum

B. Stimulated by acid and fat

C. Functions to decrease acidity → improved function of pancreatic enzymes

1. Stimulates Cl^-/HCO_3^- antiporter in pancreas → increased HCO_3^- in intestinal lumen → increased luminal pH

2. Decreased gastrin secretion from stomach and duodenum → decreased H^+ release → increased luminal pH

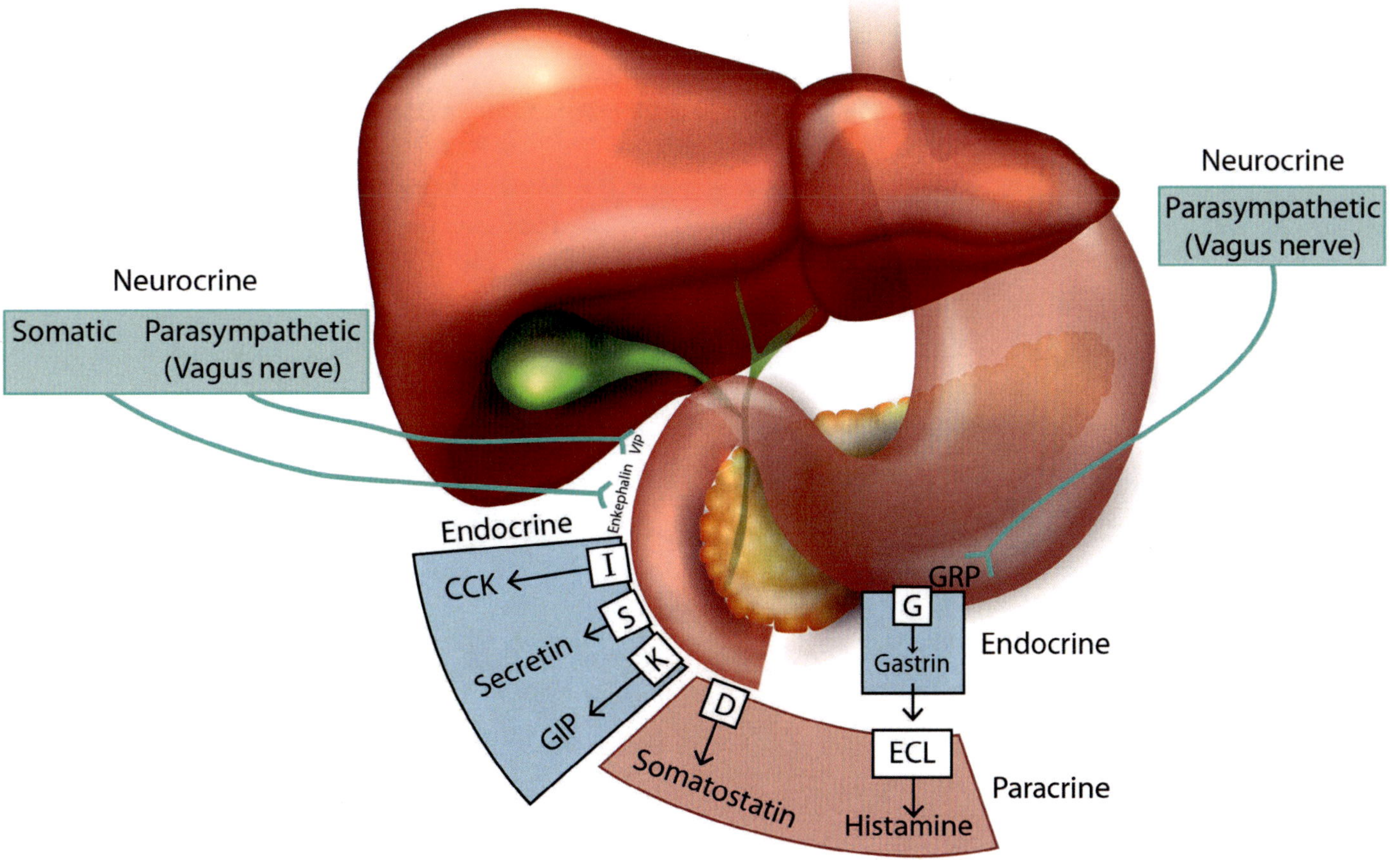

Figure 5.12 - GI Hormones

3. Increased bile production → increased fat digestion

Figure 5.12

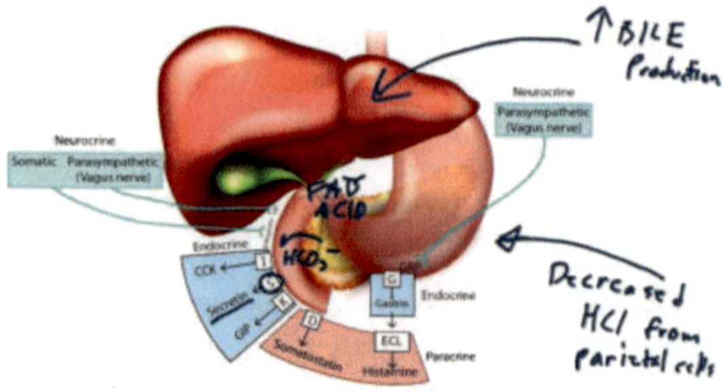

III. Glucose-dependent Insulinotropic Peptide (GIP)

A. Produced by K cells of duodenum and jejunum

B. Stimulated by fatty acids, amino acids, and oral glucose

Figure 5.12

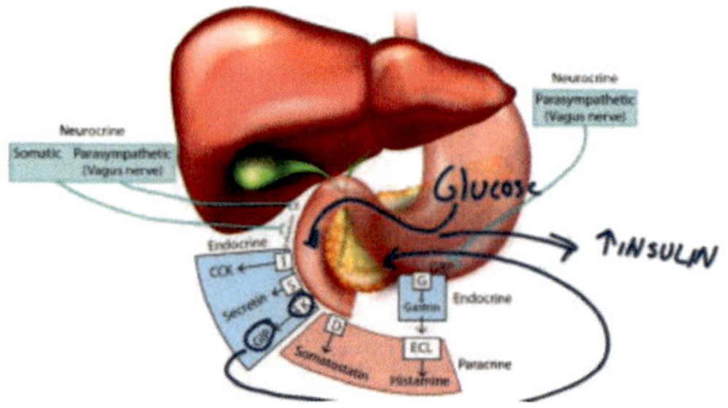

C. Aids digestion of fats and amino acids and absorption of glucose

1. Stimulates release of insulin from pancreas → increased absorption of glucose

2. Decreases H^+ secretion → improved function of pancreatic enzymes

Figure 5.12

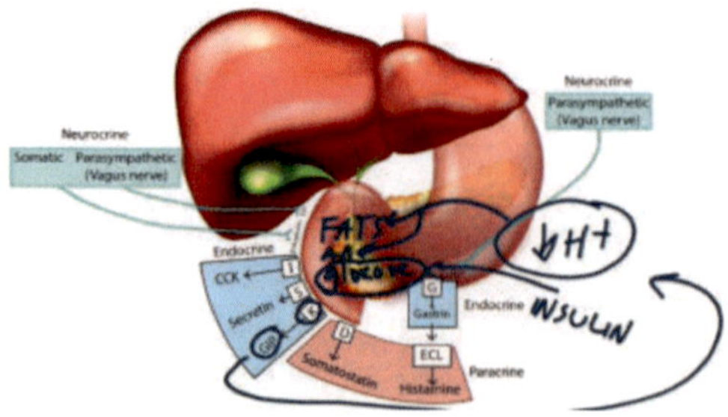

IV. Motilin

A. Released from small intestine

B. Increased while fasting

C. Functions to clear small intestines in preparation for next meal

1. Motilin = movement

2. Responsible for migrating motor complexes (MMCs)

V. Vasoactive Intestinal Peptide (VIP)

A. Released from parasympathetic ganglia (parasympathetic stimulus)

B. Functions to increase fluid and flow in intestines

1. Relaxes intestinal smooth muscle → increased electrolytes (e.g. K^+, Cl^-, and Na^+) and H_2O enter lumen

2. Relaxes sphincter of Oddi (assists CCK) → increased bile flow

C. VIPoma: Over-secretion of VIP → WDHA syndrome

Figure 5.12

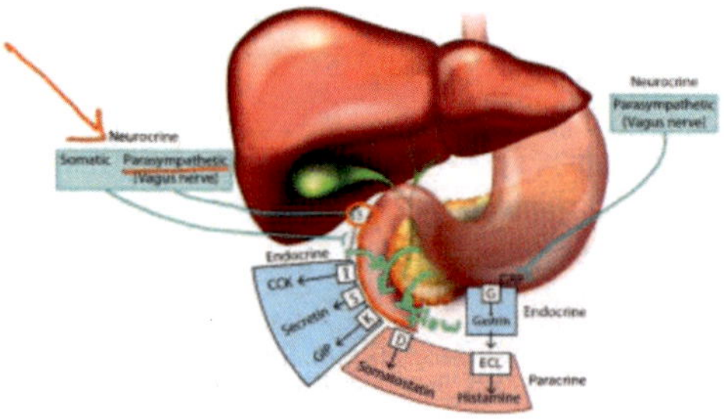

VI. Enkephalins

A. Released from neurons throughout GI tract

B. Cause constriction of smooth muscle → decreased fluid flow into intestines

C. Opiates act on enkephalin receptors → decreased fluid flow → constipation

Figure 5.12

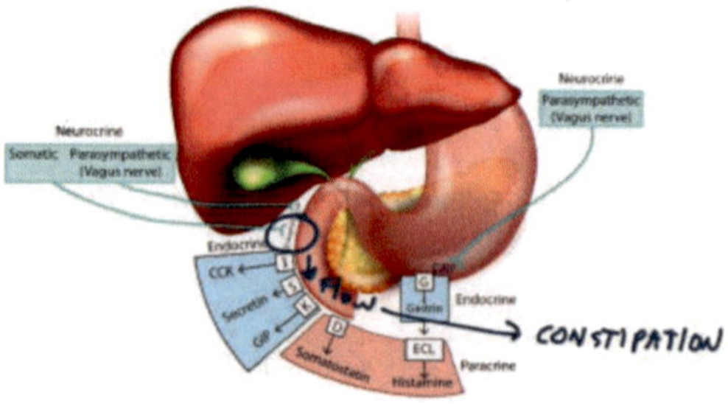

VII. Somatostatin

A. Produced by D cells (GI mucosa)

B. Stimulated by low pH

C. Inhibited by vagal stimulation (parasympathetic)

D. Inhibits release of all GI hormones and pancreatic secretions → maintains hormone balance

1. Secretin from S cells → decreased HCO_3^- from pancreas
2. Stomach hormones → decreased acid production
3. Pancreatic secretions → decreased insulin, glucagon, enzymes, HCO_3^-
4. CCK from I cells → decreased gallbladder contraction
5. GIP from K cells → decreased insulin
6. Motilin and VIP → decreased fluid and peristalsis

REVIEW QUESTIONS ?

1. A patient presents with RUQ pain after eating a meal. Ultrasound demonstrates the presence of a gallstone. The clinician deduces that the patient's pain must be caused by gallbladder contraction against the stone. What is the pathway leading to contraction of the gallbladder?

   - **Fat stimulates I cells in the duodenum to release CCK, causing gallbladder contraction**

   Fat enters duodenum → I cells → CCK ↓ contraction

2. A patient has a tumor that causes the production of excess H^+ within the stomach. What hormone will be released to counteract the acidity of the chyme? Where is it released from?

   - **Low pH stimulates S cells to release secretin (increased HCO3- from pancreas and decreased H^+ via decreased gastrin)**

   ↓ pH (high acidity) → S cell → secretin ↓ $\uparrow HCO_3^-$ $\downarrow H^+$

3. This patient has Zollinger-Ellison syndrome. What will be the serum secretin levels in this patient relative to a patient without a gastrinoma like this?

   - **Secretin is normally secreted in response to high acid (low pH)**
   - **With high levels of gastrin and acid, secretin levels will be high**

4. What is the chloride concentration in this patient's pancreatic exocrine glands, relative to normal?

   - **Secretin will stimulate the pancreas to release HCO3- in exchange for Cl^-, increasing pancreatic Cl^- levels**

   $\uparrow H^+$ → ↑ secretin → $\uparrow HCO_3^-$

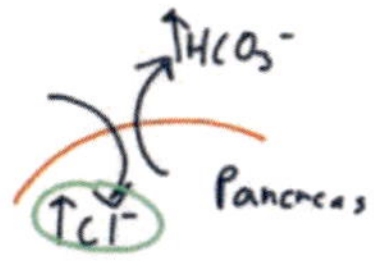

REVIEW QUESTIONS

5. A male comatose patient is receiving total parenteral nutrition (TPN). Following a feeding, his insulin levels are lower than would be expected from someone who ingested the same nutrients orally. Why would insulin be lower?

   - **Normally, fats, amino acids and glucose are ingested orally and can stimulate GIP release from the K cells**
   - **In TPN, there is decreased release of GIP, decreasing insulin release**

   Nutrients → Blood (glucose) → INSULIN
   → Oral FATS AA glucose → GIP

6. A patient is administered octreotide, a somatostatin analog to treat her variceal bleeding. At a later visit to a different clinician, several gallstones are noted incidentally on ultrasound of the patient. The patient does not note any recent RUQ pain. How might octreotide have caused these gallstones?

   - **Octreotide is a somatostatin analog and inhibits most GI hormones**
   - **High somatostatin leads to decreased CCK and gallbladder contraction, leading to bile stasis and cholesterol stones**

   ↑ somatostatin
   ↓ CCK → ↓ gallbladder contraction (↑ stasis → cholesterol stones)

7. A male patient has had chronic diarrhea for 3 months secondary to a VIP-releasing tumor. What natural hormone would normally counteract VIP?

   - **Somatostatin normally counteracts VIP**

8. A female patient eats a heavy steak with a sugary drink. What hormones would be released as a result of the fat content of her meal?

   - **Recall "Fat is SIK" (secretin, CCK, and GIP)**

   Fat is SIK → Secretin, CCK, GIP

9. What is the combined effect of Secretin, CCK, and GIP?

   - **Breakdown of fats (secretin and CCK)**
   - **Absorb glucose (GIP)**
   - **Decrease acidity (secretin and GIP)**

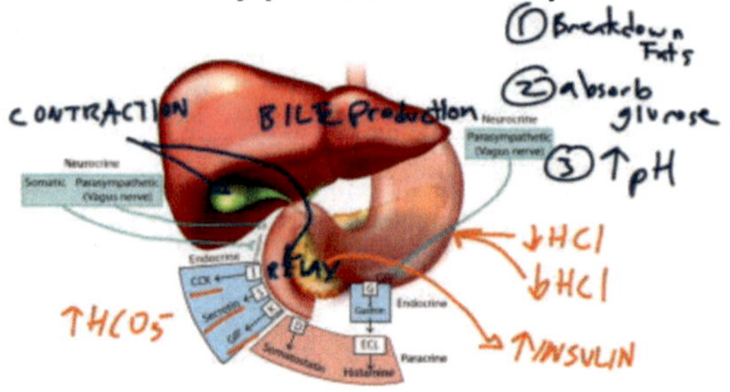

Section VI - Satiety and Hunger

I. Ghrelin

A. Released by gastric cells when the stomach is empty

B. Inhibited by stretching of stomach when food enters

C. Acts on the lateral nucleus of the hypothalamus → stimulates sensation of hunger

II. Leptin

A. Released by adipocytes continually

1. More adipocytes → more leptin secretion

B. Acts on ventromedial nucleus of the hypothalamus → stimulates satiety

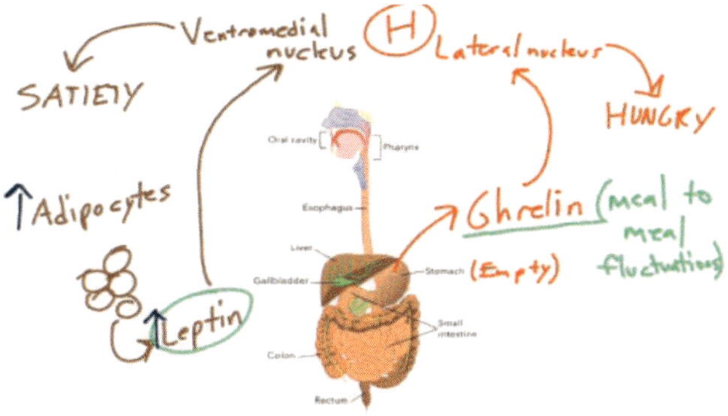

REVIEW QUESTIONS

1. A female patient eats a meal. What would happen to the level of ghrelin after her meal, compared to before?

- **An empty stomach stimulates release of ghrelin, so after eating a meal (full stomach), ghrelin levels will be lower**

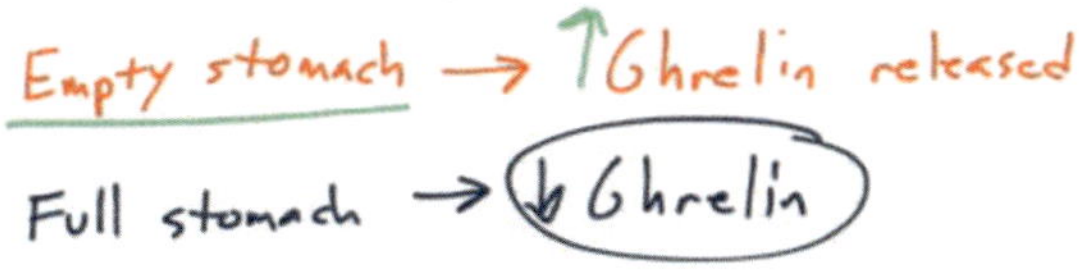

2. Referring to the same patient, what were the levels of motilin right before her meal?

- **Right before a meal (fasting), motilin will be high (growling) and ghrelin will be high (sense of hunger)**

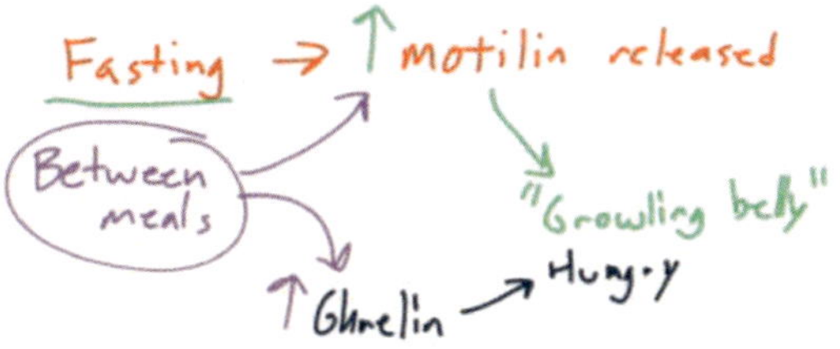

3. An obese male patient is presumed to have insensitive leptin receptors. What would be a natural and visible consequence of this defect?

- **The ventromedial nucleus houses the leptin receptors. Without these receptors, sense of satiety will be dysfunctional, leading to overeating and obesity**

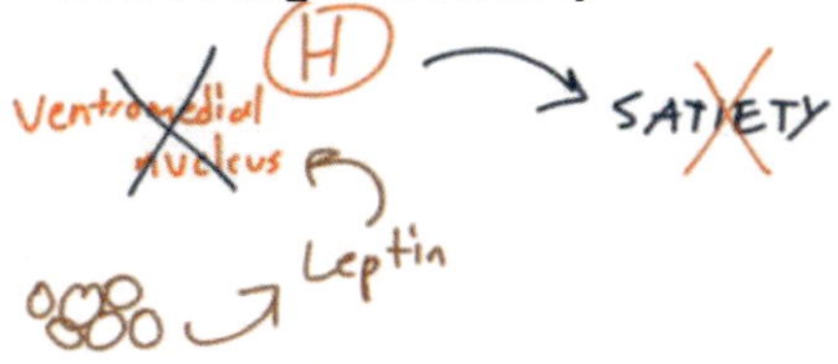

4. It was discovered that the same obese patient had fully functional leptin receptors. It was discovered that he had deficient leptin production from adipocytes. If leptin were to be administered pharmacologically, what would be a visible result?

- **The functional receptors in the ventromedial nucleus would sense the leptin, leading to a sense of satiety and weight loss**

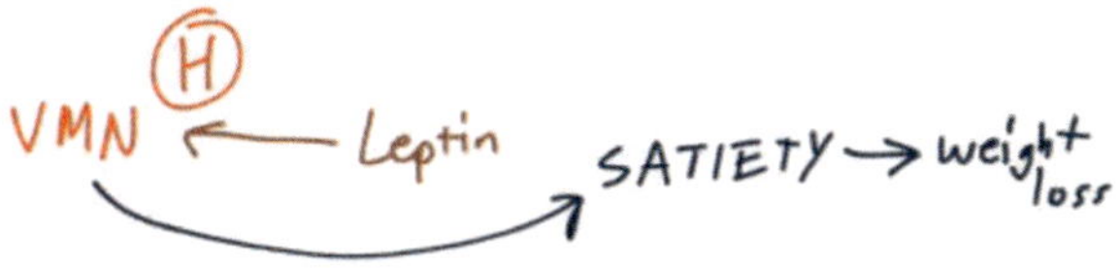

ENDOCRINOLOGY

Section I - Introduction to Endocrinology

I. Basic Principles

A. The endocrine system consists of glands that work together to maintain homeostasis.

1. A hormone is a molecule that is released from a gland into the bloodstream and modulates an aspect of physiology, typically at a distant location.
2. Figure 6.1 provides an overview of the basic anatomy.
3. Table 6.1 lists the major structures and functions of the endocrine system.

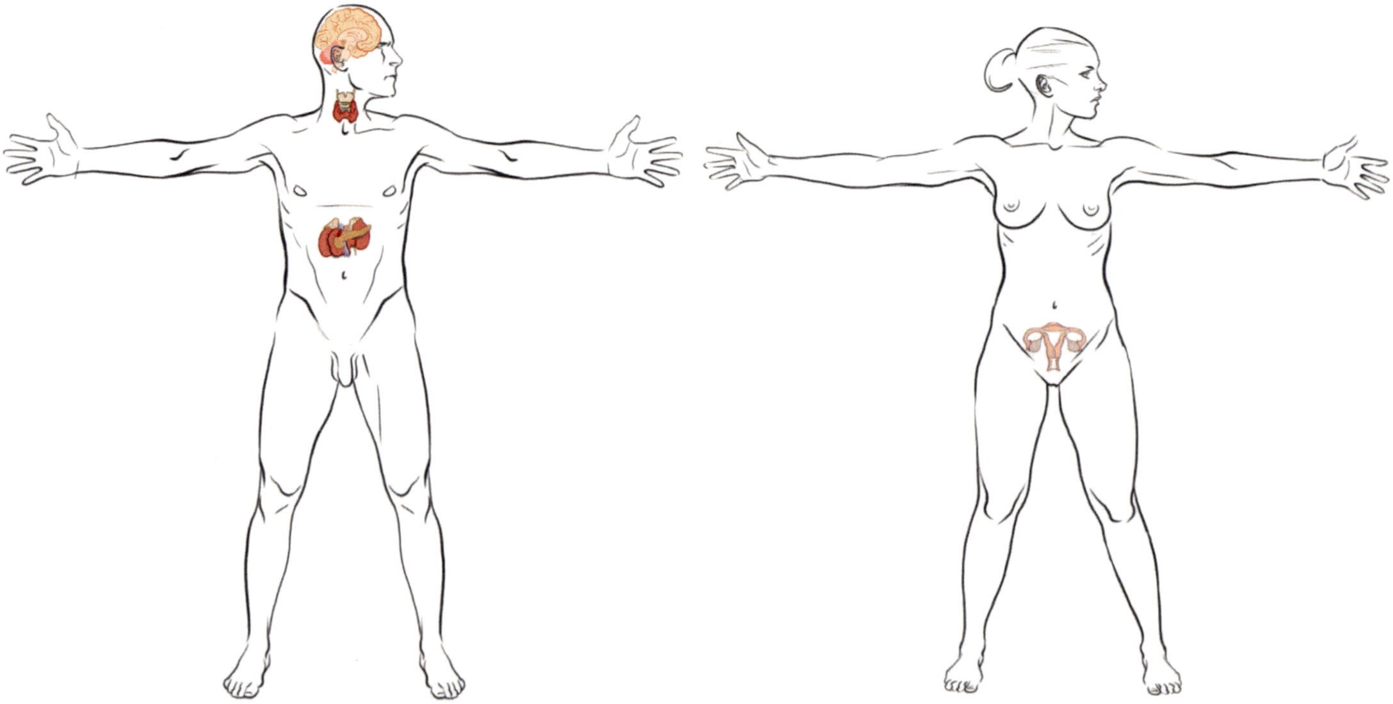

Figure 6.1 - Anatomy of the Endocrine System

Table 6.1 - Endocrine Structures and Functions

GLAND	FUNCTION
Hypothalamus	Control Center
Pituitary Gland	Control Center
Parathyroid Gland	Calcium and Bone
Skin	Calcium and Vitamin D
Thyroid Gland	Metabolism
Heart	Sodium
Adrenal Gland	Blood Pressure and Blood Volume Sexual Function (zona fasciculata) Sympathetic response (zona reticularis)
Kidneys	Blood Volume (RAAS)
Pancreas	Blood Glucose
Gonads	Sexual Function
Adipose Tissue	Appetite

II. Hypothalamic-Pituitary Axis

A. The Hypothalamus is a region in the forebrain that is responsible for regulating hormone concentrations.

1. Table 6.2 lists the hormones of the hypothalamic-pituitary axis.

Table 6.2 - Hypothalamic Hormones and Actions

Hypothalamic Hormones	Abbreviation	Major Action
Corticotropin-releasing hormone	CRH	Stimulates ACTH release
Dopamine (prolactin-inhibiting factor)	PIF	Inhibits prolactin release
Growth hormone-releasing hormone	GHRH	Stimulates GH release
Gonadotropin-releasing hormone	GnRH	Stimulates FSH and LH release
Somatostatin (somatotropin release-inhibiting hormone)	SRIF	Inhibits GH release
Thyrotropin-releasing hormone	TRH	Stimulates TSH release Stimulates prolactin (PRL) release
Antidiuretic hormone (vasopressin)	ADH	Stimulates water reabsorption at the kidneys and vasoconstriction of arterioles
Oxytocin		Stimulates milk let-down and uterine contraction

2. Most hormones made in the hypothalamus travel down the hypophyseal portal system of veins to exert their action on the anterior pituitary (adenohypophysis).
3. Oxytocin and ADH are produced in the hypothalamus and packaged into vesicles that are transported along axons to the posterior pituitary (neurohypophysis). The vesicles contain neurophysin proteins which help stabilize oxytocin and ADH.

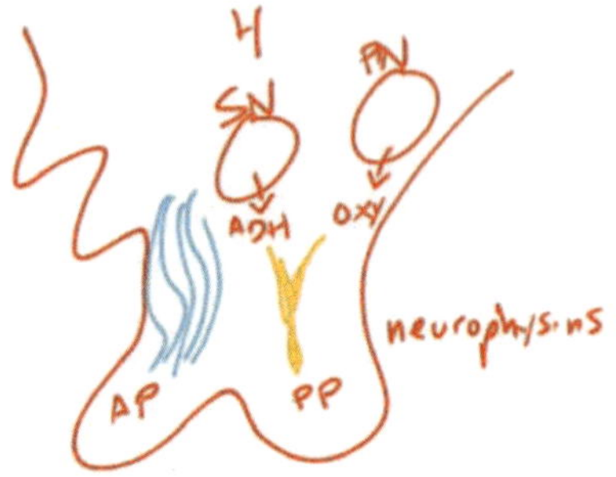

4. Drugs that act on the hypothalamus can cause an increase in ADH secretion, leading to syndrome of inappropriate antidiuretic hormone (SIADH).
5. The final hormone in the pathway of the HP axis inhibits the additional release of hormones from the hypothalamus and pituitary, a term called negative feedback.
   a) Iatrogenic use of hormones or drugs can disrupt the HP axis.

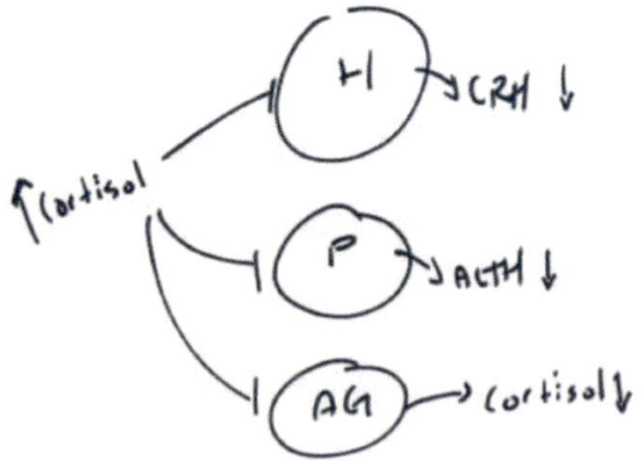

   b) Disease processes can disrupt the HP axis.

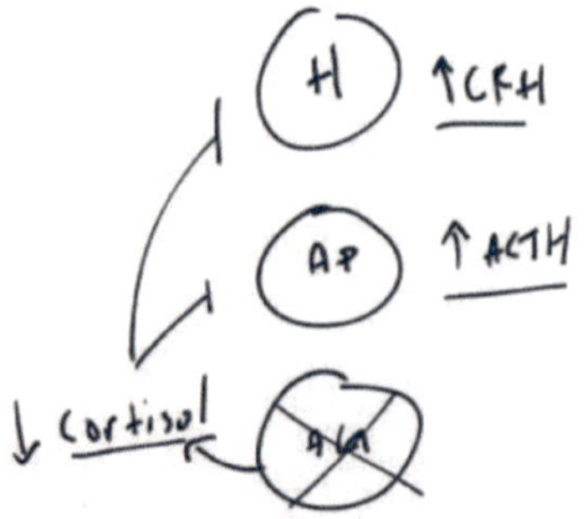

REVIEW QUESTIONS

1. What are commonly tested drugs that can cause syndrome of inappropriate antidiuretic hormone (SIADH)?
   - **SSRIs**
   - **Carbamazepine**
2. How would the hypothalamic pituitary axis be altered in a patient with rheumatoid arthritis who has a history of chronic steroid use?
   - **Exogenous cortisol would inhibit the hypothalamic pituitary axis**
   - **Endogenous CRH, ACTH, and cortisol would be decreased**
3. Why should a surgeon be cautious when operating on a patient taking exogenous cortisol?
   - **Exogenous cortisol causes atrophy of the adrenal cortex**
   - **The ability of the adrenal cortex to release cortisol during stress is diminished**
   - **Cortisol regulates blood pressure through alpha-1 receptors**
   - **During surgery the patient could become hypotensive**
4. How would Addison's disease alter the hypothalamic pituitary axis?
   - **↓ cortisol → ↑ CRH and ACTH**

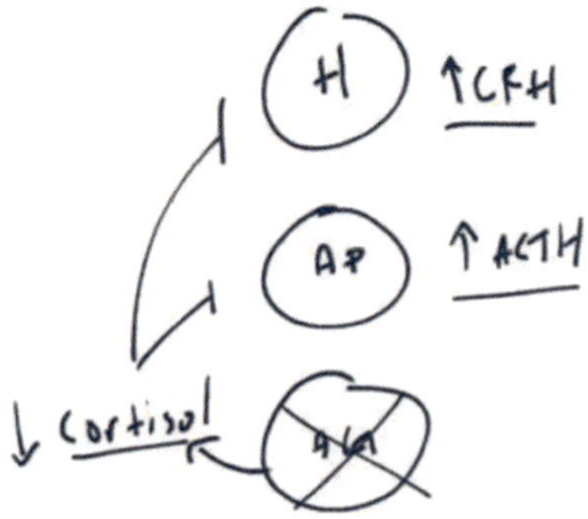

Section II - The Pituitary Gland

I. Anterior Pituitary (Adenohypophysis)

A. Table 6.3 lists the hormones produced from the anterior pituitary and their major actions.

Table 6.3 - Pituitary Hormones and Major Actions

Pituitary Hormones	Abbreviation	Major Action
Adrenocorticotropic hormone	ACTH	Production and release of the adrenal cortical hormones
Thyroid stimulating hormone	TSH	Production and release of T3/T4
Follicle stimulating hormone	FSH	Estrogen release and sperm maturation
Luteinizing hormone	LH	Androgen synthesis and ovulation
Growth hormone	GH	Protein synthesis and cell growth
Prolactin		Breast maturation and milk production
Melanocyte stimulating hormone	MSH	Production and release of melanin

B. FSH

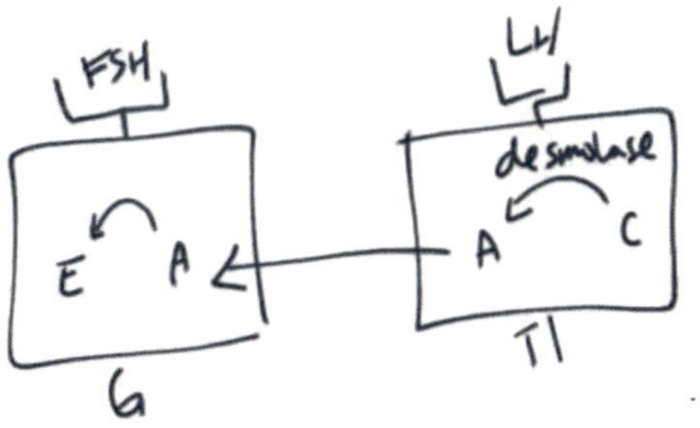

1. Acts on the sertoli cells in males to regulate sperm production. Sertoli cells release inhibin B which inhibits additional release of LH and FSH.
2. Acts on granulosa cells in females to upregulate aromatase activity which converts androgens to estrogens.

C. LH

1. Acts on leydig cells in males to regulate testosterone concentration.
2. Acts on theca interna cells in females which increases desmolase activity → increased conversion of cholesterol to androgens (testosterone and androstenedione)

D. ACTH

1. Acts on the adrenal cortex
   a) The adrenal cortex is made up three layers: glomerulosa, fasciculata, and reticularis (Figure 6.2). The three zones release aldosterone, cortisol, and sex steroids respectively.
   b) The zona glomerulosa is primarily regulated by the renin-angiotensin-aldosterone system (RAAS).
   c) The zona fasciculata and reticularis are regulated by ACTH.
2. A cosyntropin stimulation test is used to distinguish primary adrenal insufficiency (adrenal dysfunction) from secondary adrenal insufficiency (pituitary dysfunction).

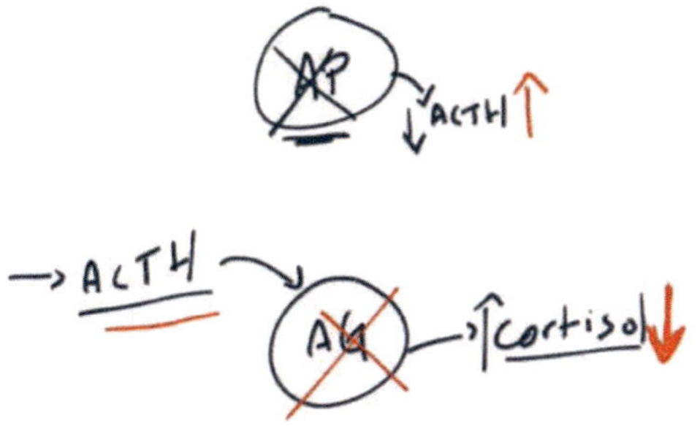

E. TSH

1. Acts on the thyroid gland to stimulate triiodothyronine (T3) and thyroxine (T4) production and release.

F. Prolactin

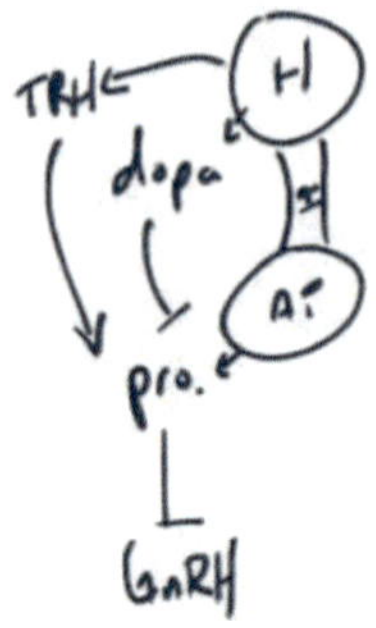

1. Acts on the mammary glands as well as the hypothalamus.
   a) In the mammary glands prolactin stimulates milk production for lactation.
   b) In the hypothalamus prolactin suppresses GnRH → decreased FSH and LH → decreased estrogen and testosterone → decreased sexual function and fertility
2. TRH increases prolactin release from the anterior pituitary.
3. Dopamine
   a) Dopamine is released from the hypothalamus and constitutively blocks the release of prolactin from the anterior pituitary.
   b) Dopamine antagonist medications can cause hyperprolactinemia.

G. GH

1. Acts on the liver and causes release of insulin-like growth factor (IGF-1). IGF-1 binds to receptor tyrosine kinases → cellular growth via increased protein synthesis (bones, muscles, and most organs)
2. Increased GH decreases tissue sensitivity to insulin (makes patient insulin-resistant) → hyperglycemia → subsequent hyperinsulinemia
3. GH release is inhibited by IGF-1, glucose, and other complex factors.
4. Excess GH can result in gigantism in children or acromegaly in adults.

II. Intermediate Pituitary

A. Melanocyte-stimulating hormone (MSH) is produced from the precursor molecule pro-opiomelanocortin (POMC).

1. POMC is cleaved to produce ACTH and MSH.
2. MSH stimulates melanocytes to produce and release melanin.

III. Posterior Pituitary

A. ADH and oxytocin are made in the hypothalamus but released from the posterior pituitary gland.

B. Oxytocin

1. Acts on the uterus (contractions) and mammary glands (milk let-down).

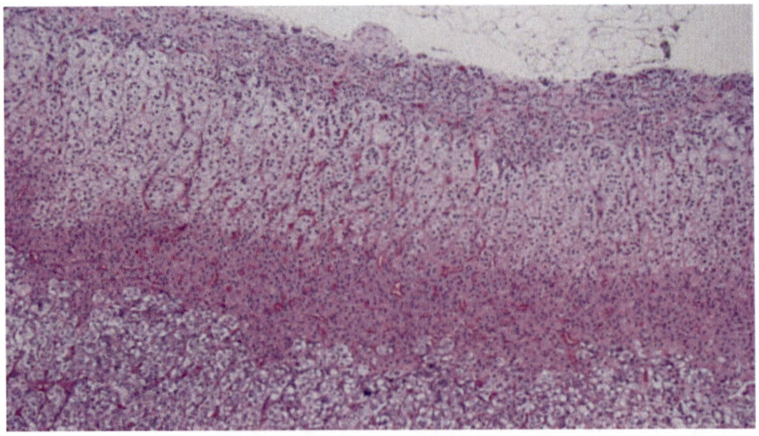

Figure 6.2 - The Adrenal Gland
(Courtesy of Roberto Alvaro A. Taguibao, M.D.; University of California Irvine Medical Center)

C. ADH

1. Acts on the V_1 receptors on vascular smooth muscle
   a) Results in vasoconstriction and subsequent increased blood pressure.
2. Acts on the V_2 receptor on the principal cells of the collecting duct
   a) Increases aquaporin channels on the cell membrane → increased H_2O reabsorption
   b) Primary regulator of plasma sodium concentration

D. Diabetes insipidus (DI)

1. Excessive loss of diluted urine
2. A water deprivation test is used to distinguish central and nephrogenic diabetes insipidus as well as primary polydipsia.
3. Primary (psychogenic)
   a) Urine osmolarity will correct with water deprivation test.
   b) Treat with water restriction.
   c) Commonly associated with psychiatric history.
4. Central
   a) Due to hypothalamic/pituitary dysfunction → decreased ADH release
   b) Urine osmolarity will not normalize with water deprivation test.
   c) Administration of ADH will normalize urine osmolarity.
   d) Treat with a synthetic ADH analog (desmopressin).
5. Nephrogenic
   a) Due to V_2 receptor inhibition (lithium) or defect (genetics).
   b) Urine osmolarity will not normalize with water deprivation test.
   c) Administration of ADH will not normalize urine osmolarity.
   d) Treat with hydrochlorothiazide and indomethacin

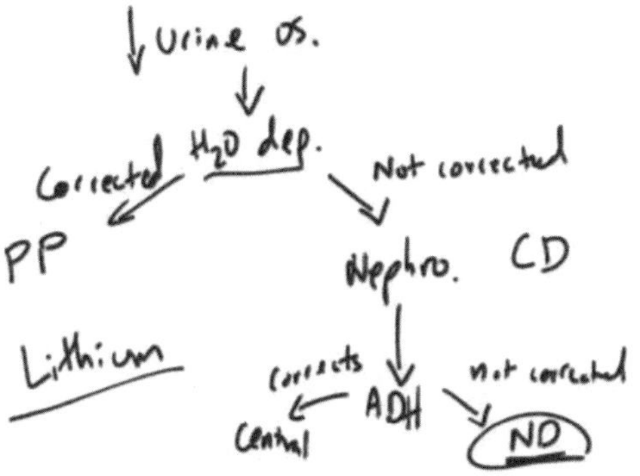

REVIEW QUESTIONS

1. How would the hypothalamic pituitary axis be altered in a patient with Klinefelter's syndrome?
   - **Klinefelter's syndrome → extra X chromosome (XXY) → testicular fibrosis → ↓ inhibin B, ↓ testosterone, ↑ FSH, and ↑ LH**

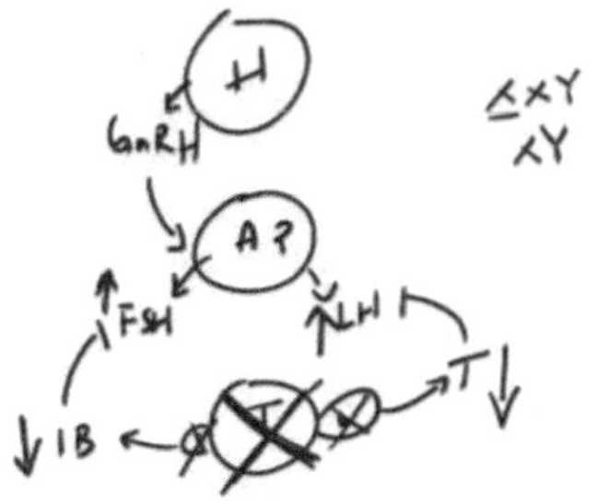

2. How would the prolactin concentrations change in a patient with a severed infundibulum after a car accident?
   - **Dopamine travels through the infundibulum to inhibit prolactin at the anterior pituitary.**
   - **A lack of dopamine signaling would result in increased prolactin concentrations**

3. What can be used to treat a prolactinoma?
   - **Bromocriptine (a dopamine agonist)**
   - **Dopamine normally inhibits prolactin**

4. A 23-year-old woman with a history of schizophrenia presents to your office with concerns of infertility. What should be on your differential?
   - **Antipsychotic medications used to treat schizophrenia are dopamine antagonists**
   - **As dopamine decreases, prolactin rises which inhibits GnRH**
   - **Low GnRH results in low FSH and LH which disrupts the menstrual cycle**

5. What is the name of the disease caused by excess growth hormone (GH)?
   - **Acromegaly (adults) and gigantism (children)**

6. How is acromegaly diagnosed?
   - **Initial diagnosis is made by detecting elevated IGF-1 as growth hormone (GH) normally acts on the liver to increase IGF-1**
   - **Diagnosis confirmed with glucose tolerance test**
   - **Glucose normally inhibits GH**
   - **If glucose is administered and GH doesn't decrease, the patient must have a GH secreting tumor**

7. In what disease would you expect a patient to have excess pro-opiomelanocortin (POMC)?
   - **Addison's disease**

8. What is a commonly tested cancer that secretes ADH?
   - **Small cell lung cancer**

9. How would the sodium and blood volume change in a patient with small cell lung cancer resulting in the ectopic production of ADH?
   - **ADH → ↑ H_2O reabsorption → ↓ renin → ↓ aldosterone → Na^+ loss**
   - **ADH → ↑ blood volume → ↑ atrial natriuretic peptide (ANP)→ ↑ Na^+ loss**
   - **The ↑ ADH and opposing forces of aldosterone and ANP result in euvolemic hyponatremia**

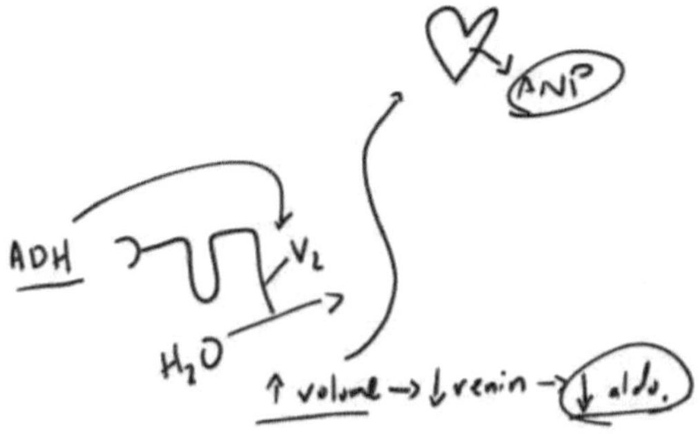

10. What drug is commonly associated with nephrogenic diabetes insipidus?
    - **Lithium**

Section III - The Thyroid Gland

I. Thyroid Hormone Synthesis

A. Synthesis

1. Iodide is brought into the follicle (Figure 6.3) with Na^+ through the sodium-iodide symporter (NIS).
2. Within the follicular cell, thyroglobulin is synthesized from tyrosine → secretory vesicles export thyroglobulin into lumen
3. Within the lumen, iodine and thyroglobulin are combined via the enzyme peroxidase to form monoiodotyrosine (MIT) and diiodotyrosine (DIT). This process is known as "organification."
   a) 2 DIT molecules make thyroxine (T_4).
   b) 1 DIT molecule and 1 MIT molecule make triiodothyronine (T_3).

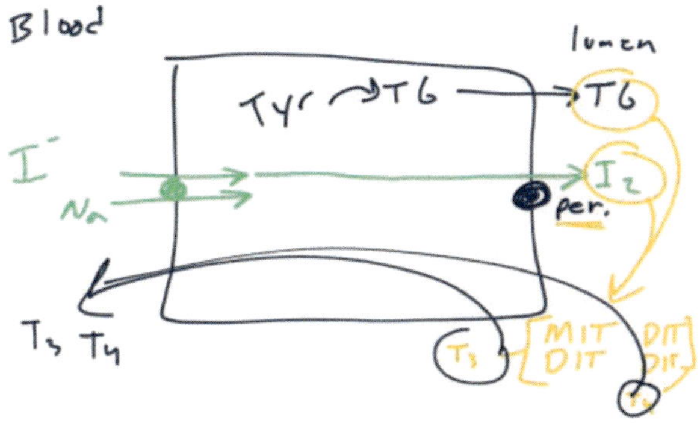

II. Export and Peripheral Activation

A. When the thyroid follicle is stimulated by TSH, molecules of T_4 and T_3 will be brought from the lumen into the cell by endocytosis.

B. The thyroid produces four times more T_4 than T_3 (80:20). T_4 is considered the pre-hormone, while T_3 is the active and more potent hormone.

1. When T_4 enters a cell in the peripheral tissues it will be converted to T_3 by 5'-iodinase.
2. T_4 can also be converted to reverse T_3 (rT_3) which is inactive. This mechanism is utilized in states when less hormone is required (i.e. during illnesses).

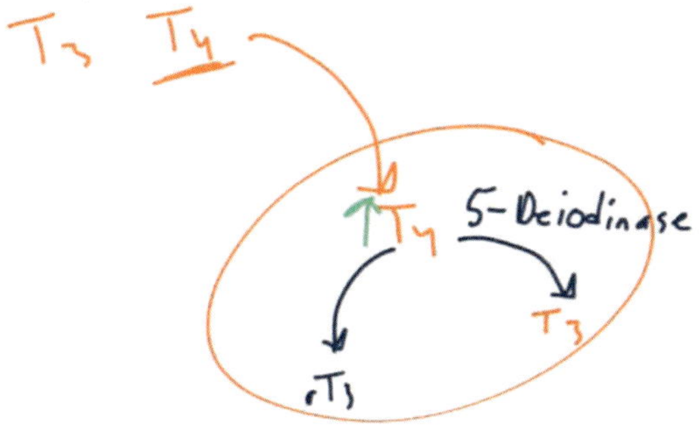

C. T_3 acts on target cell nucleus and alters gene expression.

D. T_4 is transferred through the placenta.

1. A fetus with thyroid dysgenesis can have normal thyroid levels.

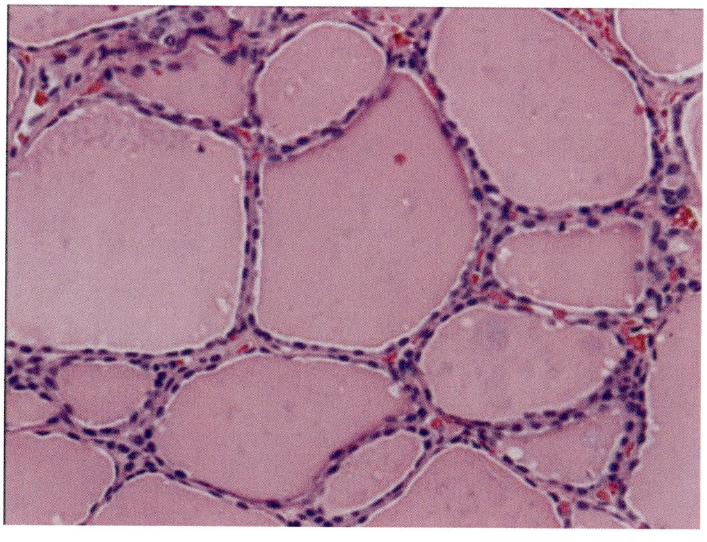

Figure 6.3 - Thyroid Follicles.
(Courtesy of Roberto Alvaro A. Taguibao, M.D.; University of California Irvine Medical Center)

III. Thyroid Binding Globulin (TBG)

A. The liver synthesizes TBG which binds T_3 and T_4. Only the free T_3 and T_4 are active.

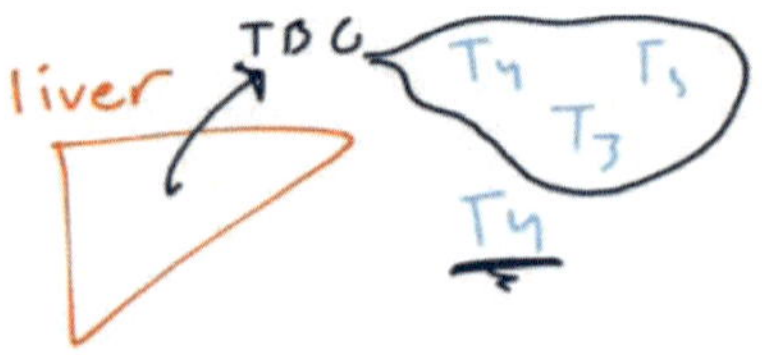

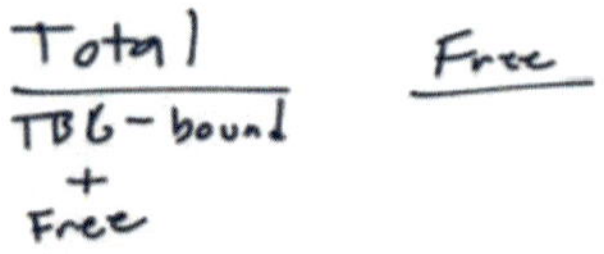

B. Estrogen increases TBG synthesis → increased binding of T_3 / T_4 by TBG → transiently decreased free T_3/T_4 (hypothyroid state) → transiently increased TSH to stimulate release of T_3 / T_4 from thyroid → net result is normal **free** T_3 / T_4 with increased **total** T_3 / T_4 (TBG-bound T_3 / T_4 + free T_3/T_4)

1. Pregnancy and Oral contraceptive pills (OCPs) can increase levels of TBG due to increased levels of estrogen.

C. TBG synthesis is decreased in liver dysfunction → increased **free** T_3 and T_4 → transiently increased T_3 / T_4 (hyperthyroid state) → transiently decreased TSH to compensate for excess T_3 / T_4 → net result is **normal** free T_3 / T_4 and **decreased** total T_3 / T_4 (TBG-bound T_3 / T_4 + free T_3 / T_4).

D. T3 and T4 can also be bound by thyroid binding globulin (TBG) and albumin, which has less affinity than TBG.

IV. Radioactive Iodine Uptake (RAIU) Test

A. The uptake of iodine should be proportional to the activity of TSH receptor activity → hyperthyroidism (excess thyroid hormone production) would have a high uptake of iodine, while thyroiditis (leakage of thyroid hormone) would have low iodine uptake.

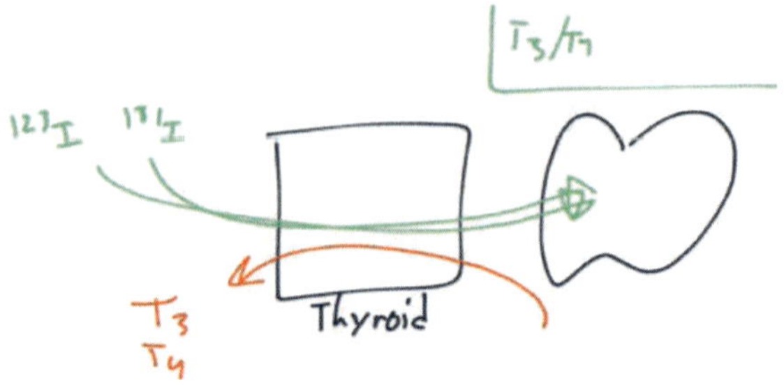

V. Actions of Thyroid Hormone

A. Acts to upregulate the actions of many organs and processes

1. Bones growth. T3/T4 have a synergistic effect on bone growth with GH. This is an example of a permissive effect.
2. Central nervous system (CNS) development.
3. Metabolism upregulated: Increased Na^+/K^+ ATPase → O_2 consumption (O_2 required to make ATP) → increased respiratory rate and ventilation. The electron transport chain is upregulated to make ATP, of which, heat is a by-product → increased heat production.

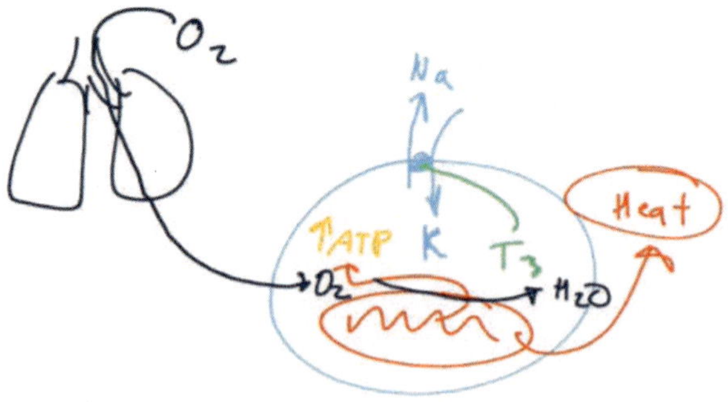

4. Autonomic nervous system (ANS) stimulation. T3/T4 stimulate β1 adrenergic receptors on the heart → increased heart rate and contractility

VI. Hyperthyroidism

A. Due to high levels of thyroid hormone.

B. Primary hyperthyroidism is caused by excessive production and release of thyroid hormone from the thyroid gland → excessive stimulation of T3/T4 receptors in peripheral tissues

1. High T_3 and T_4
2. Low TSH

C. Secondary hyperthyroidism is caused by excessive release of TSH from the anterior pituitary → excessive stimulation of thyroid gland → excessive production of thyroid hormone

1. High T_3 and T_4
2. High TSH (or inappropriately normal)

VII. Hypothyroidism

A. Due to low levels of thyroid hormone.

B. Primary hypothyroidism is caused by decreased function of the thyroid gland.

1. Low T_3 and T_4
2. High TSH

C. Secondary hypothyroidism is caused by decreased function of the anterior pituitary gland.

1. Low T_3 and T_4
2. Low TSH (or inappropriately normal)

REVIEW QUESTIONS ?

1. A child has been exposed to radioactive iodine, which enters and circulates the blood. You are concerned about the radioactive iodine entering the thyroid and increasing the child's risk of developing thyroid cancer. Pharmacologically what could you do to prevent the thyroid from absorbing the radioactive iodine?

- **Potassium iodide (KI) will overwhelm the Na-I pump, blocking uptake of radioactive iodine**
- **Alternatively, perchlorate can be used to block the function of the Na-I pump**

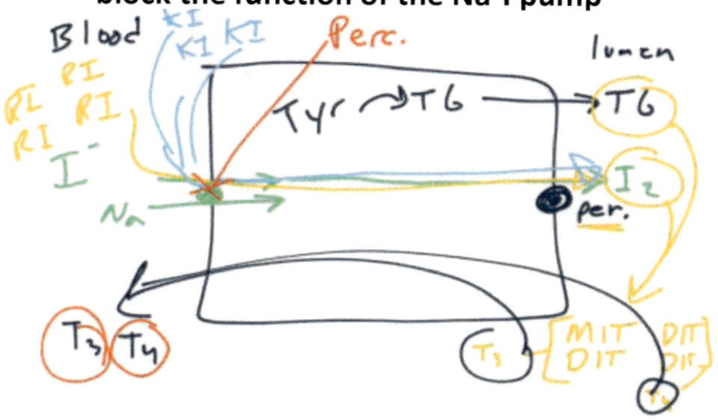

2. A female patient with a history of psychiatric illness is abusing levothyroxine to lose weight. Given her excess ingestion of T4, what would happen to levels of T3, T4, TSH, and rT3?

- **High exogenous T4 would negatively feedback to decrease TRH and TSH function**
- **High T4 would cause increased production of rT3**

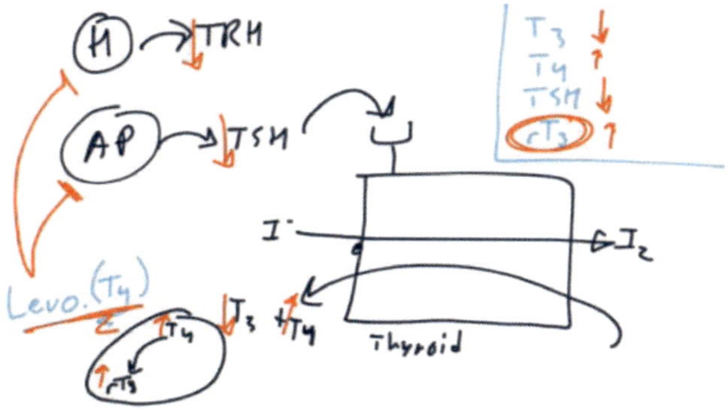

REVIEW QUESTIONS

3. A patient comes in with chronic fatigue, thinning hair and weight gain and a family history of Hashimoto's hypothyroidism. You suspect that this patient has primary hypothyroidism. If this is the case, what would the levels of TSH, T_3, T_4 and rT_3 be in this patient?

- **Primary hypothyroidism would have decreased thyroid hormone production**
- **Low thyroid hormone would cause high TRH and TSH levels**
- **rT_3 would be low since there is minimal T_4**

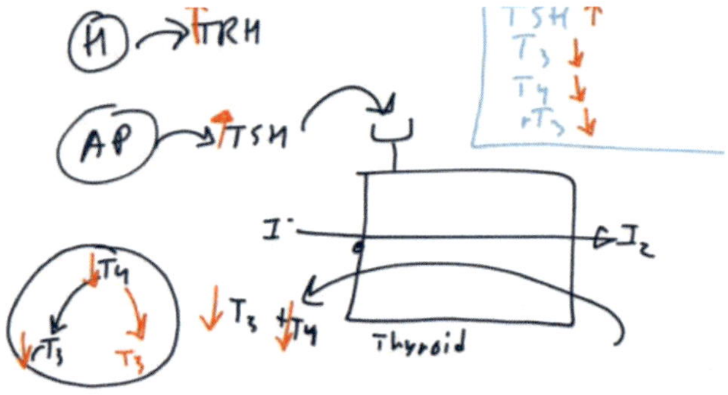

4. A patient with liver failure has low levels of thyroid binding globulin (TBG), what would happen to the total thyroid and free T_3/T_4 levels?

- **Low TBG means decreased thyroid hormone binding and normal free T_3 and T_4**
- **Total thyroid hormone = free + bound**
- **Normal free + low bound = low total**

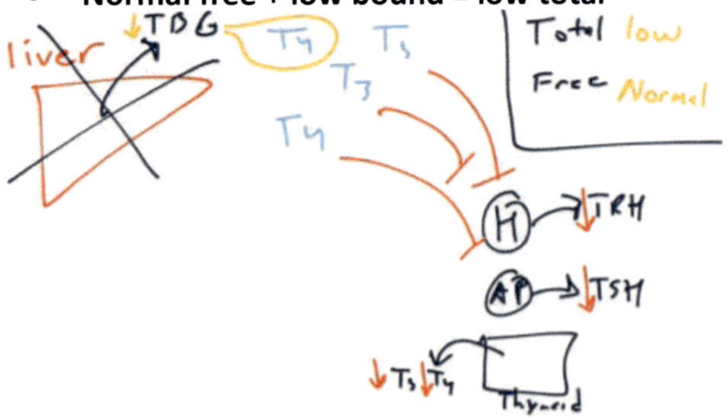

5. A pregnant patient has normal, physiologically elevated estrogen. This increase in estrogen can increase the amount of thyroid-binding globulin (TBG) produced. what would the increased TBG do to *free* T_3/T_4 and *total* T_3/T_4?

- **High TBG means increased binding, leading to low free hormone initially**
- **Decreased hormone leads to increased TRH and TSH, leading to normalization of T_3 and T_4**
- **Total thyroid hormone = free + bound. Normal free + high bound = high total**

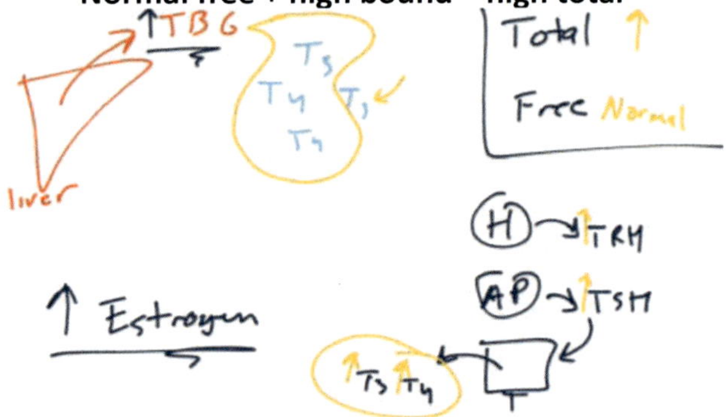

6. A patient has low T_4 and low TSH. Does this patient have primary or secondary hypothyroidism?

- **In the presence of low T_4, TSH should increase. If TSH remains low, the pituitary gland must be dysfunctional (secondary hypothyroidism)**

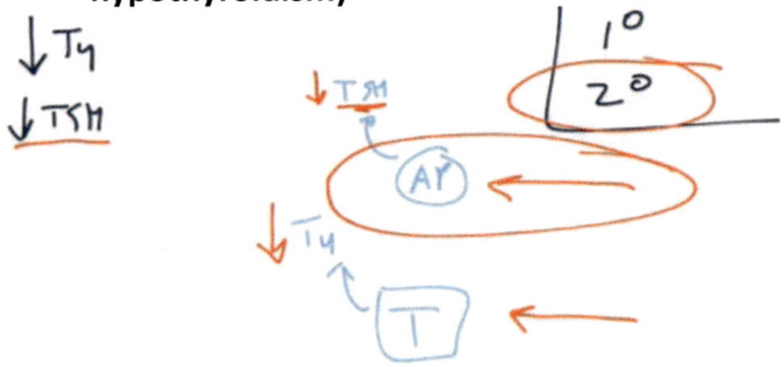

Section IV - Calcium Homeostasis

I. Calcium Homeostasis

A. Calcium levels are primarily maintained by 3 organs (bone, kidney and small intestine) and three molecules (Vitamin D, PTH, and calcitonin).

II. Parathyroid Hormone (PTH)

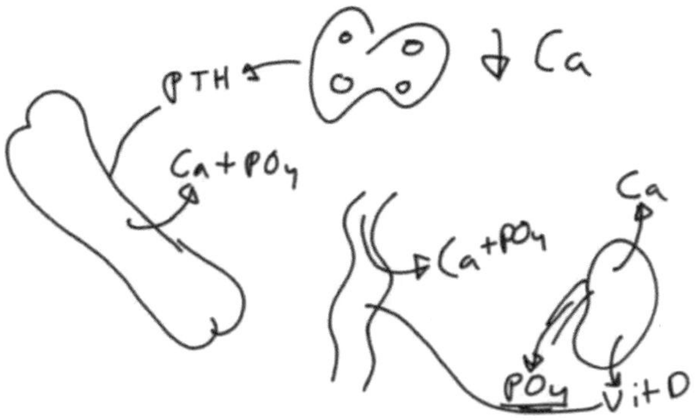

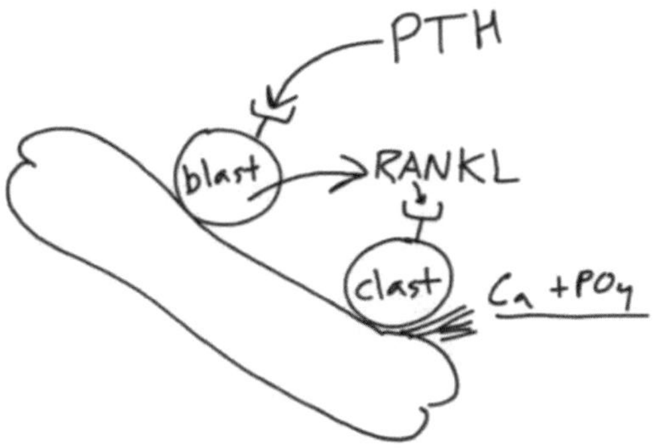

A. Stored in chief cells

B. Released from the parathyroid glands in response to low levels of calcium via negative feedback mechanism involving calcium-sensing receptors (CaSR).

C. The actions of PTH are to maintain the level of serum calcium. It does this by acting on several tissues via the G-protein coupled receptors on the osteoblasts, renal tubules and gut epithelial cells.

1. Bone: A constant level of PTH inhibits the osteoblasts (bone-forming cells) which in turn stimulates the osteoclasts (bone-resorptive cells) via the RANK receptors to increase osteoclast activity → increased Ca_2^+ and PO_4^{3-} release from bone into circulation. Intermittent PTH will stimulate osteoblasts promoting skeletal health

2. Kidneys: PTH acts on distal tubules and promote reabsorption of calcium and hydrogen while decreasing the reabsorption of phosphate and bicarbonate.

3. Gut: PTH increases 1α-hydroxylase activity which converts the 25 (OH) vitamin D to the active 1, 25 (OH)2 Vitamin D, which promotes small intestinal absorption of calcium and phosphate.

D. PTH increases 1α-hydroxylase activity in the kidney, the final step in producing active vitamin D.

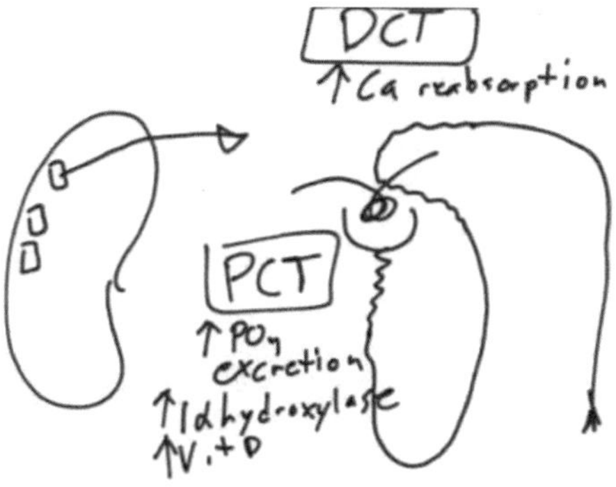

E. Hypoparathyroidism

1. Low levels of PTH cause low serum calcium.

2. Common causes include surgery (esp thyroidectomy or parathyroidectomy), Congenital (DiGeorge syndrome) and autoimmune conditions (MEN 1).

3. Familial hypoparathyroidism

a) Calcium sensing receptors are overly sensitive → decreased serum levels of PTH

F. Hyperparathyroidism

1. Primary hyperparathyroidism causes high serum calcium. It is caused by tumors (mostly benign) of the parathyroid gland resulting in over secretion of PTH. 4 gland hyperplasia is seen in Multiple Endocrine Neoplasia Type 1.

2. Symptoms of hyperparathyroidism include kidney stones (from hypercalcemia), abdominal pain (from hypercalcemia), bone loss (osteopenia/osteoporosis) from increased osteoclast activity, and fatigue and depression (from hypercalcemia).

3. Secondary hyperparathyroidism is caused by persistently low serum levels of calcium which stimulate the parathyroid glands to release PTH. Common causes are low vitamin D status, low calcium intake, and chronic kidney disease.

III. Vitamin D

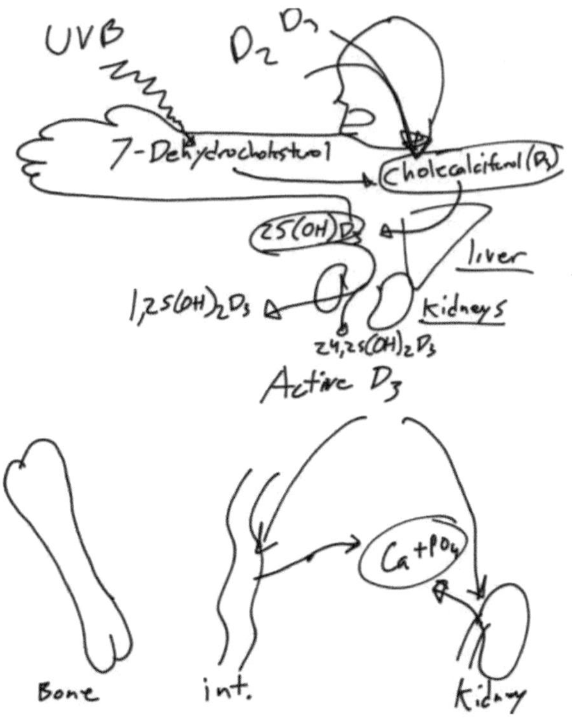

A. 7-Dehydrocholesterol is present in the skin and becomes converted to cholecalciferol (vitamin D_3) in the presence of UV-B sunlight.

B. Cholecalciferol (vitamin D3) can also be ingested.

C. Cholecalciferol is then hydroxylated to 25-hydroxyvitamin D3 (25-hydroxycholecalciferol) by 25-hydroxylase in the liver. 25 (OH) Vit D3 is the storage form.

1. Liver failure would cause an increase of cholecalciferol (precursor) and a decrease in 25-hydroxyvitamin D3 (product).

D. The kidney then converts the 25-hydroxyvitamin D3)to 1,25-dihydroxyvitamin D3 (1,25 (OH)2 D3) via the enzyme 1α-hydroxylase. 1, 25 (OH)2 D3 is the active form.

1. Kidney failure would cause an increase of 25-hydroxyvitamin D3 (25-hydroxycholecalciferol) and decrease levels of 1, 25 (OH)2 D3 .

2. In states of excess production of vitamin D, the kidney can convert 25-hydroxyvitamin D to an inactive product called 24,25-hydroxyvitamin D.

E. 1, 25 (OH)2 D_3 promotes calcium and phosphate absorption from the small intestine. An excess of vitamin D would result in hypercalcemia and hyperphosphatemia. A deficiency in vitamin D would result in hypocalcemia and hypophosphatemia.

1. Increases in calcium would increase serum levels of 24,25 hydroxyvitamin D_3, the inactive form.

2. Granulomatous diseases (Sarcoidosis, Tuberculosis) involve macrophages which have 1α-hydroxylase activity, leading to increased 1,25 Vitamin D_3 production and subsequent hypercalcemia. This can also occur in Lymphomas.

IV. Calcitonin

A. Produced by the parafollicular C cells of the thyroid

B. Antagonizes the effects of PTH (↓ serum Ca^{2+})

C. Not clinically significant in lowering serum Ca^{2+}

D. FNA stains positive for calcitonin in medullary carcinoma of the thyroid.

REVIEW QUESTIONS ?

1. If the sensitivity of the calcium-sensing receptors on the parathyroid gland decreased, what would happen to serum levels of PTH and calcium, and the urinary levels of phosphate and cAMP?

- **Decreased calcium sensitivity → decreased negative feedback mechanism → increased PTH → increased PTH activity on bone (increased serum Ca^{2+}) and kidney (increased Ca^{2+} reabsorption, PO_4^{3-} excretion and cAMP production**

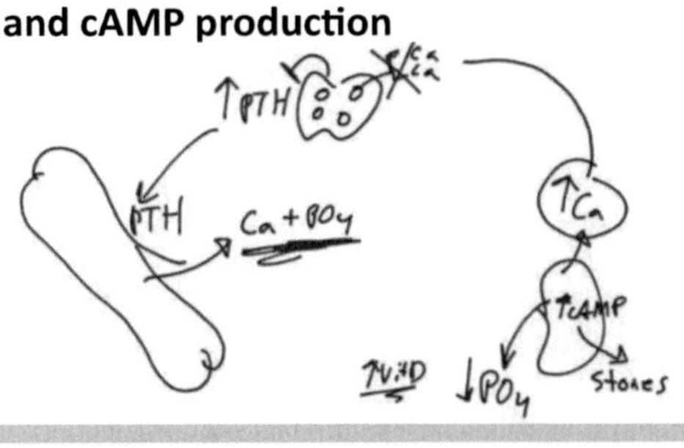

REVIEW QUESTIONS

2. A patient had total removal of the thyroid. What would happen to levels of PTH, calcium, phosphate and vitamin D?

- **Loss of parathyroid glands → decreased PTH**
- **Low PTH → decreased Ca^{2+} and PO_4^{3-} from bone**
- **Low PTH → decreased Ca2+ reabsorption, PO_4^{3-} excretion and decreased vitamin D production from kidney**

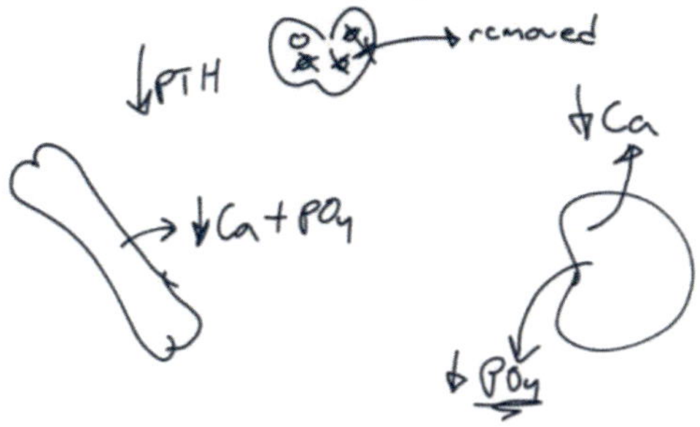

3. What would happen to the vitamin D levels in patients not exposed to sun? Why?

- **Decreased UVB rays decreases 7-Dehydrocholesterol conversion to cholecalciferol (D_3)**

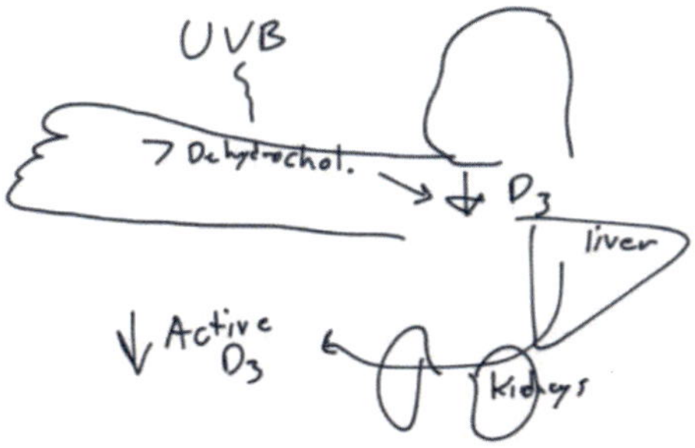

4. What would happen to the level of PTH if the patient has a malabsorption problem in the small intestines?

- **Decreased vitamin D absorption means decreased absorption of Ca^{2+} and PO_4^{3-}, triggering increased PTH release**

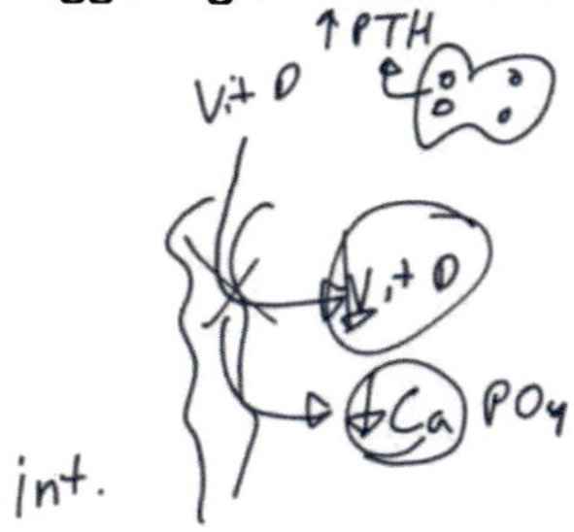

5. What would happen to serum levels of calcium and PTH and urinary cAMP in a patient taking excess oral vitamin D?

- **High oral vitamin D would lead to increased intestinal absorption of Ca^{2+} and PO_4^{3-} (less would be excreted as waste)**
- **Increased Ca^{2+} leads to decreased PTH release, leading to decreased PTH activity on the kidney, leading to decreased cAMP**

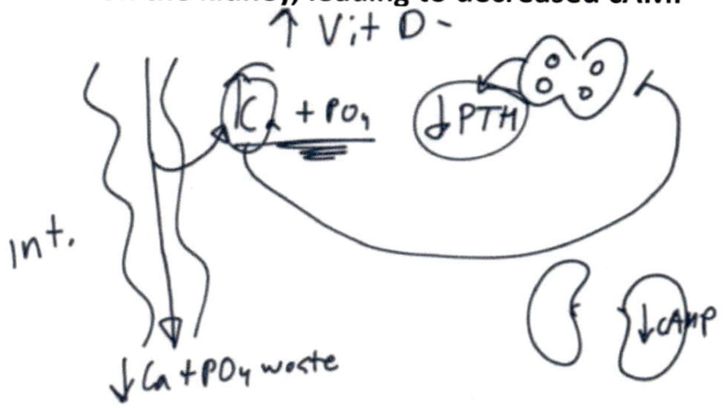

6. What would happen to serum levels of calcium, phosphate, PTH, and vitamin D in a patient with kidney disease?

- **Kidney dysfunction leads to decreased vitamin D production as well as decreased Ca^{2+} reabsorption from the kidney**
- **Decreased vitamin D leads to decreased to Ca^{2+} and PO_4^{3-}**
- **PTH would be increased**

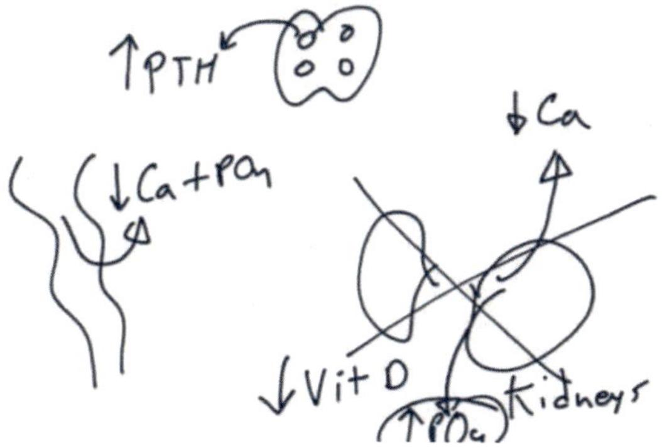

Section V - Insulin and Glucagon

I. Insulin is the major anabolic hormone of the body.

A. Actions

1. Increases lipogenesis in adipose tissue.
2. Increases glycolysis in muscle and hepatic tissues.
3. Increases protein synthesis in muscle tissue.
4. Increases glucose uptake by increasing GLUT-4 expression on the surface of adipose and skeletal muscle tissues.

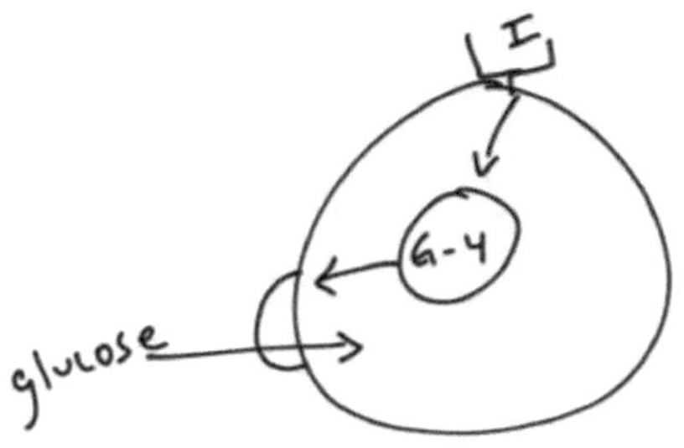

B. Synthesis

1. Produced by the beta cells of the pancreatic islets (Figure 6.4).
   a) Preproinsulin (ER) → proinsulin (secretory vesicles) → C-peptide and insulin are released into the blood in equal amounts.

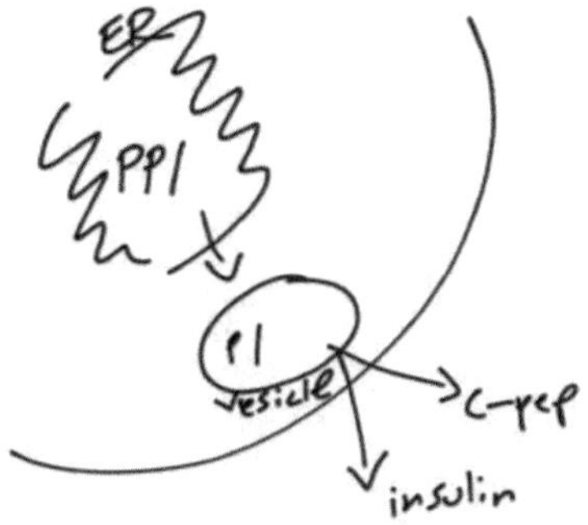

C. Regulation

1. Secreted in response to glucose entering the beta cells → increase ATP → inhibits K channels → activates Ca^{2+} channels → exocytosis of insulin granules.
2. Incretins (GLP-1 and DPP-4) are hormones that work together to control insulin release.

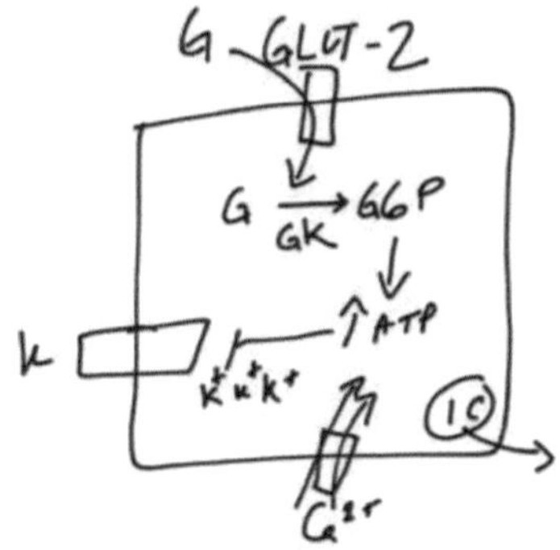

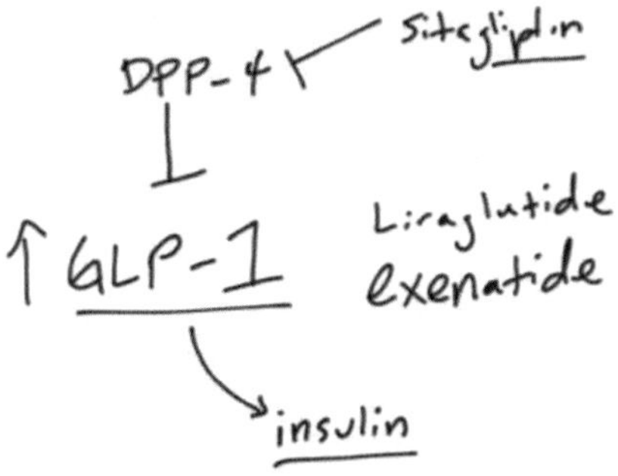

II. Glucagon is the major catabolic hormone of the body and prevents hypoglycemia by antagonizing the action of insulin in the fasting state.

A. Actions

1. Promotes glycogenolysis as well as gluconeogenesis to increase blood glucose.
2. Up-regulates the enzyme glycogen phosphorylase.
3. Activates hormone sensitive lipase within adipose tissue.
   a) Fat is mobilized into the bloodstream which can then be taken to the liver and converted into ketones.

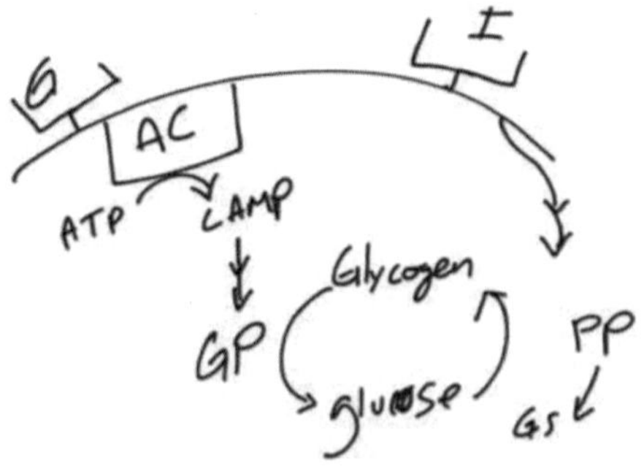

B. Synthesis

1. Produced in the alpha cells of the pancreatic islets

C. Regulation

1. Secreted in response to hypoglycemia

III. Fasting and Starvation

A. Glycolysis primarily occurs during a well-fed state.

B. Hepatic glycogenolysis and then gluconeogenesis primarily occur several hours after the last meal.

C. Lipolysis and ketone production primarily occur after a day of fasting.

D. Proteolysis occurs last and will ultimately result in death.

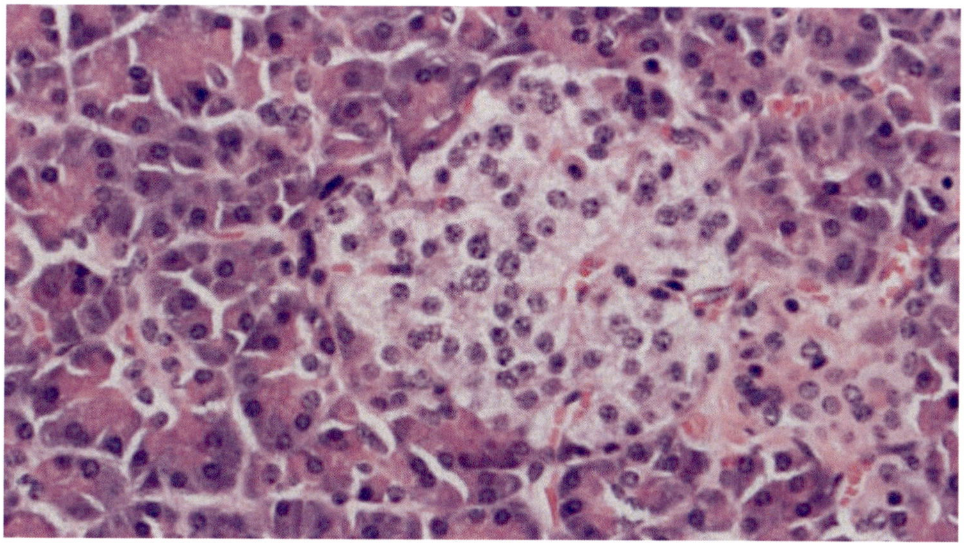

Figure 6.4 - Pancreatic Islet (Courtesy of Roberto Alvaro A. Taguibao; University of California Irvine Medical Center)

REVIEW QUESTIONS

1. How does insulin alter the concentration of free fatty acids in the serum?
   - **Insulin increases lipogenesis within adipose tissue → low free fatty acids in the serum**
2. Aside from insulin, what else increases the translocation of GLUT-4 vesicles to the cell surface?
   - **Exercise**
3. A 12-year-old boy presents to the emergency department with symptoms of hypoglycemia. As the attending you are unsure if the boy has developed an insulinoma or if he is abusing his sister's insulin who happens to be a type I diabetic. How could you distinguish the two?
   - **Insulinoma: high c-peptide and high endogenous insulin**
   - **Abuse: low c-peptide and low endogenous insulin**
4. How would decreased expression or function of glucokinase within pancreatic beta cells alter blood glucose levels?
   - **Glucokinase acts as a sensor by triggering insulin release in response to hyperglycemia**
   - **If the enzyme is not optimally functioning then higher glucose concentrations are necessary to trigger the release of insulin.**
   - **This is called maturity onset diabetes of the young (MODY)**
5. What drugs used to treat type II diabetes act by inhibiting the potassium channels within pancreatic beta cells?
   - **Sulfonylureas**
6. What are some drugs that block dipeptidyl peptidase-4 (DPP-4)?
   - **Sitagliptin**
7. What are some drugs that act as glucagon-like peptide-1 (GLP-1) analogs?
   - **Liraglutide and exenatide**
8. What other organ(s) in addition to the liver participates in gluconeogenesis?
   - **The kidneys**

Section VI - Diabetes

I. Diabetes

A. Hyperglycemia due to insufficient insulin (type 1) of inadequate insulin action (type 2)

B. In type I diabetes the beta cells are damaged by auto-antibodies and do not produce insulin.

1. Diabetic ketoacidosis (DKA)

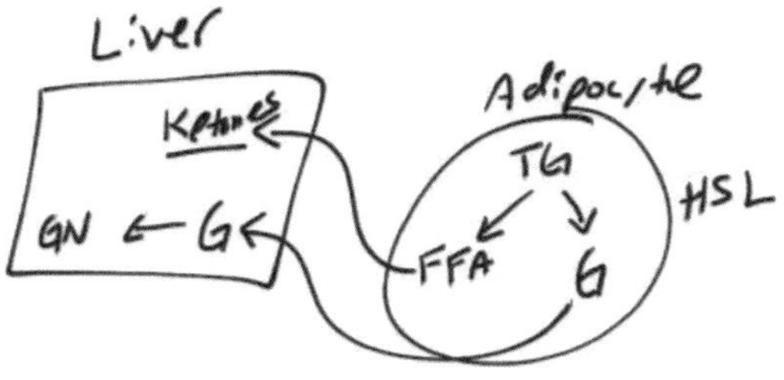

a) Insulin deficiency results in lipolysis and subsequent ketoacidosis.

b) Acidosis stimulates the respiratory center in an attempt to reduce CO_2.

c) The area postrema is stimulated resulting in nausea and vomiting.

d) Potassium

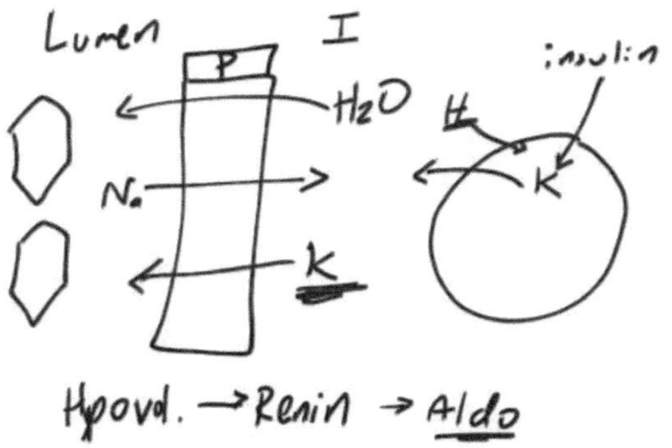

(1) Hyperglycemia results in osmotic diuresis, hypovolemia, and activation of the renin-angiotensin-aldosterone system (RAAS).

(2) Aldosterone increases K excretion, resulting in a total body hypokalemia.

(3) Insulin deficiency results in a decreased intracellular K.

(4) Acid stimulates the H/K exchanger, resulting in an increased extracellular K.

(5) Treatment includes IV fluids, K^+ replacement, and insulin.

C. In type II diabetes there is insufficient insulin (despite an increased insulin compared to baseline) to counteract the hyperglycemia.

1. Insulin resistance

a) Early in the pathogenesis of type II diabetes the baseline insulin is very high due to chronic hyperglycemia.

b) Cells become resistant to the insulin by decreasing the number of insulin receptors on the surface.

c) Insulin resistance results in increased activity of hormone sensitive lipase and subsequent hyperlipidemia.

D. Gestational diabetes

1. Hyperglycemia during the second and third trimesters of pregnancy.

2. Glucose can cross the placenta, but insulin cannot.

3. Maternal hyperglycemia results in excessive fetal production of insulin.

4. After birth the maternal supply of glucose is terminated and excessive fetal insulin results in transient hypoglycemia in the neonate.

II. Hypoglycemia

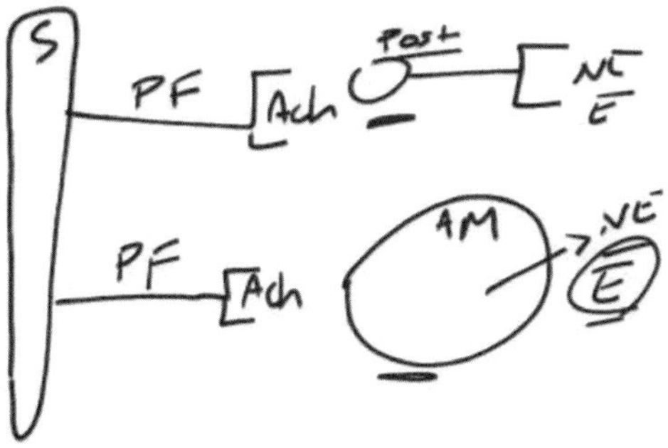

A. Causes include excess insulin use, other antidiabetic meds, excess physical activity, or inadequate food (glucose) intake.

B. Glucagon, epinephrine, and cortisol protect against hypoglycemia.

1. Glucagon
   a) In acute hypoglycemia alpha cells of the pancreas are activated → increased glucagon → glycogenolysis
2. Epinephrine
   a) In acute hypoglycemia the ANS stimulates the adrenal medulla to release epinephrine.
   b) Acts on the beta-2 receptors of the liver to upregulate glycogenolysis.
3. Cortisol
   a) In chronic hypoglycemia the HP axis is upregulated → increased ACTH → increased release of cortisol → increased gluconeogenesis

REVIEW QUESTIONS

1. How would the plasma sodium concentrations be altered in a patient with diabetic ketoacidosis (DKA)?
   - **Glucose within the lumen of the nephron exerts an osmotic force on sodium resulting in sodium loss and hyponatremia.**
2. What would happen to the serum and urine osmolarity in a patient with DKA?
   - **Glucose within the lumen of the nephron pulls water from the plasma into the urine → decreased urine osmolarity and increased plasma osmolarity.**
3. What would be the endogenous serum fasting insulin concentration of a 60-year-old woman with a 40 year history of poorly controlled type II diabetes?
   - **Prolonged poorly controlled diabetes → damage to the pancreas → low serum fasting insulin concentration**
4. So how does hyperlipidemia alter GLUT-4 channels?
   - **Impairs GLUT-4 insulin-dependent glucose uptake → exacerbation of insulin resistance**
5. A 21-year-old female presents to the emergency department after she was found unconscious by her friend. She is a known type I diabetic with a suicidal history. What should you suspect and what should you administer as soon as possible?
   - **The patient likely overdosed on insulin → hypoglycemia → syncope**
   - **Administer glucagon**

Section VII - Adrenal Glands

I. Adrenal Glands

   A. Superior to the kidneys

   B. Two parts: Cortex (outside) and Medulla (inside)

II. Adrenal Medulla

   A. Stimulated by acetylcholine from the sympathetic nervous system

   B. Secretes epinephrine and norepinephrine

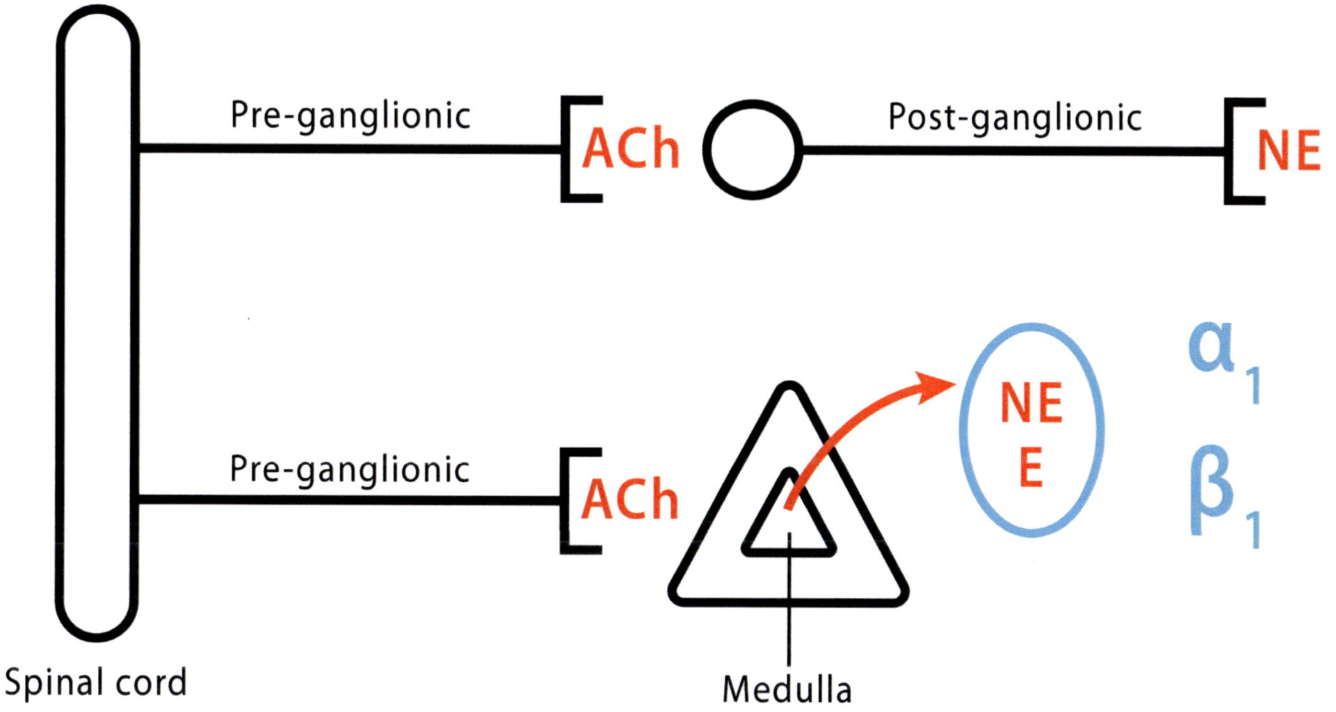

Figure 6.5 - Pre and Post ganglionic

III. Adrenal Cortex

   A. The adrenal cortex has 3 sections:

      1. Zona glomerulosa

      2. Zona fasciculata

      3. Zona reticularis

   B. All cortex hormones are derived from cholesterol

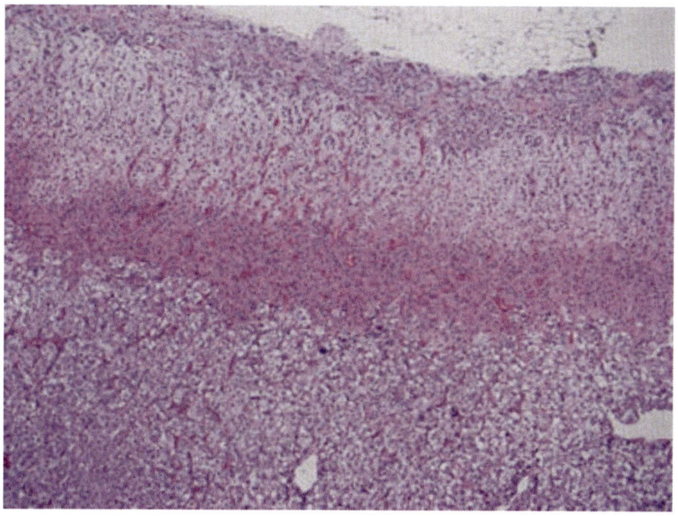

Figure 6.6 - The Adrenal Gland
(Courtesy of Roberto Alvaro A. Taguibao, M.D.; University of California Irvine Medical Center)

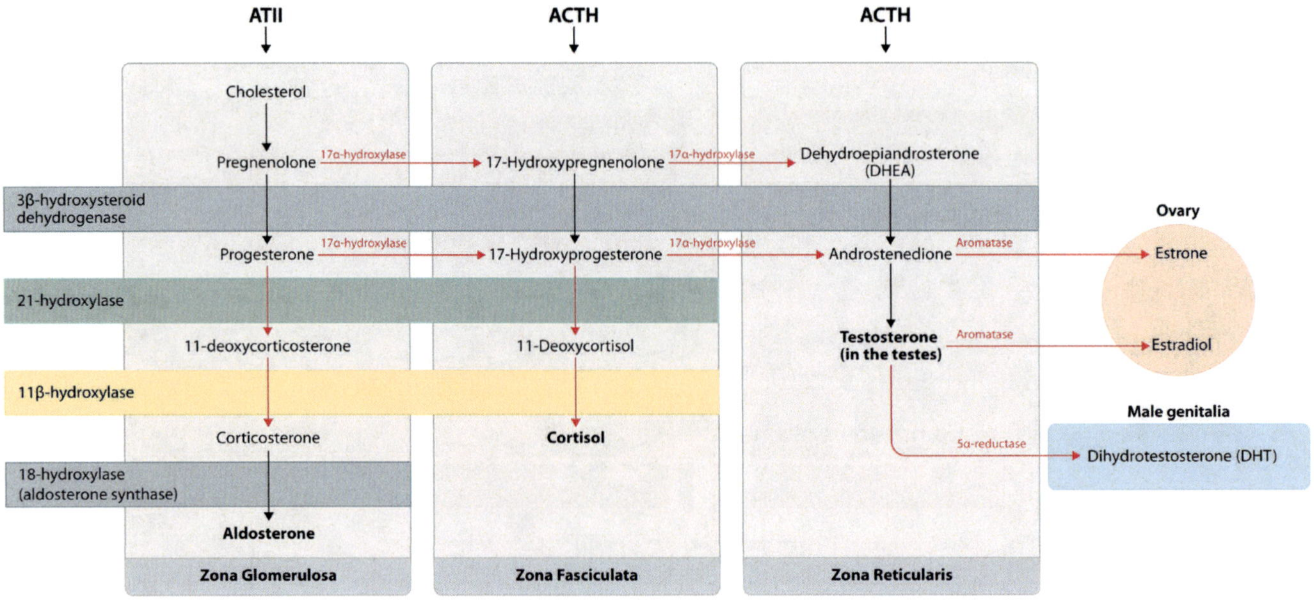

Figure 6.7 - Congenital Adrenal Hyperplasias

Name	Stimulus	Hormone Product	Hormone Product Action	Pathology
Zona glomerulosa	Angiotensin II	Aldosterone	• Acts on collecting duct • Reabsorbs Na^+ and H_2O → increase blood pressure • Secretes K^+ and H^+	• 1° hyperaldosteronism • 2° hyperaldosteronism • 1° hypoaldosteronism • 2° hypoaldosteronism
Zona fasciculata	ACTH	Cortisol	Important for stress response • α1 vasoconstriction (↑ blood pressure) • ↑ gluconeogenesis/lipolysis (diabetogenic and adipocyte growth) • ↑ proteolysis (weak extremities) • ↓ IL-2 (immunosuppression) • ↓ phospholipase A2 (anti-inflammatory) • ↓ osteoblast activity (bone weakness) • ↓ fibroblast activity (thin skin; striae) • Inhibits CRH, ACTH and GnRH	• 1° hypercortisolism • 2° hypercortisolism • 1° adrenal insufficiency • 2° adrenal insufficiency • 3° adrenal insufficiency
Zona reticularis	ACTH	Testosterone	• Converted to estrogen and DHT • Sexual differentiation in utero • Many other functions	• Congenital adrenal hyperplasias

Table 6.4 - Adrenal cortex zones and hormone productst

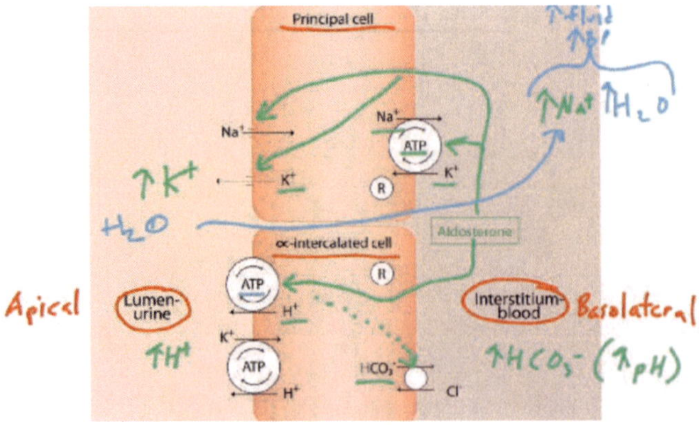

IV. Aldosterone Escape

A. High levels of aldosterone ↑ serum $Na+/H_2O$ and ↓ serum K^+ ↑ Na^+/H_2O → ↑ BP → ↑ ANP → ↑ GFR → ↑ Na^+/H_2O excretion → hypertensive effects of aldosterone are diminished

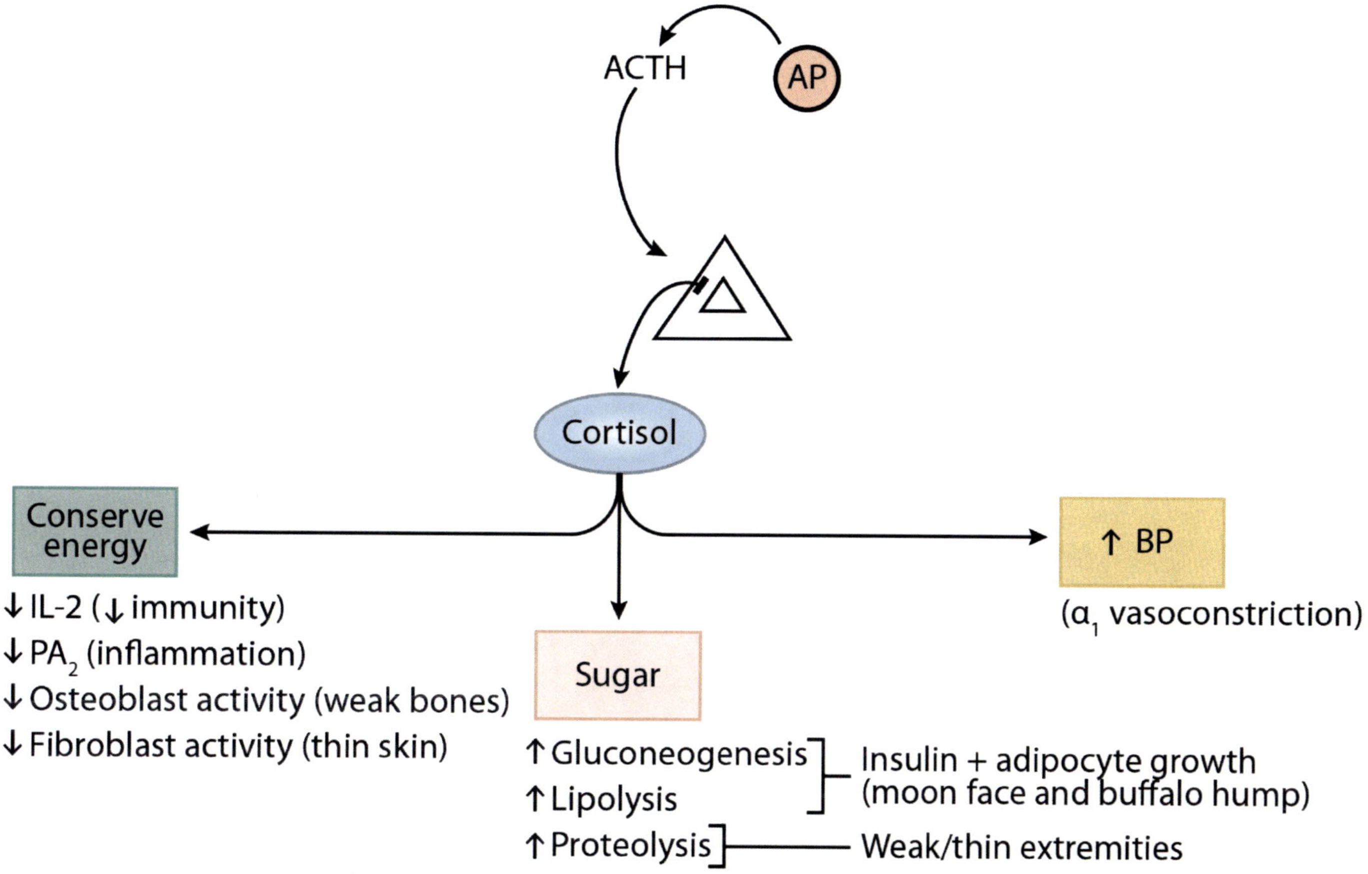

Figure 6.8 - Cortisol Functions

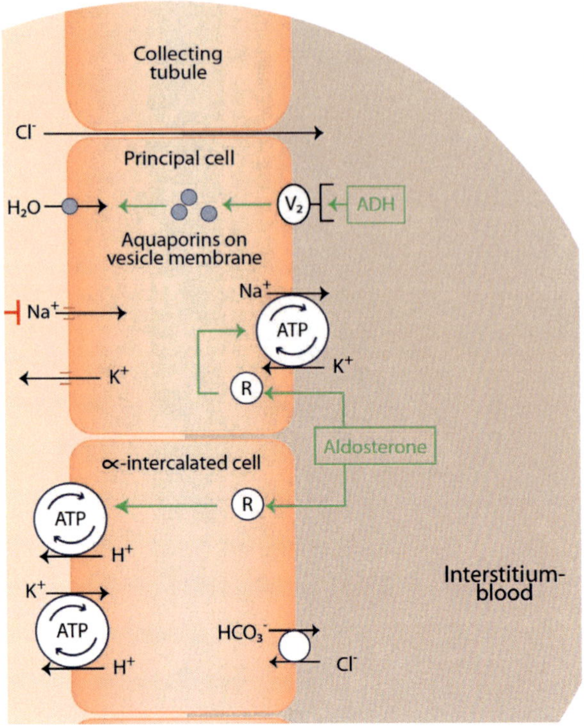

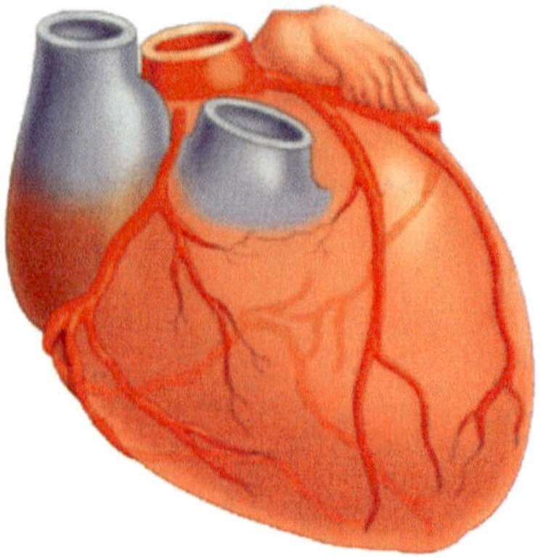

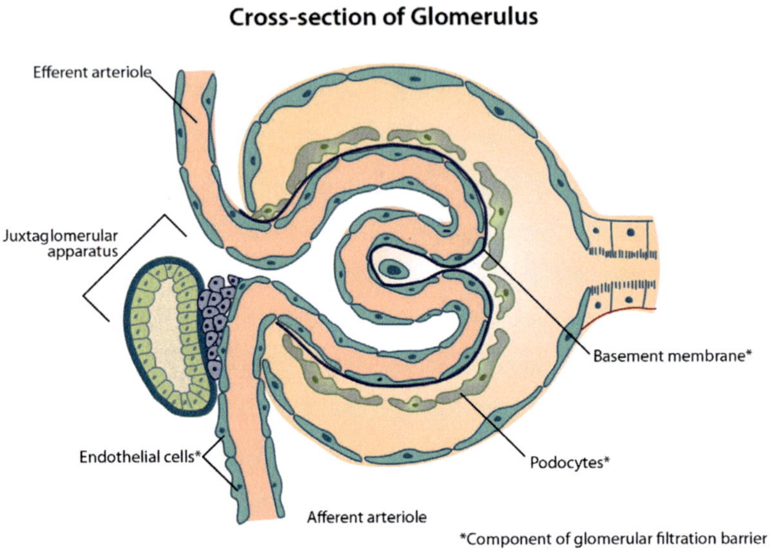

Figure 6.9 - Aldosterone Escape Mechanism

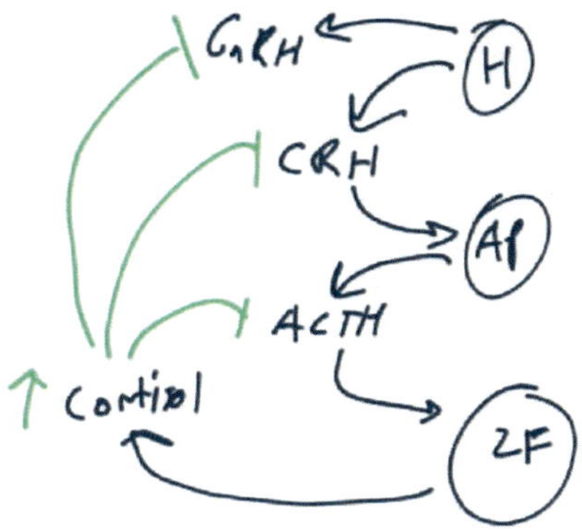

(↓LH + FSH)

REVIEW QUESTIONS ?

1. The anterior pituitary was severely damaged in a patient. What would happen to the levels of hormones produced by the adrenal cortex?

- **Low cortisol and androgens**
- **The anterior pituitary gland produces ACTH which normally stimulates the zona fasciculata and the zona reticularis. Without stimulation from ACTH, production of cortisol and androgens would be decreased**
  - **The zona glomerulosa is regulated by the renin-angiotensin-aldosterone system, not ACTH → aldosterone production will not be inhibited**

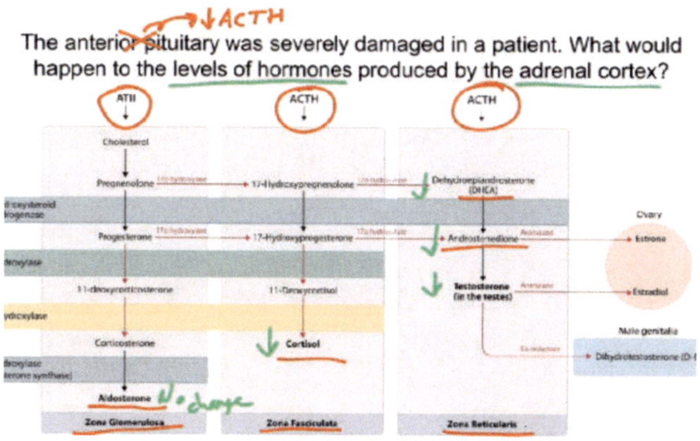

2. A patient with an aldosterone-secreting tumor has low potassium, high serum pH and normal blood pressure. Explain why the pressure is normal instead of high?

- **Aldosterone escape has reduced the hypertensive effects of aldosterone**
- **Within a few weeks of elevated aldosterone levels, aldosterone escape will take effect**
  - **Aldosterone escape: ↑ blood pressure → ↑ atrial natriuretic peptide release from atria → ↑ GFR → ↑ excretion of Na^+ and H_2O → normalized fluid volume and blood pressure**

Na^+/H_2O → ↑BP → ↑ANP → ↑GFR → ↑$Na + H_2O$ excretion

Aldosterone escape

REVIEW QUESTIONS

3. A 33-year-old female presents with severe emotional distress. Further discussion with the patient reveals she has been pulling all-nighters regularly for several months and recently lost her 1-year-old infant. What would happen to the levels of FSH and LH in this patient and why?

   - **FSH and LH would be decreased**
   - **Physical or emotional stress → CRH release from hypothalamus → ACTH release from anterior pituitary → cortisol release from the zona fasciculata**
   - **Cortisol will negatively feedback and not only inhibit CRH and ACTH release, but also inhibit GnRH release → ↓ FSH and LH → loss of many reproductive functions (problems conceiving, cessation of menses)**

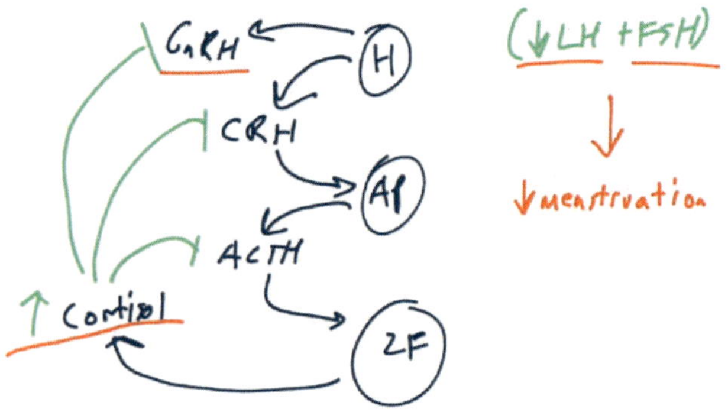

Section VIII - Congenital Adrenal Hyperplasia

I. Congenital Adrenal Hyperplasia

A. 3 types:

1. 17α-hydroxylase deficiency
2. 21-hydroxylase deficiency
3. 11β-hydroxylase deficiency

B. Decreased cortisol → ↑ ACTH → adrenal hyperplasia

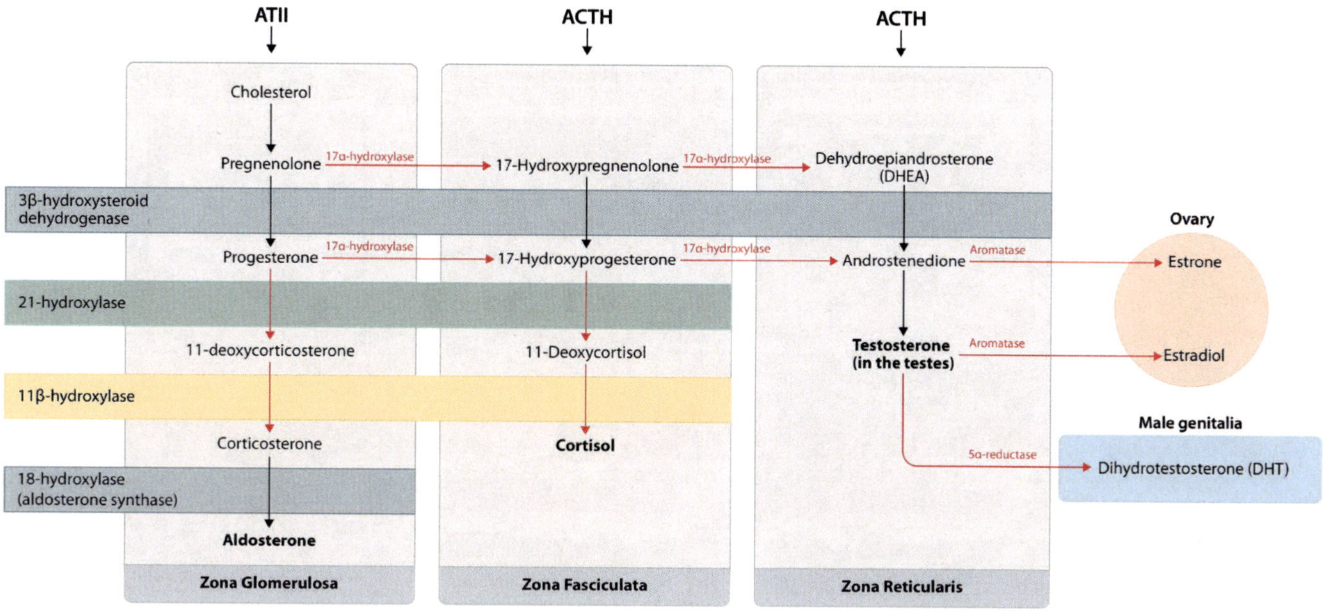

Figure 6.10 - Congenital Adrenal Hyperplasias

II. Steps for Evaluating Congenital Adrenal Hyperplasias

A. Step 1: assess androgen levels

B. Step 2: assess mineralocorticoid levels

Enzyme deficiency	Hormone levels	Metabolic findings	Female manifestations	Male manifestations	Memory hook
17α-hydroxylase	↑ aldosterone ↓ cortisol ↓ androgens and estrogens	↑ BP (↓ renin) → aldosterone escape within a few weeks of birth → normal BP ↑ pH ↓ K^+ ↑ ACTH/MSH	Birth: normal Puberty: no 2° traits	Birth: ambiguous Puberty: ambiguous	"Access androgens through alpha"
21-hydroxylase	↓ aldosterone ↓ cortisol ↑ androgens and estrogens ↑ progesterone and 17-OH progesterone	↓ BP (salt wasting) ↓ pH ↑ K^+ ↑ ACTH/MSH	Birth: ambiguous Puberty: precocious	Birth: normal Puberty: precocious	"People do shocking things at 21"
11β-hydroxylase	↓ aldosterone ↑ 11-deoxycorticosterone ↓ cortisol ↑ androgens and estrogens	↑ BP (↓ renin) → aldosterone escape within a few weeks of birth → normal BP ↑ pH ↓ K^+ ↑ ACTH/MSH	Birth: ambiguous Puberty: precocious	Birth: normal Puberty: precocious	"Beta than nothing"

Table 6.5 - Congenital Adrenal Hyperplasias

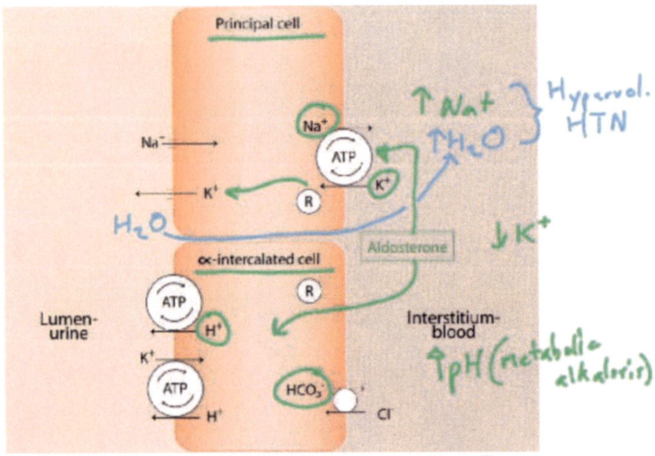

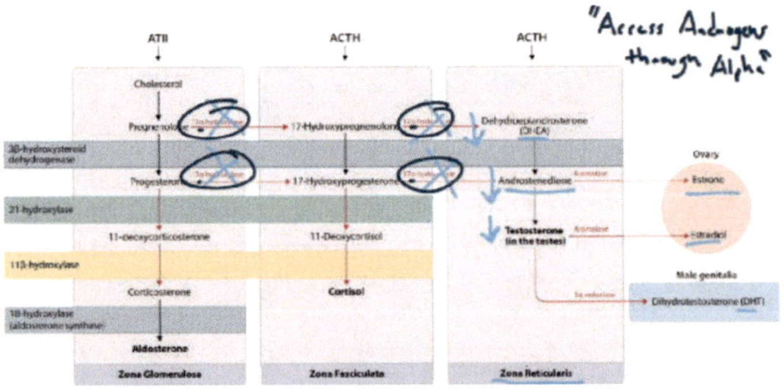

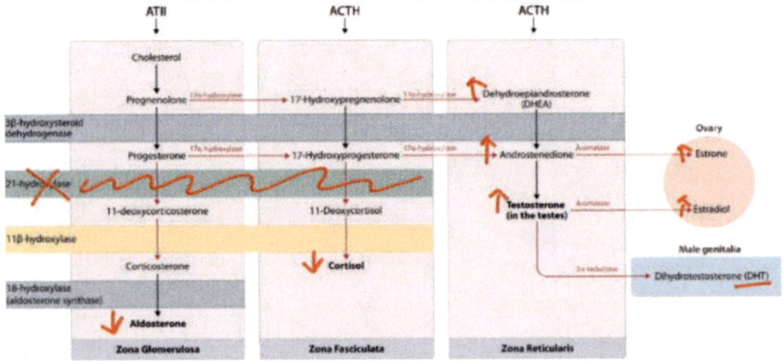

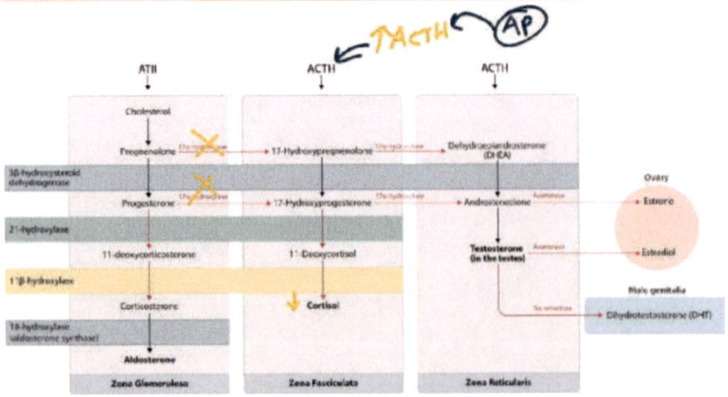

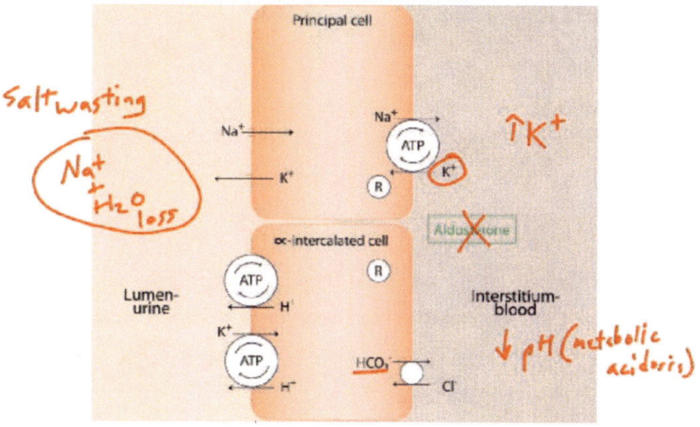

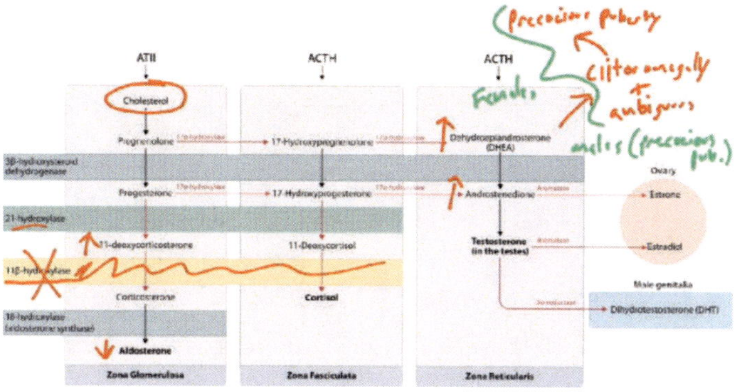

REVIEW QUESTIONS ?

1. A 2-hour-old male has a deficiency of the enzyme 17 α-hydroxylase. What abnormalities would be expected with regard to serum pH, blood pressure, and electrolytes?

- **↑ blood pressure, ↑ serum pH, hypokalemia**
- **Recall the two steps:**
    - **Step 1: assess the androgens**
    - **Step 2: assess the mineralocorticoids**

- **Step 1: With 17 α-hydroxylase deficiency, androgen production would be blocked because androgen precursors are unable to reach the zona reticularis → ↓ androgens**
    - **Recall the memory hook: "Access androgens through alpha"**
- **Step 2: Less substrate reaching the zona glomerulosa means more substrate accumulating in the zona glomerulosa → ↑ aldosterone (mineralocorticoid)**
    - **High aldosterone will cause the following:**
        - **↑ Na^+ and H_2O reabsorption → ↑ blood pressure**
        - **↑ HCO^{3-} production and absorption → ↑ serum pH**
        - **↑ K^+ excretion → hypokalemia**

An 2-hour-old male has a deficiency of the enzyme 17 α-hydroxylase. What abnormalities would be expected with regard to serum pH, blood pressure, and electrolytes?

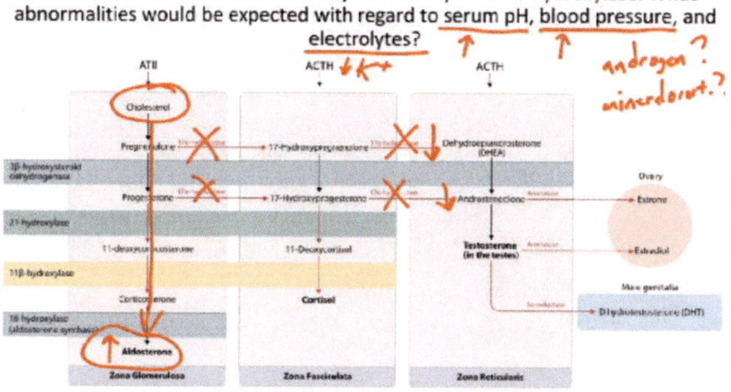

REVIEW QUESTIONS

2. A 7-year-old girl is brought to clinic by her mother due to concerns regarding early menstruation. An abdominal CT is obtained and reveals enlarged adrenal glands bilaterally. Her serum pH is elevated. What is the likely potassium level in this girl's serum?

- **Potassium level should be low**
- **Recall the two steps:**
    - **Step 1: assess the androgens**
    - **Step 2: assess the mineralocorticoids:**
- **Step 1: In the context of congenital adrenal hyperplasia, precocious puberty indicates high androgen levels → 17α-hydroxylase is functional**
    - **Recall the memory hook: "Access androgens through alpha"**
- **Step 2: Increased serum pH indicates mineralocorticoid (11-deoxycorticosterone) levels are high → excess secretion of K^+ → hypokalemia**
    - **Recall the memory hook: "Beta than nothing" → 11β-hydroxylase must be the deficient enzyme**
    - **If 21-hydroxylase were deficient, not even the weak mineralocorticoid 11-deoxycorticosterone would be produced**

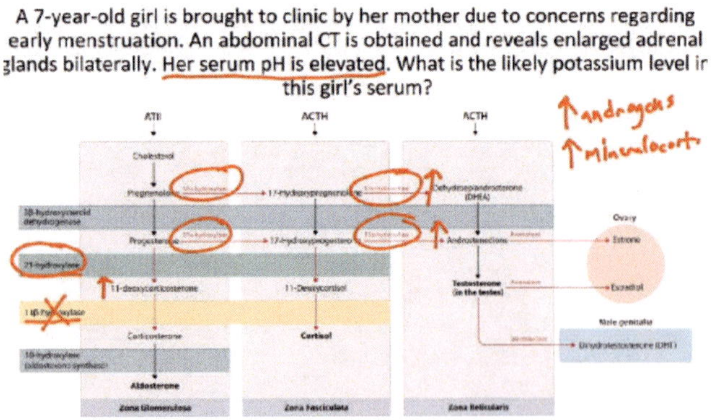

3. A 2-day-old neonate with congenital adrenal hyperplasia appears lethargic and dehydrated. What enzyme deficiency should be suspected?

- **21-hydroxylase deficiency**
- **A dehydrated and lethargic infant in the context of congenital adrenal hyperplasia is suspicious for salt-wasting and shock → 21-hydroxylase deficiency**
    - **Recall the memory hook: "People do shocking things at 21"**

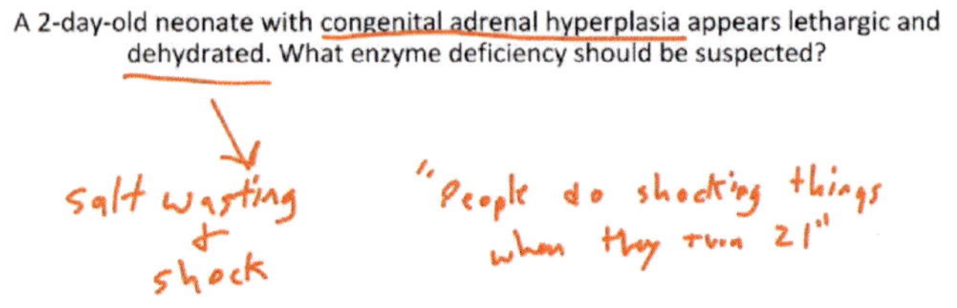

REPRODUCTION

Section I - Male Anatomy Overview

I. Male Anatomy (Figure 7.1)

A. Urinary pathway

1. Urethra (bilateral) → bladder → prostatic urethra (central) → membranous urethra (central) → penile urethra (central)

B. Ejaculation pathway

1. Seminiferous tubules (bilateral) → epididymis (bilateral) → ductus (vas) deferens (bilateral) → ejaculatory duct (bilateral) → prostatic urethra (central) → membranous urethra (central) → penile urethra (central)

C. Seminiferous tubules (Figure 7.2)

1. Responsible for producing sperm
2. Composed of:
   a) Sertoli cells (stimulated by FSH)
      (1) Secrete inhibin B, MIF, and androgen-binding protein
         (a) Nourish spermatozoa
   b) Leydig cells (stimulated by LH)
      (1) Secrete testosterone
   c) Spermatogonia (stimulated by testosterone)

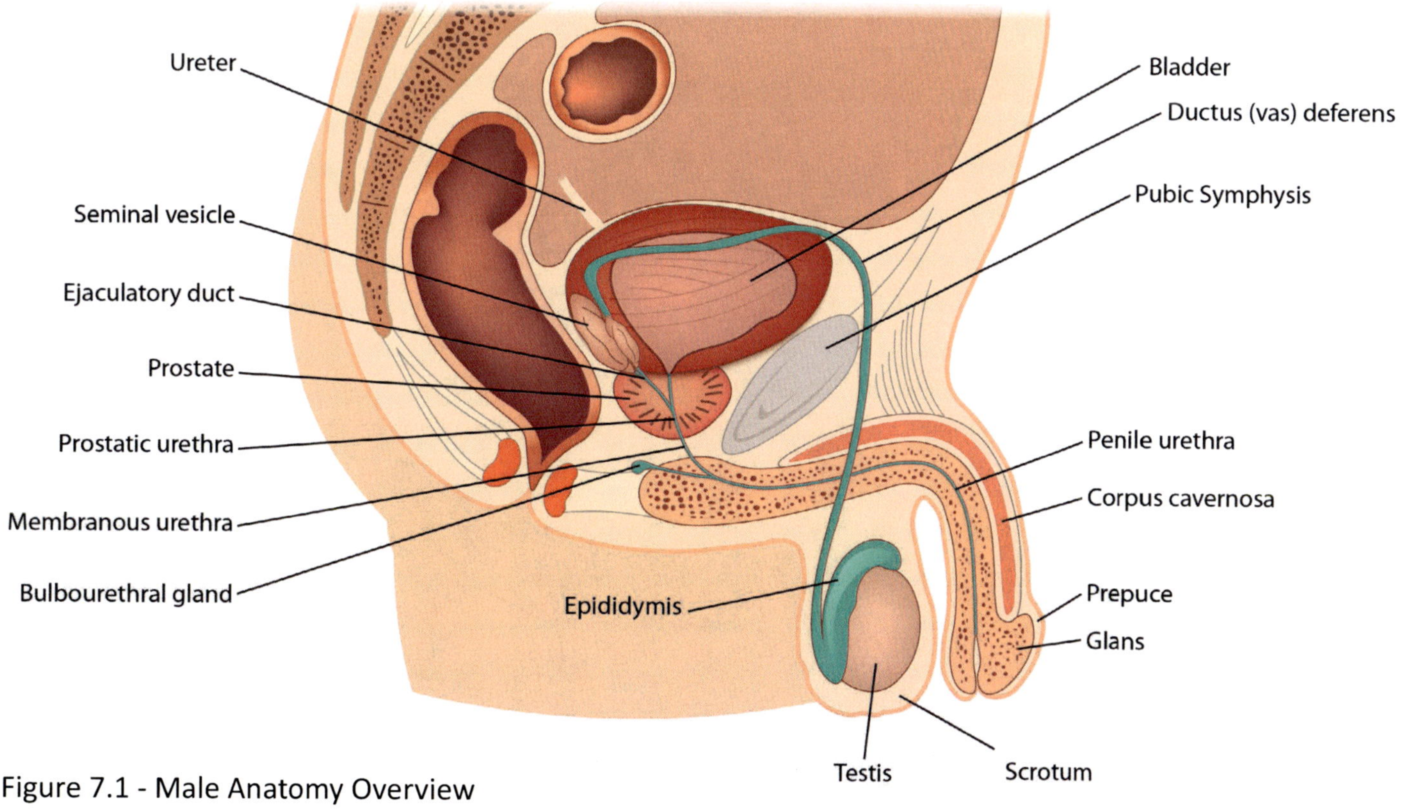

Figure 7.1 - Male Anatomy Overview

II. Spermatogenesis (Figure 7.3)

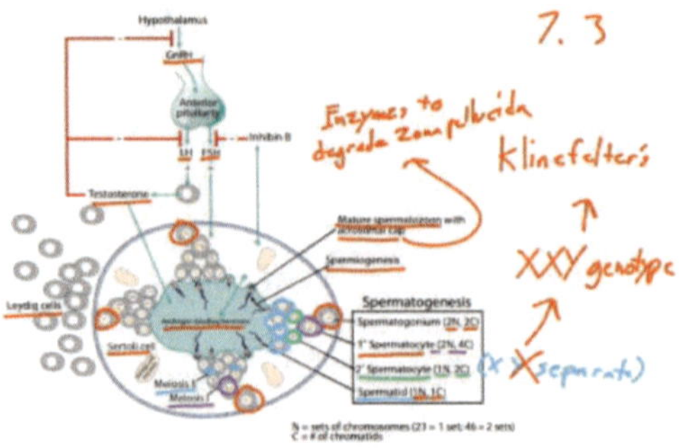

A. Occurs in seminiferous tubules

B. Begins at puberty (pulsatile GnRH release → increased LH and FSH → increased testosterone)

C. Spermatogonium (2N, 2C; present at birth) → Primary spermatocyte (2N, 4C) → Meiosis I → Secondary spermatocyte (1N, 2C) → Meiosis II → Spermatids (1N, 1C) → Spermiogenesis (loses cytoplasmic contents and gains acrosome) → Mature spermatozoon (1N, 1C)

D. Takes 2 months to complete

III. Sperm Location

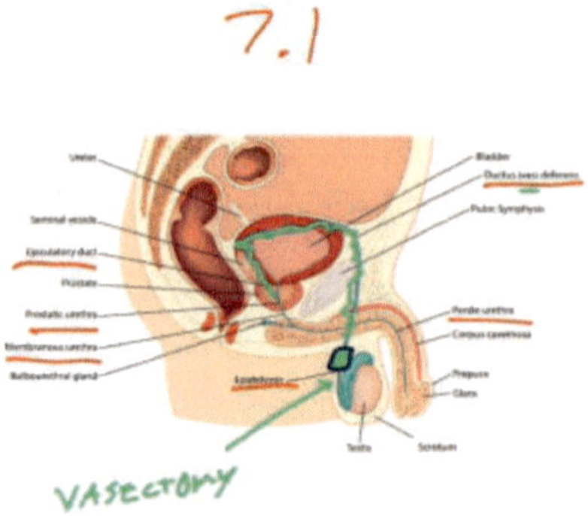

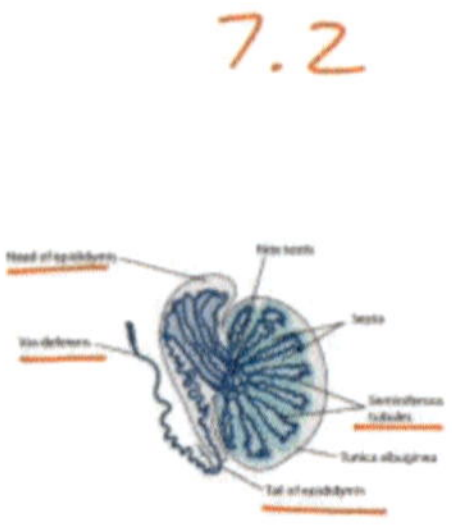

A. Before ejaculation

1. Sperm resides in seminiferous tubules, vas deferens, and ejaculatory ducts (vasectomy will not clear this sperm out of these locations)

B. Emission

1. Sperm enters the prostatic urethra

C. Ejaculation

1. Sperm travels from the prostatic urethra through the membranous and penile urethra

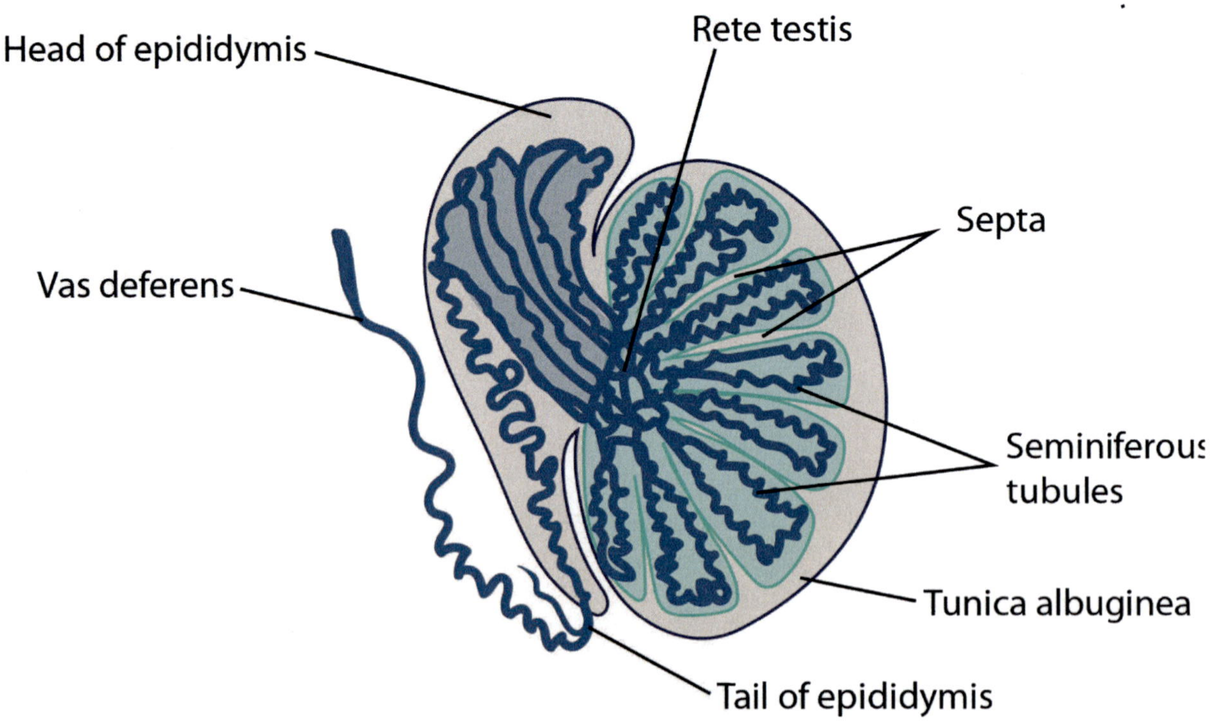

Figure 7.2 - Testis

IV. Semen Composition

A. Seminal vesicles (70%):

1. Fructose (energy for sperm)
2. Alkaline environment (pH of 7.2-7.8: neutralize acidic vaginal tract)

B. Prostate gland (30%):

1. Proteolytic enzymes
2. Prostate specific antigen (PSA; liquefies semen)

C. Bulbourethral gland (1%):

1. Alkaline secretions (neutralize acid in male urethra)

D. Testicles (4%): sperm

V. Innervation of Male Anatomy (Figure 7.4)

A. Somatic stimulation: pudendal nerve (sacral plexus: L4-S4)

B. Parasympathetic stimulation: pelvic nerve (S2-S4) → nitric oxide (NO) → guanylate cyclase stimulation → cGMP production (smooth muscle relaxation) → arteriole dilation corpus cavernosum → erection

C. Sympathetic stimulation: hypogastric nerve (T10-L2) → emission (sperm enters the prostatic urethra)

D. Stimulation of the pudendal nerve (L4-S4) → ejaculation

VI. Erectile Dysfunction

A. Inability to reliably obtain or maintain an erection

B. Vascular: decreased blood flow (e.g. DM, HTN, smoking)

C. Neurological:

1. Damage pelvic splanchnic nerves (e.g. prostatectomy)
2. Damage to hypogastric nerves (e.g. spinal cord injury)
3. Damage to pudendal nerve → no penile stimulation

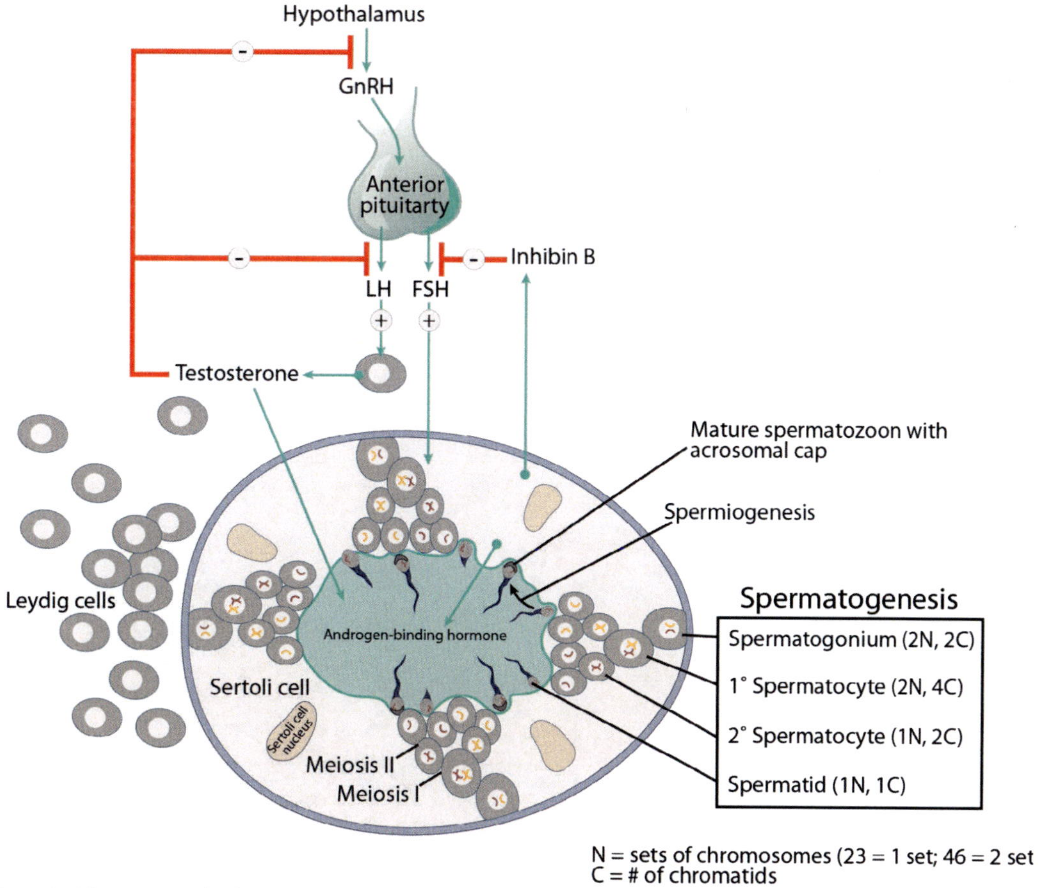

Figure 7.3 - Seminiferous Tubules and Spermatogenesis

D. Psychological: fear, stress → ED with morning erections intact

E. Endocrine: low testosterone → low libido

F. Impact of drugs

1. PDE inhibitors prevent breakdown of cGMP → erection promotion
2. Norepinephrine will constrict arterioles and inhibits erection. Think of sympathetic responses leading to increased norepinephrine.

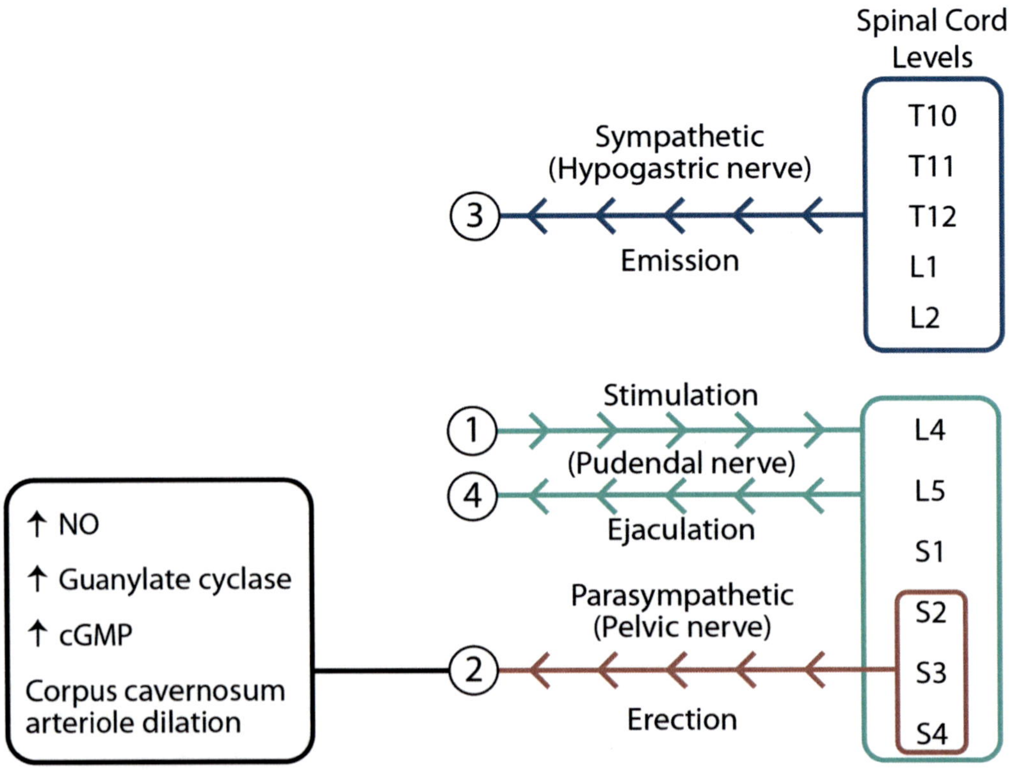

Figure 7.4 - Erection Pathway

REVIEW QUESTIONS ?

1. A male patient has defective sertoli cells and functional leydig cells. What would be the expected level of testosterone within the seminiferous tubules, relative to normal?

- **Leydig cells will continue to produce testosterone**
- **Sertoli cells will not produce sufficient androgen-binding protein (ABP), which normally binds testosterone, keeping it within the tubules. With low ABP, testosterone will be lower in the tubules**

Leydig Cells normal → Normal testosterone production

Sert~~oli~~ cells → ↓inhibin B + ↓ABP

2. A couple has been experiencing infertility. Upon analyzing the male's semen, the clinician identifies an immature sperm cell with 23 chromosomes without sister chromatids. At what stage in spermatogenesis is this cell likely in?

- **23 chromosomes (haploid) indicates 1N**
- **No sister chromatids indicates 1C**
- **1N, 1C indicates spermatid stage of spermatogenesis**

3. A man presents with a mild discomfort deep in his groin. A digital rectal exam is performed and bilateral blockage of the seminal vesicles is suspected. Upon semen analysis, what would be the suspected pH?

- **Normal semen pH is alkaline (7.2-7.8)**
- **Seminal vesicles contribute significantly to creating alkaline semen**
- **Blockage or dysfunction of seminal vesicles results in lower semen pH (acidic)**

4. During a prostatectomy, the surgeon accidentally severs the pelvic nerve. The pudendal nerve remains fully functional. Following stimulation of his penis, what would the level of cGMP be, relative to a normal response?

- **Loss of pelvic nerve function leads to decreased parasympathetic activity (and decreased cGMP)**
- **Note: Functions of the hypogastric nerve (emission) and pudendal nerve (stimulation and ejaculation) will remain functional**

Para~~symp~~athetic → ↓cGMP

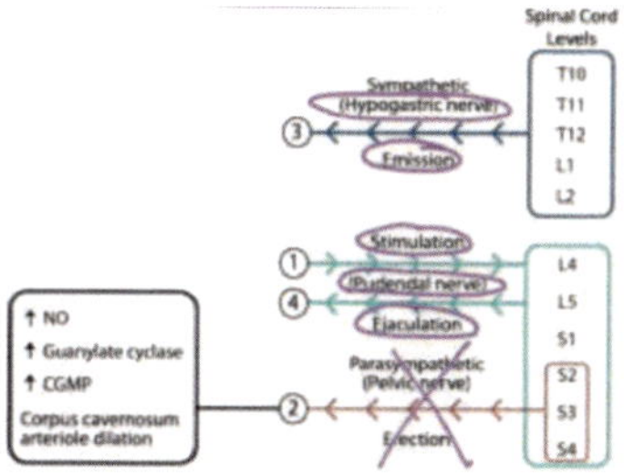

5. A man presents with symptoms of erectile dysfunction. He claims he has been very uninterested in sex recently but continues to have morning erections. What is the likely cause of his erectile dysfunction?

- **Morning erections rule out neurologic and vascular pathologies**
- **Decreased libido raises suspicion for low testosterone**

morning erections → erection pathway is functional

↓blood flow or nerve damage unlikely

↓Testosterone or Psychological stress

Section II - Androgens

I. Testosterone (Figure 7.5)

A. Responsible for differentiation of vas deferens, seminal vesicles and epididymis (internal genitalia).

B. Causes growth of penis, seminal vesicles, sperm, muscle, RBCs, and deepening of voice (puberty).

C. GnRH → LH → Leydig cell release of testosterone

D. Small amounts of testosterone are made in the zona reticularis of the adrenal cortex.

1. The adrenal cortex also produces androstenedione (weak androgen).

II. Dihydrotestosterone (DHT) (Figure 7.5)

A. Responsible for differentiation of penis, prostate and scrotum (external genitalia).

B. Causes the growth of the prostate.

C. Testosterone → dihydrotestosterone (DHT) via 5α-reductase

D. 5α-reductase is located in hair follicles, prostate, penis and scrotum

1. 5α-reductase deficiency → lack of differentiation of prostate, penis, scrotum (ambiguous external genitalia until puberty when testosterone levels increase)

III. Exogenous Testosterone

A. Increased activation of nuclear transcription factors → increased protein synthesis → increased muscle mass

B. Inhibition of GnRH

1. Decreased LH release → decreased production of testosterone → atrophy of Leydig cells (smaller testicles)

2. Decreased FSH release → decreased spermatogenesis in Sertoli cells → azoospermia (infertility)

C. Excess testosterone can be converted to estrogen via aromatase → gynecomastia

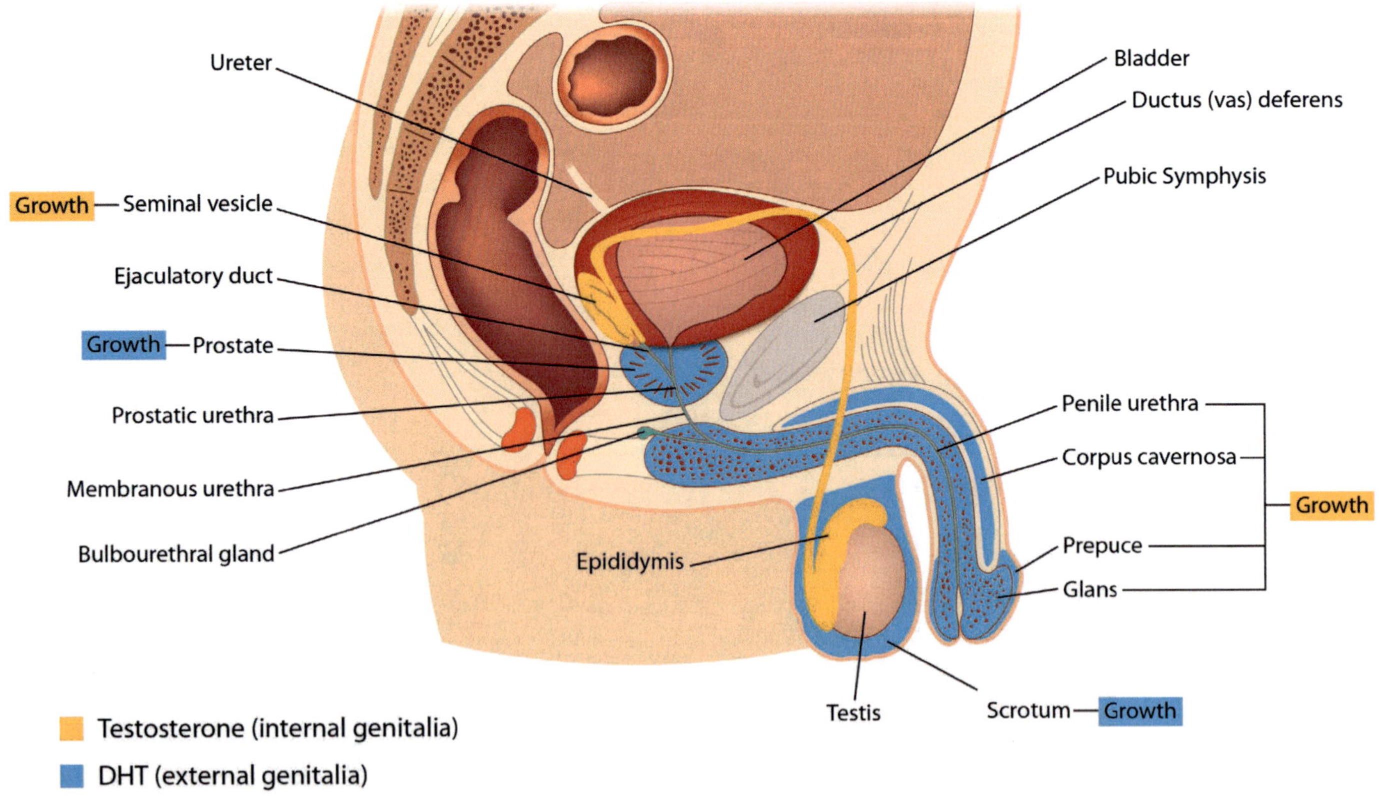

Figure 7.5 - Roles of Testosterone and DHT in Development

REVIEW QUESTIONS

1. A male newborn has 5α-reductase deficiency and normal testosterone levels. What structures would be developed upon birth?

    - **Internal genitalia does not rely on DHT and will therefore be formed at birth (i.e. epididymis, vas deferens, and seminal vesicles)**

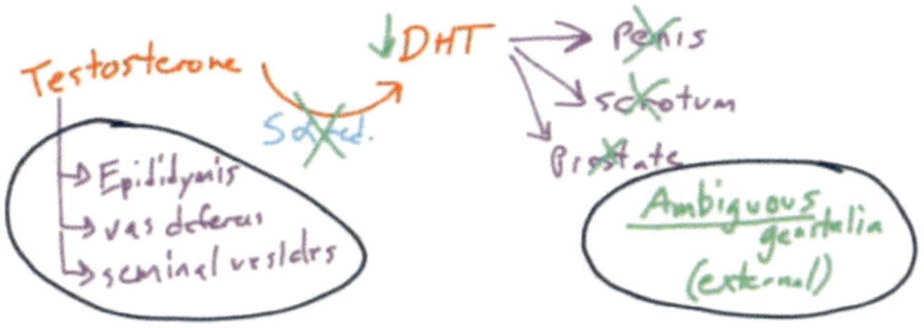

2. An infant with an XY genotype has androgen insensitivity syndrome. What will be the levels of FSH, LH, MIF, and testosterone, relative to normal?

    - **Insensitivity to androgens includes the hypothalamus and anterior pituitary, so high testosterone will not negatively feedback to these structures, leading to increased GnRH, FSH and LH**
    - **FSH will continue to stimulate the sertoli cells, leading to high MIF**
    - **LH will continue to stimulate the leydig cells, leading to high testosterone**

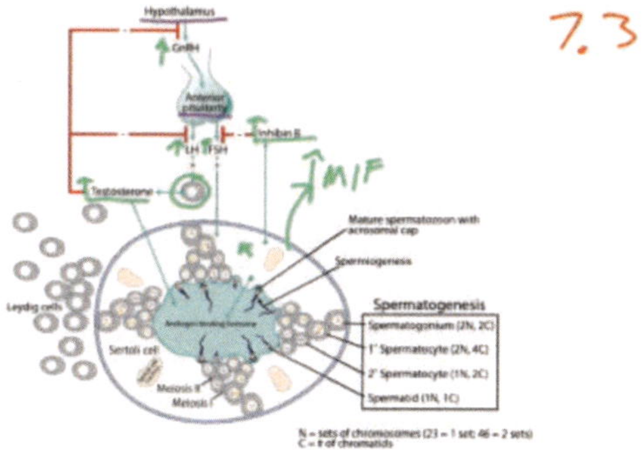

3. A man is taking exogenous testosterone to build muscle mass. What would be the levels of inhibin B, testosterone, and LH in his serum?

    - **Testosterone → ↓ GnRH + ↓ LH + ↓ inhibin B**

Section III - Menstrual Cycle and Oogenesis

I. Figure 7.6 provides an overview of the female reproductive anatomy.

II. Ovaries

A. Oogenesis (Figure 7.7 & 7.8)

1. Oogonia (N = 2, C = 2) are immature female reproductive cells that are destined to become mature ova.
2. Females are born with a limited number of oogonia.
3. By the time the child is ready to be delivered, all of the oogonia have replicated their DNA and are primary oocytes (N = 2, C = 4).
4. Primary oocytes are arrested in prophase of meiosis I until ovulation.
5. Close to the time of ovulation, the primary oocyte undergoes a division resulting in a secondary oocyte (N =1, C = 2), and the first polar body.
6. The secondary oocyte is arrested in metaphase II until it comes in contact with sperm.
7. Once the sperm penetrates the egg, the secondary oocyte completes the final meiotic division resulting in a polar body and a mature ovum (N = 1, C = 1).

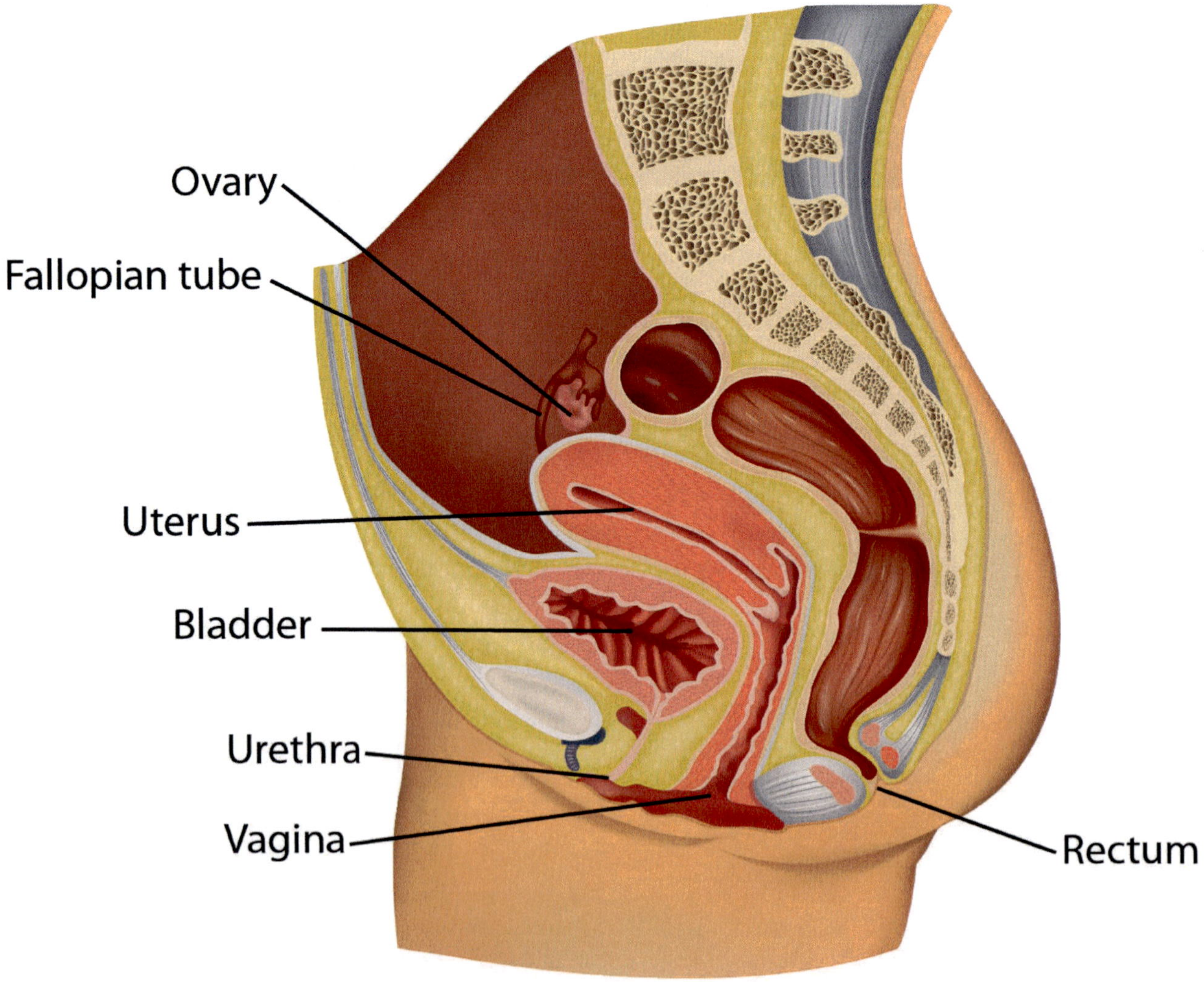

Figure 7.6 - Female anatomy

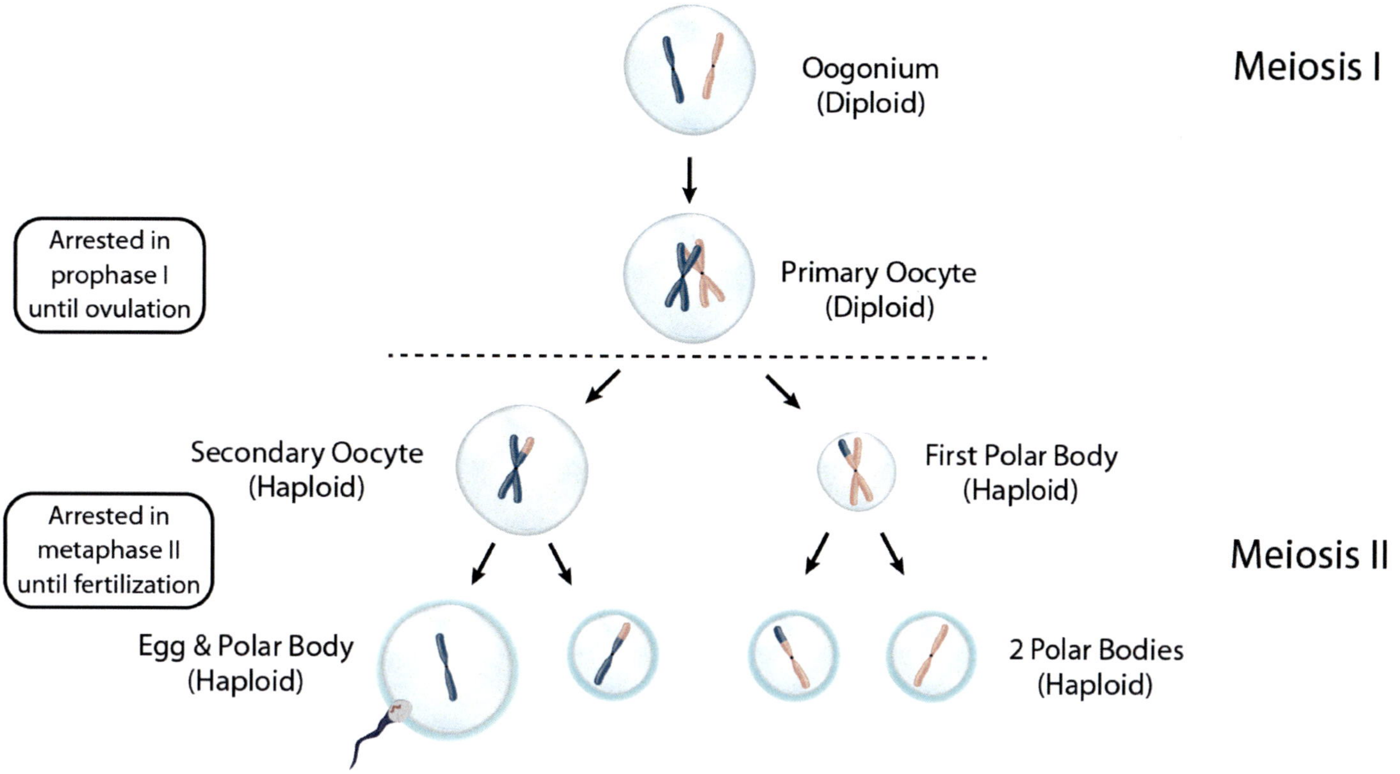

Figure 7.7 - Oogenesis

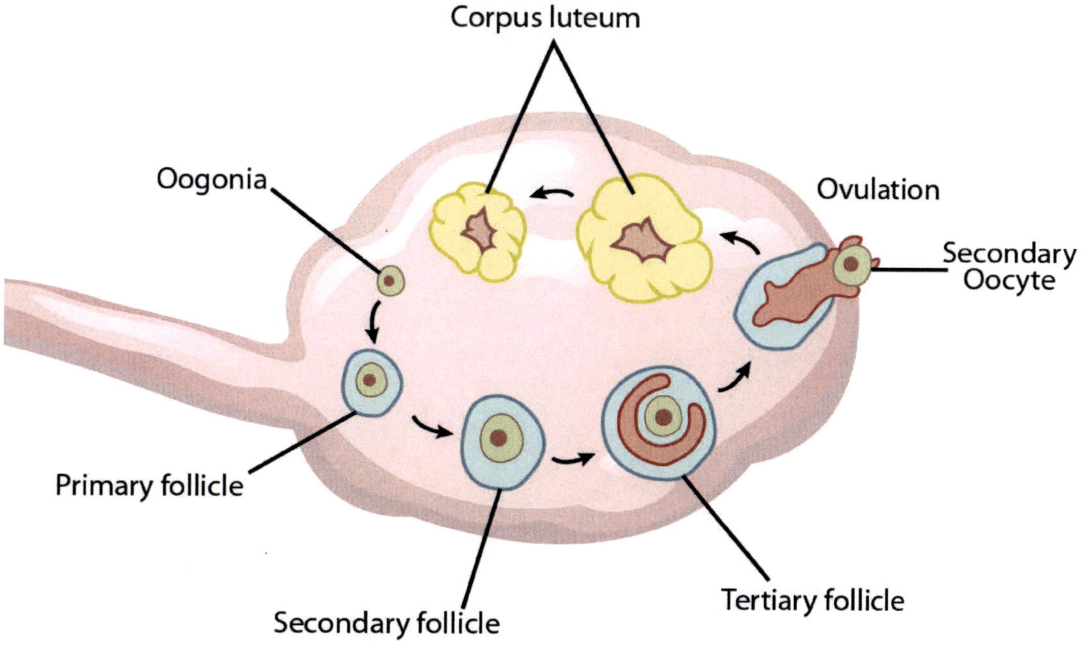

Figure 7.8 - Ovarian oogenesis

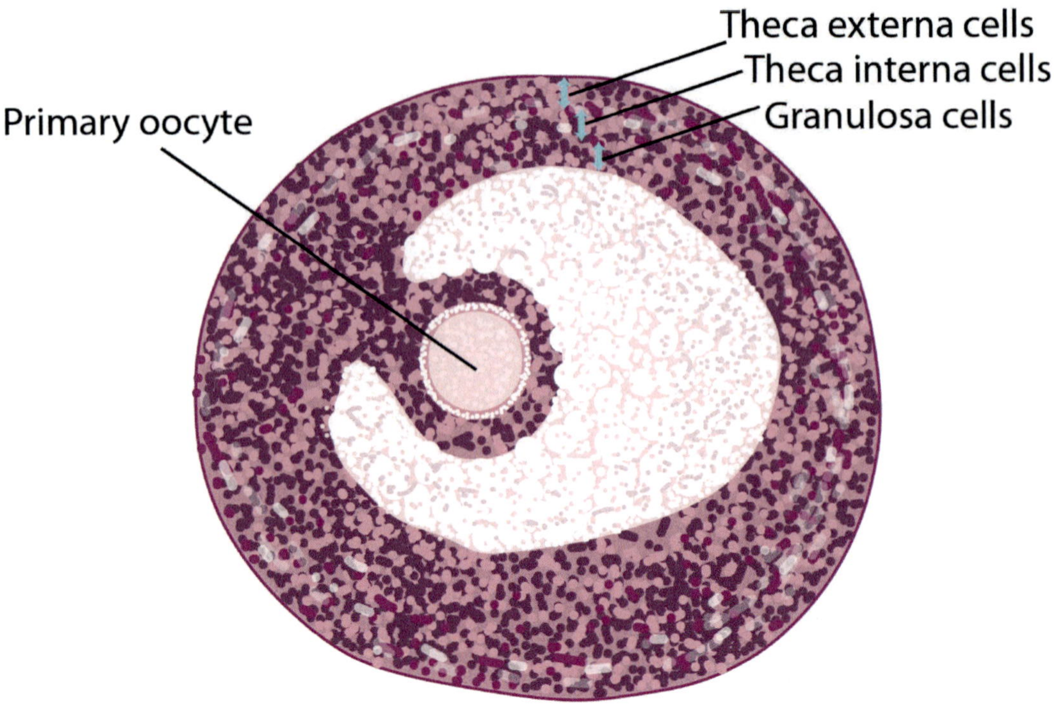

Figure 7.9 - Tertiary follicle

B. Ovarian follicles (Figure 7.9) are the functional unit of the ovaries.
   1. Follicles contain granulosa cells, theca cells, and the primary oocyte.
   2. Granulosa cells produce estrogens from androgens via aromatase.
      a) Estrogen stimulates endometrial proliferation.
   3. Theca interna cells produce androgens from cholesterol via desmolase.
   4. The corpus luteum is the product of a ruptured follicle.
      a) Produces progesterone which acts on the endometrium to stimulate proliferation and glandular secretion.

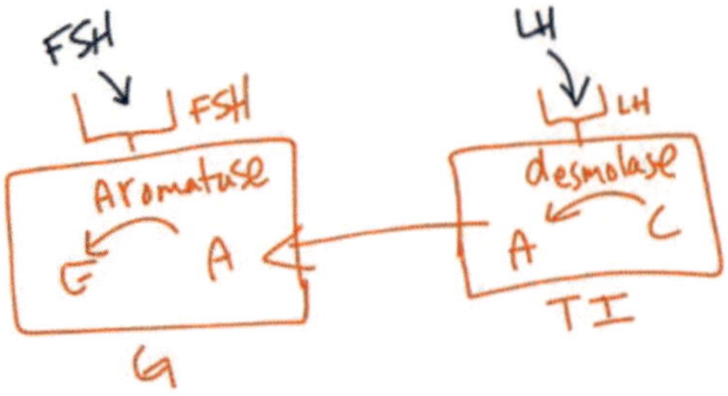

III. Menstrual Cycle (Figure 7.10)

A. The menstrual cycle is split into the follicular phase and the luteal phase.

B. The hypothalamus secretes GnRH which causes the anterior pituitary to secrete FSH and LH.

C. FSH and LH act on the granulosa cells and theca interna cells to produce estrogen.

D. Estrogen induces proliferation of the endometrium and is responsible for the LH surge.

E. The surge in LH causes the follicle to rupture.

F. After rupture, the follicle forms the corpus luteum which produces progesterone.

G. Progesterone acts on the endometrium to stimulate proliferation and glandular secretion. It's important in maintaining the endometrium and preventing menstrual flow.

H. If the oocyte is not fertilized, then the corpus luteum degenerates and the levels of estrogen and progesterone drop resulting in menstrual flow.

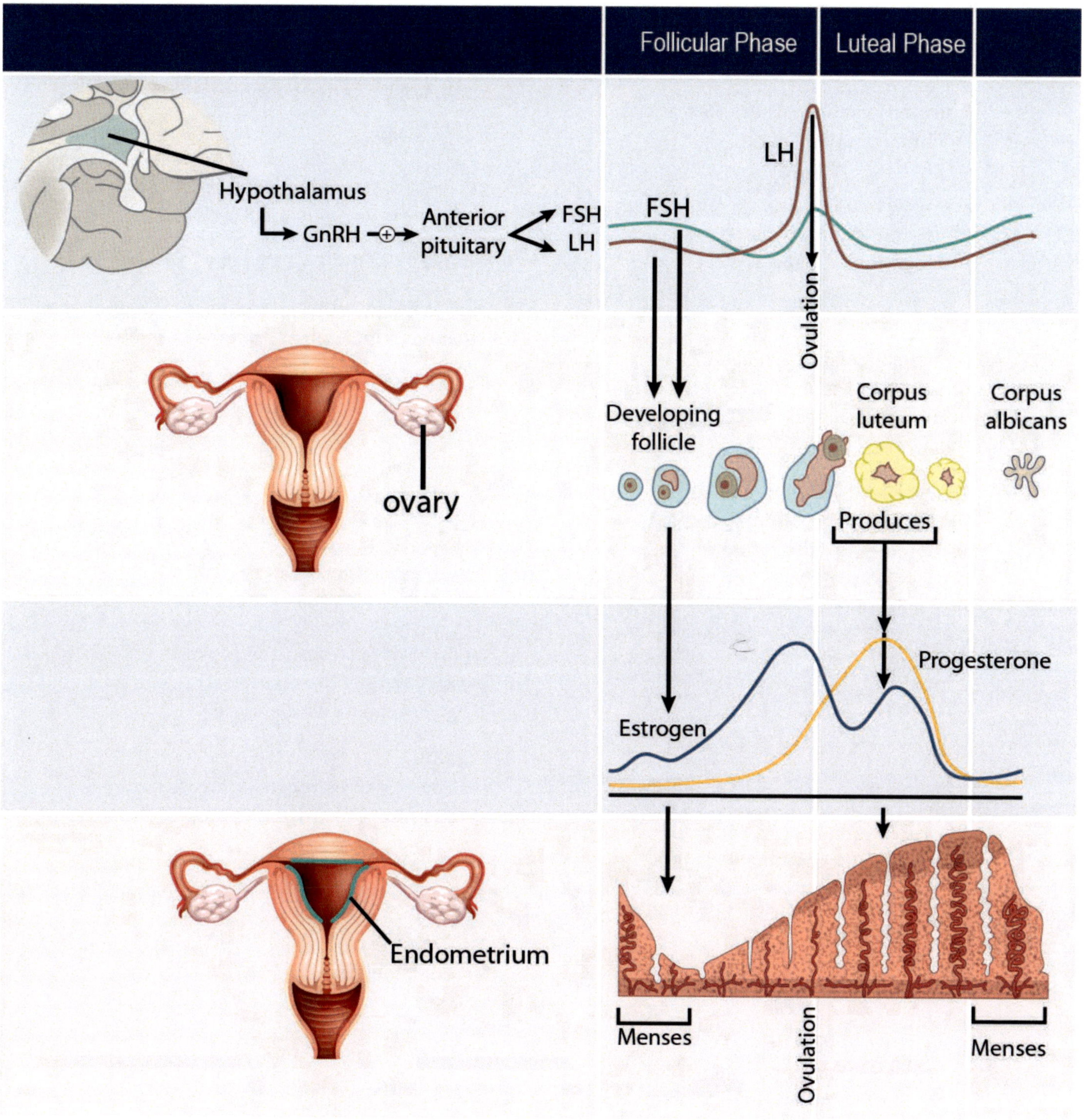

Figure 7.10 - Menstrual cycle overview

REVIEW QUESTIONS

1. Why does breastfeeding reduce the likelihood of pregnancy?

    - **↑ prolactin inhibits GnRH, FSH, and LH → ↓ likelihood of pregnancy**

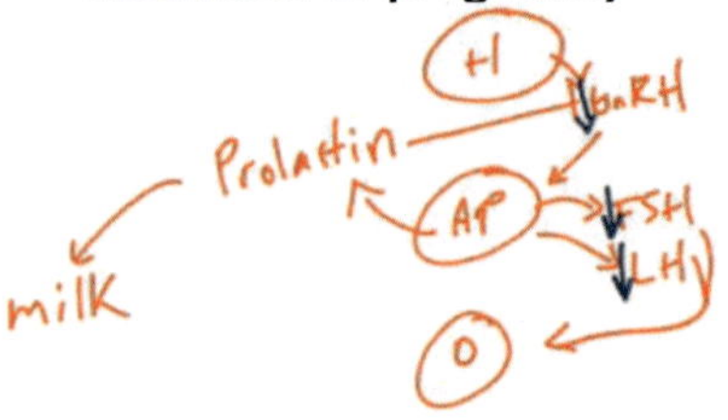

2. A 26-year-old female has had difficulty becoming pregnant and also complains of very heavy menstrual bleeding. What is the most likely diagnosis?

    - **Anovulatory cycle**
    - **The hypothalamic pituitary axis is disrupted → no corpus luteum forms → ↓ progesterone and ↑ estrogen → fragile endometrium**

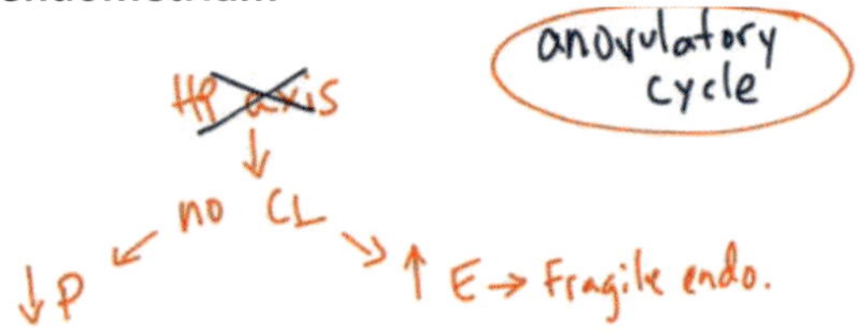

3. How is the hypothalamic pituitary axis altered in an extremely athletic woman?

    - **Exercise inhibits GnRH → ↓ FSH and LH**

↑exercise/diet → ↓GnRH → ↓FSH & LH → ↓E ↓P

4. What are the actions of pulsatile GnRH compared to continuous GnRH?

    - **Pulsatile: ↑ LH and FSH**
    - **continuous: ↓ LH and FSH**

pulsatile → ↑LH & ↑FSH
continuous → ↓LH & ↓FSH

Leuprolide

5. What drug is a GnRH analog and can have varying results depending on if it is administered continuously or in a pulsatile fashion?

    - **Leuprolide**

6. On what day does ovulation occur in a typical 28 day cycle of the menstrual cycle?

    - **Day 14 (28 - 14 = 14)24 day - 14 = day 10**

7. How is the hypothalamic pituitary axis altered in a patient with Turner syndrome?

    - **Turner syndrome → ovarian failure → ↓ estrogen → ↑ GnRH, FSH, and LH**

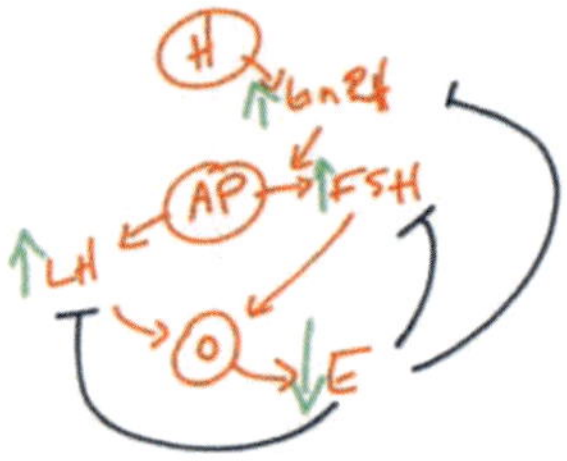

8. What would estrogen and progesterone levels be on day 12 of the menstrual cycle relative to day 19 of the menstrual cycle?

    - **28**
    - **day 12 = ↑ estrogen, ↓ progesterone**
    - **day 19 = ↓ estrogen, ↑ progesterone**

9. What medication can be helpful in treating patients who are unable to ovulate due to a lack of an LH surge?

    - **Clomiphene**

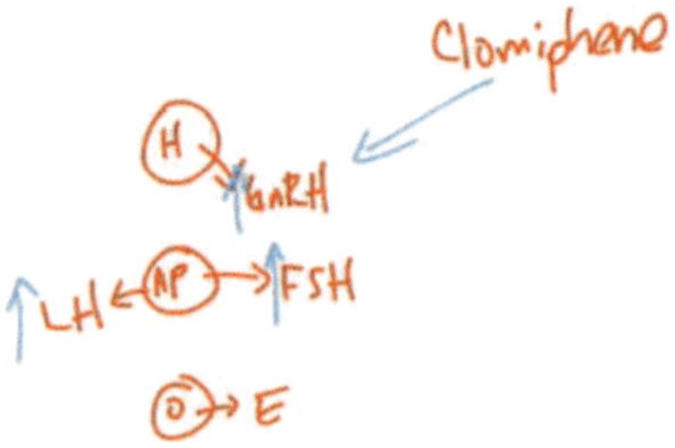

REVIEW QUESTIONS

10. A 5-year-old girl has symptoms of precocious puberty. The physician believes the symptoms may be due to a tumor. What hormone normally stimulates the likely tumor?

    - **Estrogen normally induces puberty in young females**
    - **Granulosa cell tumors can produce high levels of estrogen and induce precocious puberty**
    - **FSH stimulates granulosa cells to produce estrogen**

11. A woman with a normal 28 day menstrual cycle has high levels of estrogen and peaked levels of progesterone. What event is likely to occur in the next several days?

    - **On a typical 28 day menstrual cycle, ovulation occurs on day 14 and menstruation occurs on day 1**
    - **Several days before menstruation occurs, progesterone is at a peak and estrogen is also somewhat high**
    - **The patient is likely around day 24-25 in her menstrual cycle which means menstruation is likely to occur in the next several days**

12. How does progesterone impact lactation?

    - **Progesterone inhibits prolactin which inhibits breast milk production**
    - **The placenta produces progesterone so after delivery prolactin levels rise allowing lactation to occur**

Section IV - Pregnancy

I. Conception

A. Fertilization occurs on day 1 of ovulation → implantation 6 days later

B. First 8-10 weeks the syncytiotrophoblasts of embryo release hCG → corpus luteum continues to release progesterone and estradiol

C. Human Chorionic Gonadotropin

1. Maintains corpus luteum → continued release of progesterone for 8-10 weeks
2. Structurally similar to LH (as well as TSH and FSH) → hCG can act on leydig cells (increased testosterone) and theca interna cells (increased androgens)
3. Higher than non-pregnant patients, but lower than normal pregnancy
   a) Ectopic pregnancy
   b) Edward and Patau syndrome
   c) Non-viable pregnancy
4. Higher than normal pregnancy
   a) Pregnancy with down syndrome
   b) Hydatidiform moles/choriocarcinoma (follow-up by measuring serum hCG)
   c) Multiple gestations

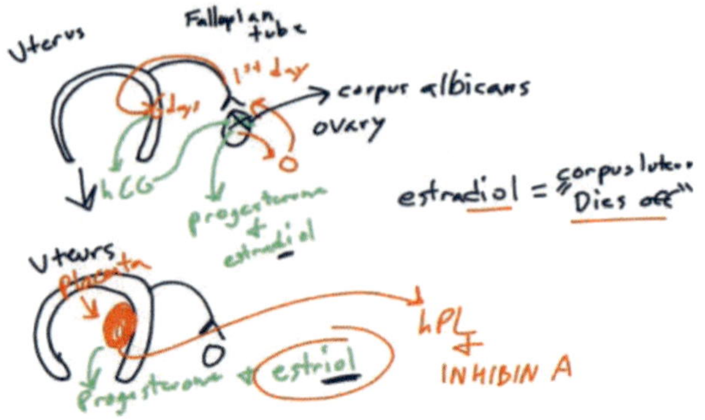

II. Pregnancy (Figure 7.11)

A. After 8-10 weeks the placenta will release:

1. Progesterone
   a) Released from corpus luteum and placenta
   b) Endometrial gland and spiral artery development (maintains endometrium)
   c) Breast development

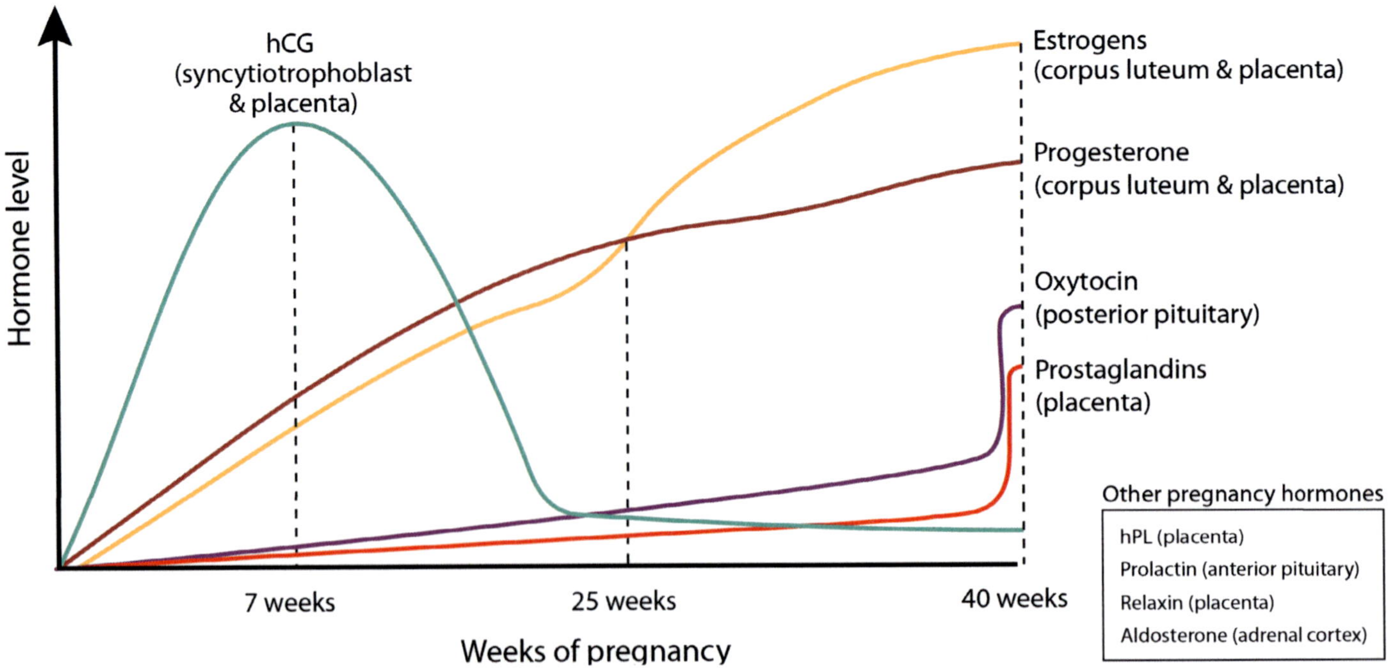

Figure 7.11 - Pregnancy Hormones

d) Decreases estrogen receptor stimulation (prevents uterine contractility)

e) Decreases myometrial excitability (contractions)

f) Causes vasodilation (↓ BP and ↓ PVR) → dilated carotid sinus and aortic sinus → decreased vagal tone → slightly increased heart rate

g) Acts centrally on the brainstem to increase respiratory rate.

2. Estrogens

a) Released from corpus luteum (estradiol) and placenta (estriol)

b) Endometrial proliferation

c) Increases myometrial excitability (inhibited by progesterone)

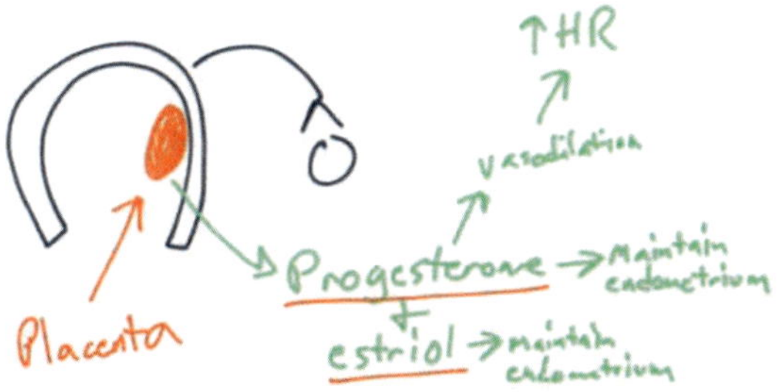

3. Human placental lactogen (hPL)

a) Human placental lactogen (hPL) → decreases maternal insulin sensitivity and increases maternal lipolysis → increased nutrients for fetus

b) Gestational diabetes: increased maternal serum glucose → excess glucose in fetus → increased insulin release in fetus → insulin acts as growth factor leading to enlarged fetus (macrosomia)

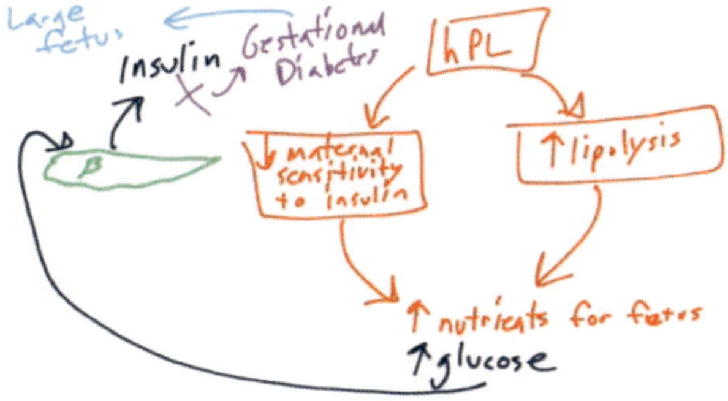

4. The placenta also releases:

a) Inhibin A (used in maternal quadruple screen)

b) Relaxin

(1) Relaxes pubic symphysis and pelvic ligaments → easier passage of fetus

(2) Cervical dilation during labor

c) Renal changes

(1) Renal arteriole vasodilation → increased GFR → increased urinary frequency and decreased Cr

d) Prostaglandins (see Delivery)

III. Other Hormones of Pregnancy

A. Aldosterone

1. Released from adrenal cortex

2. Increased water reabsorption from collecting duct → increased plasma volume → increased cardiac output

B. Prolactin is released from the anterior pituitary

1. Prepares mammary glands for milk production

IV. Physiologic Changes During Pregnancy

A. Hematologic

1. Increased plasma volume and decreased viscosity (aldosterone → reabsorption)

2. Upregulation of clotting factors

3. Lower HCT (↑ RBC mass < ↑ plasma volume)

B. Cardiovascular

1. Slightly increased heart rate (progesterone → vasodilation)

2. Increased cardiac output (increased plasma volume, preload)

3. ↓ BP and ↓ PVR

C. Renal

1. Increased urinary frequency (relaxin → renal arteriole dilation → increased GFR)

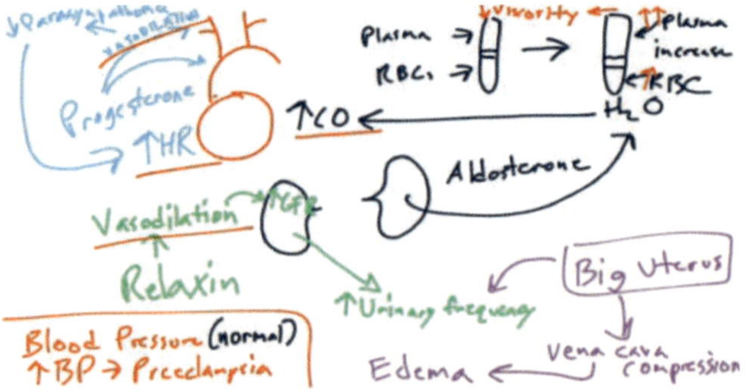

2. ↓ Cr

3. Physiologic hydronephronism R>L

D. Pulmonary

1. ↑ TV → respiratory alkalosis (↓ CO_2)

2. ↓ FRC

E. GI

1. Relaxation of LES → reflux

2. ↑ ALP from placenta

V. Maternal Quadruple Screen (Table 7.1)

A. Includes 3 hormones produced by the placenta:

1. ß-hCG

2. Estriol

3. Inhibin A

B. Includes one hormone produced by the fetal GI tract, liver and yolk sac:

1. Alpha fetoprotein (AFP)

C. All four should increase throughout pregnancy

1. If different than expected → think dating error or pathology

VI. Delivery (Parturition)

A. Pre-labor

1. Increased estrogen:progesterone ratio → increased uterine stretching → oxytocin released from posterior pituitary → mild uterine contractions (false labor/Braxton-Hick contractions)

B. Labor

1. Fetal stress → fetal release of cortisol → prostaglandin release from placenta → uterine and cervical stretch → maternal release of oxytocin → increased uterine contractions → increased release of prostaglandins → perpetuation of uterine contractions

Table 7.1 - Genetic Disorders

Genetic Disorder	AFP	β-hCG	Estriol	Inhibin A
Trisomy 13 (Patau Syndrome)	Normal	↓	Normal	Normal
Trisomy 18 (Edward Syndrome)	↓	↓	↓	Normal
Trisomy 21 (Down Syndrome)	↓	↑	↓	↑

REVIEW QUESTIONS

1. A researcher is performing a study and evaluates the levels of hCG, progesterone, and estrogen in a patient at 8 weeks gestation and a woman at 35 weeks gestation. What will be the relative levels of these hormones for both patients?

    - **At 8 weeks gestation: hCG > progesterone > estrogen**
    - **At 35 weeks gestation: estrogen > progesterone > hCG**

2. A 22-year-old, sexually active female presents with sharp abdominal pain and elevated β-hCG. What is the likely diagnosis?

    - **Elevated β-hCG should make you think of several conditions. The abdominal pain raise the suspicion of ectopic pregnancy**

ectopic pregnancy → lower than normal pregnancy
Edwards Syndrome →
Patau Syndrome →

multiple gestations
hydatidiform mole
choriocarcinoma
Down Syndrome

3. A pregnant 30-year-old female presents at 7 weeks gestation. Serum analysis demonstrates abnormally low hCG. What risks does this pose to the developing fetus?

    - **Without corpus luteum, there will not be enough progesterone to maintain the pregnancy**

↓hCG → Corpus luteum degenerates to corpus albicans
↓
Progesterone (8-10 weeks) → spontaneous abortion

28 weeks
↓
placenta provides progesterone

4. A pregnant female at 30 weeks gestation demonstrates a recent onset of elevated blood sugar. What would be the expected insulin level in her and what would be the expected insulin level in the fetus?

    - **High amounts of glucose will cross the placenta, stimulating fetal release of insulin**
    - **Note: Maternal insulin is too large to cross the placenta**

5. Following birth, the infant becomes hypoglycemic. Why?

    - **Upon birth, transplacental glucose will decrease, but fetal insulin levels are slow to decrease, leading to fetal hypoglycemia**

6. A pregnant woman at 18 weeks gestation states that she read online that some pregnant women develop dilated cardiomyopathy. This is her first pregnancy and she wants to make sure she and the baby are healthy. Her vitals are all within normal limits. Why might pregnancy increase the risk for dilated cardiomyopathy?

    - **Increased plasma volume can lead to increased stretch on the heart**
    - **Disequilibrium of fluid and cardiac function can result in HF**

↑Aldosterone → ↑plasma volume → ↑EDV → SV → CO
→ stretching of heart → HF

7. A pregnant woman develops a deep vein thrombosis (DVT). Why was she more likely to develop a blood clot than a non-pregnant individual? Is her blood more viscous?

    - **Although clotting factors increase in pregnancy, increasing risk of DVT, plasma volume is increased and results in decreased viscosity of blood**

8. A pregnant patient at 21 weeks gestation has sufficient levels of progesterone. How will this affect her heart?

    - **Progesterone increases vasodilation and decreases vagal tone, resulting in an overall sympathetic effect on the heart (increased heart rate)**

VASODILATION → ↓vagal tone
↓
↑sympathetic → ↑HR

REVIEW QUESTIONS

9. A woman is 33 weeks pregnant and the maternal quadruple screen test is administered. Results show that everything is normal except β-hCG. The clinician notes that the β-hCG is higher than for non-pregnant individuals but is lower than expected for a patient at 33 weeks gestation. What does this scenario indicate?

- **AFP, estradiol and inhibin A are all normal**
- **β-hCG is low for someone at 33 weeks gestation (though still high for a non-pregnant individual)**
- **Suspect trisomy 13**

A(B)E − I (B ↓)
Trisomy 13 "B-low 13"

10. A clinician administers the maternal quadruple screen test to a pregnant patient at 26 weeks gestation. The levels of each of the 4 components are higher than what would be expected at 26 weeks gestation. What is the cause of the high levels?

- **If all are elevated, aneuploidy is unlikely.**
- **Suspect that she is higher along in gestation than 26 weeks**

↑ (A B E − I)
likely >26 weeks gestation

13 − "B-low 13"
18 − "ABE is 18"
21 − "BI is high"

11. A pregnant female presents concern about having a baby with Down syndrome. You order a maternal quadruple screen. If the screen indicates a positive result, what would be the levels of each of the 4 components?

- **High β-hCG and inhibin A**
- **Low AFP and estradiol**

12. A female at 34 weeks gestation says that she is experiencing mild contractions that occur every few days. She has never been pregnant before this pregnancy and she is concerned she is about to deliver. If she is experiencing false labor contractions, how would you describe the oxytocin and prostaglandin levels?

- **False labor would not have elevated oxytocin and prostaglandins, as in true labor**

false labor/Braxton-Hicks (↑E/P)
↓oxytocin + ↓Prostaglandins

13. A female patient at 39 weeks gestation would like to induce labor. She is given the option of having a vaginal prostaglandin-releasing sepository, which she accepts. How would the prostaglandin sepository induce labor?

- **Cervical ripening increases oxytocin release, leading to contractions and further release of prostaglandins**

Prostaglandins → vagina → cervical ripening → Oxytocin → ↑ contractions → Prostaglandins

Section V - Integrated Female Physiology

I. Menopause is the time in a woman's life when menstruation ceases.

   A. Caused by a decrease in estrogen due to a depletion of oocytes

      1. Estrogen

         a) Primary female sex hormone

         b) Necessary for the development of primary and secondary sexual characteristics

         c) Increases glandular secretions of the vagina and cervix resulting in increased vaginal lubrication

         d) Acts on the epiphyseal growth plate to stimulate bone growth

         e) Inhibits osteoblast apoptosis and promotes osteoclast apoptosis

         f) Increases HDL and decreases LDL

         g) Acts on the liver resulting in increased concentrations of many coagulation proteins. Also decreases antithrombin III which can result in an overall increased risk of thrombosis if estrogen concentrations become excessive

         h) Acts on the uterus to stimulate endometrial proliferation

         i) Upregulates HMG-CoA reductase → increased cholesterol synthesis

II. Polycystic ovarian syndrome (PCOS) is a disorder caused by excess androgens.

   A. Although the exact mechanism is not entirely clear, there is evidence suggesting that adrenal enzymes (i.e. 17α-hydroxylase and 17,20-lyase) that convert cholesterol to androgens are upregulated.

   B. Genetic, environmental, and other factors may also contribute to disruption of the hypothalamic pituitary axis resulting in elevated levels of FSH and LH.

   C. Excess LH stimulates the theca interna cells to convert cholesterol to androgens.

   D. Excess androgens from the theca interna cells and the adrenal glands interfere with the normal development of follicles resulting in anovulatory cycles.

   E. Because the corpus luteum is unable to form, progesterone concentrations are decreased resulting in an imbalance of estrogen and progesterone.

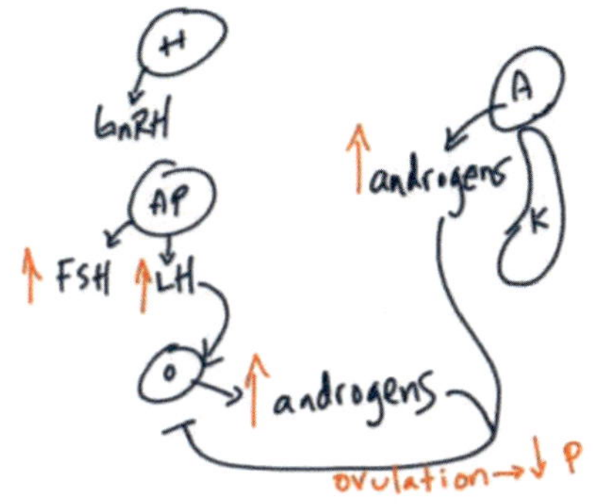

III. Aromatase Deficiency

   A. Aromatase converts androgens to estrogens in the gonads and peripheral tissues.

   B. A deficiency in females results in accumulation of androgens, resulting in infantile virilization.

   C. Males are unaffected.

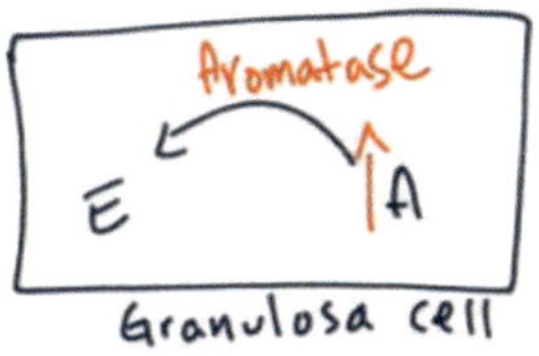

REVIEW QUESTIONS ?

1. How can oral contraceptive pills reduce the risk of developing ovarian tumors?

   - **OCPs inhibit ovulation → ↓ cellular damage and repair → ↓ risk of cancer**

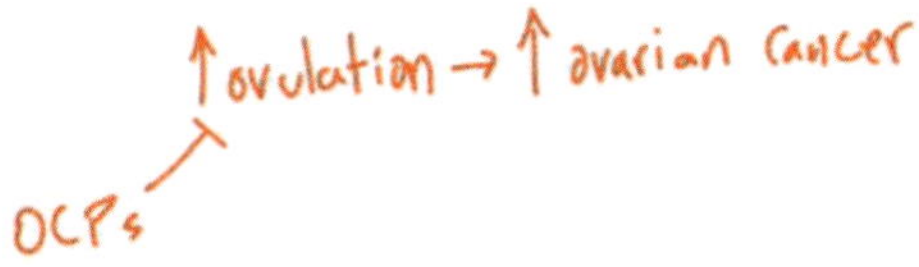

REVIEW QUESTIONS

2. What causes hot flashes in menopausal women?

- **A drop in estrogen**

↓E → H → ↑ vasodilation

3. A newborn baby has ambiguous genitalia. A detailed history is taken from the mother who states that during pregnancy her voice deepened and dark hair began to develop on her face. What is the most likely diagnosis?

- **Aromatase deficiency**
- **Excess androgens from the fetus crossed through the placenta resulting in maternal symptoms**

4. A 50-year-old female presents with amenorrhea and vaginal dryness. How will the levels of GnRH, FSH, LH, inhibin B, and estrogen likely compare to a healthy 23-year-old female?

- **Menopause → ↓ estrogen and inhibin B → ↑ GnRH, LH, and FSH**

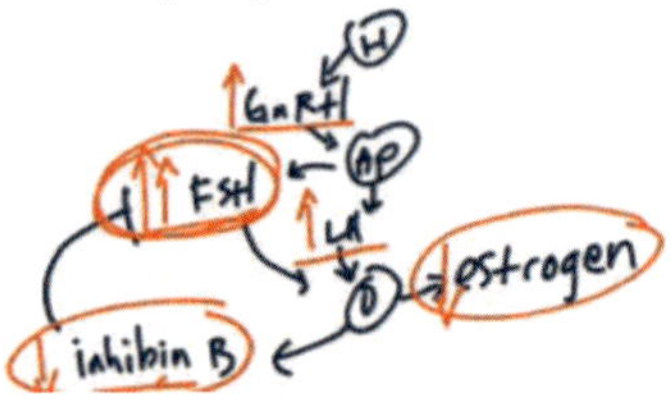

5. What changes would likely occur to the uterus as a result of using tamoxifen? Why can this drug increase the risk for thrombosis?

- **Tamoxifen is an estrogen receptor antagonist in breast tissue and an agonist in uterine and liver tissue → ↑ risk of uterine cancer and ↑ risk of thrombosis**

(breast = antagonist)
(uterus = agonist)
(liver = agonist)
↳ ↑ thrombosis

6. A 24-year-old obese female presents to the office due to concerns of infertility. Upon exam you notice she has dark hair around her lips and neck. How will the plasma concentration of LH, androgens, and progesterone compare to that of a healthy 24-year-old woman?

- **PCOS → ↑ androgens from adrenal glands → inhibition of ovulation**
- **PCOS → ↑ insulin → ↑ FSH and LH → ↑ androgen production from theca interna cells → inhibition of ovulation**
- **Ovulation doesn't occur → no corpus luteum → ↓ progesterone**

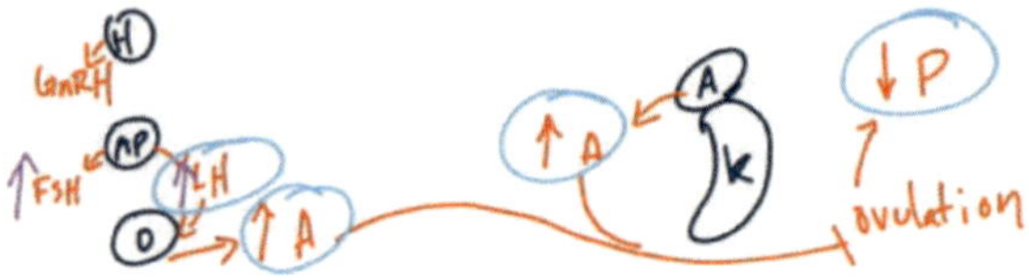

7. What type of oral contraception may be helpful in reducing the risk of osteoporosis?

- **OCPs containing estrogen**
- **Estrogen inhibits osteoblast apoptosis → ↑ osteoblasts → ↑ bone**
- **Estrogen promotes osteoclast apoptosis → ↓ osteoclasts → ↓ bone**
- **What ovarian tumor would likely cause hyperplasia of the endometrium?**

OCP ⊣ LH & FSH
(estrogen)
↑ osteoblasts → ↑ bone
↓ osteoclasts → ↓ bone

8. What ovarian tumor would likely cause hyperplasia of the endometrium?

- **A granulosa cell tumor**
- **Production of excess estrogen → hyperplasia of the endometrium → increased risk for endometrial cancer**

9. A 65-year-old female presents for a routine physical. How will her lipid panel likely compare to a healthy 25-year-old woman?

- **↑ HDL**
- **↓ LDL**

↓ estrogen → ↑HDL ↓
↳ ↓LDL ↑

NEUROLOGY

Section I - Cerebral Hemispheres

I. Cerebral Hemispheres and Landmarks

A. Sulci and fissures are the grooves of the brain.

1. Longitudinal fissure (Figure 8.1)
2. Lateral sulci
3. Central sulci (Figure 8.2)
4. Parieto-occipital sulci (Figure 8.3)

B. Lobes

1. Frontal lobe
   a) This region of the brain is responsible for judgement, concentration, orientation, and primitive reflexes.
   b) The primary motor cortex is the location of all of the upper motor neurons that are responsible for movement.
   c) The frontal eye field region is associated with eye movement.
   d) Broca's area is responsible for motor speech.
2. Parietal lobe
   a) The primary sensory cortex processes all sensory input from the contralateral side of the body.
   b) The angular gyrus is involved in performing mathematical calculations, writing, distinguishing left from right, and identifying fingers on the hand.
   c) Damage to the dominant parietal cortex results in Gerstmann syndrome.
   d) Damage to the non-dominant parietal cortex results in hemispatial neglect.
3. Temporal lobe
   a) Superior temporal gyrus
      (1) Contains the primary auditory cortex
      (2) Contains Wernicke's area
   b) The hippocampus is responsible for memory formation (Figure 8.4 and 8.5).

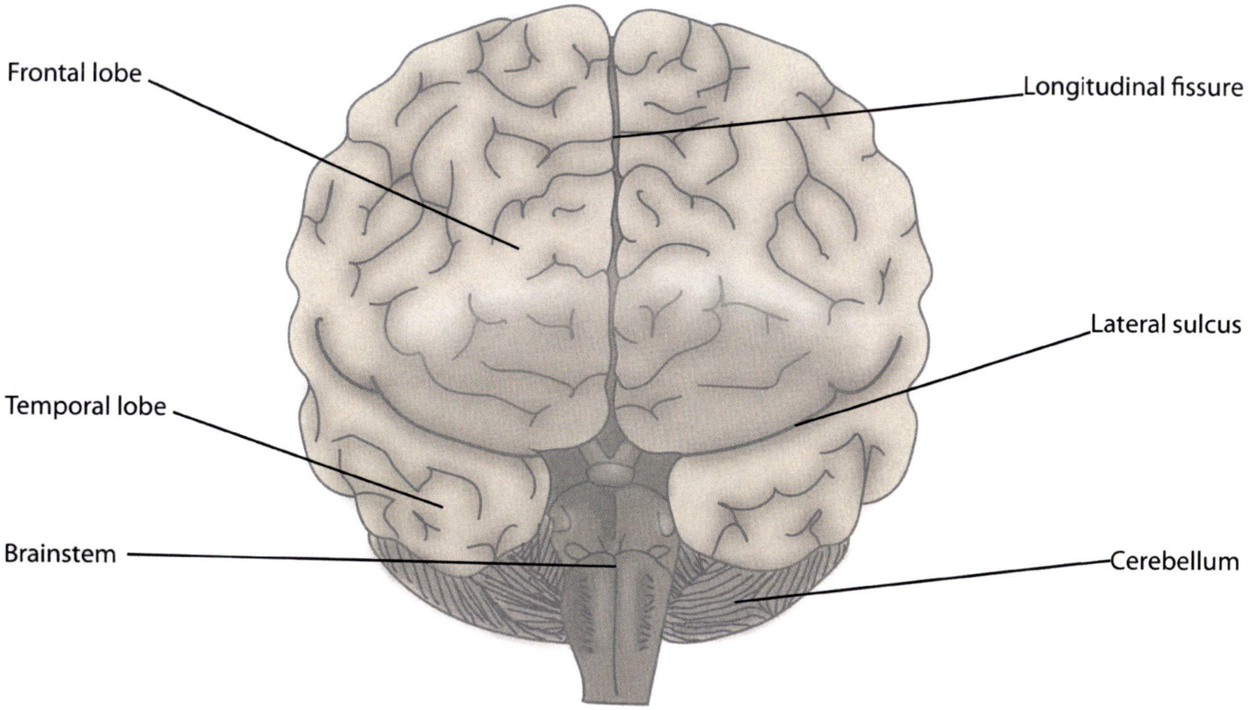

Figure 8.1 - Anterior view of the brain

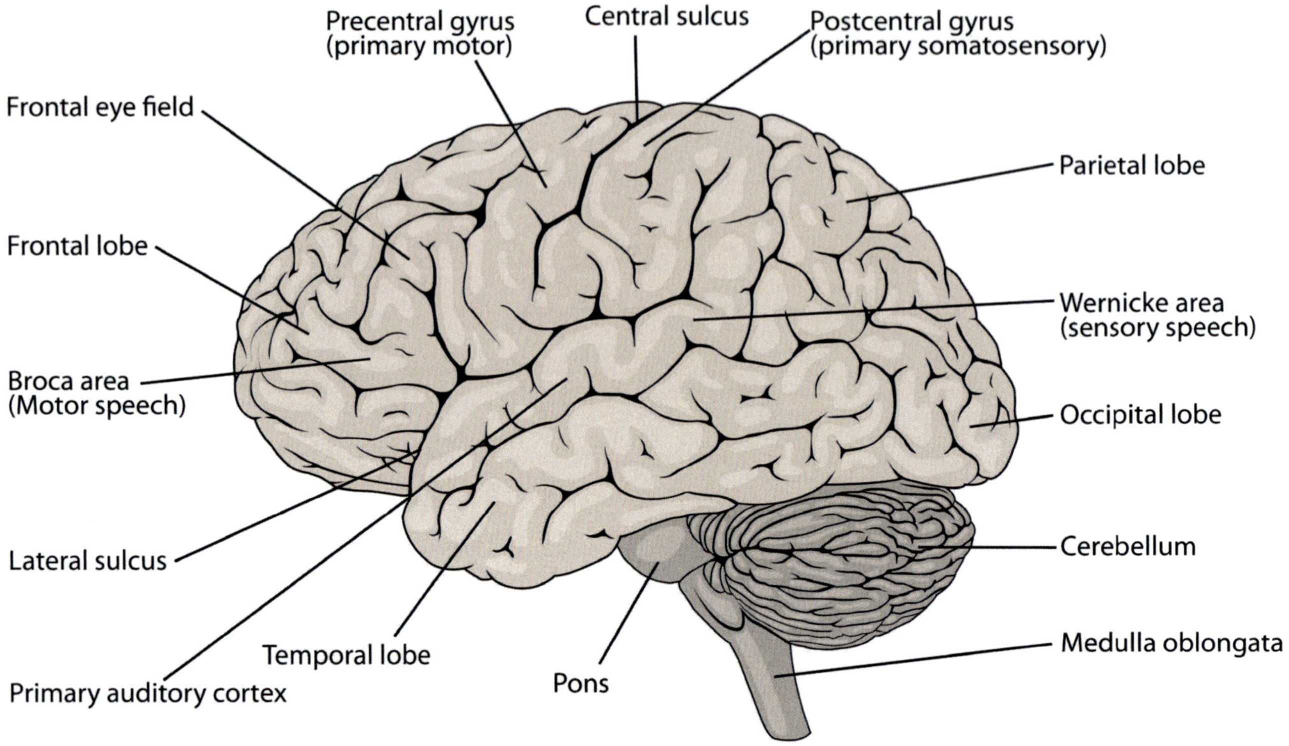

Figure 8.2 - Lateral view of the brain

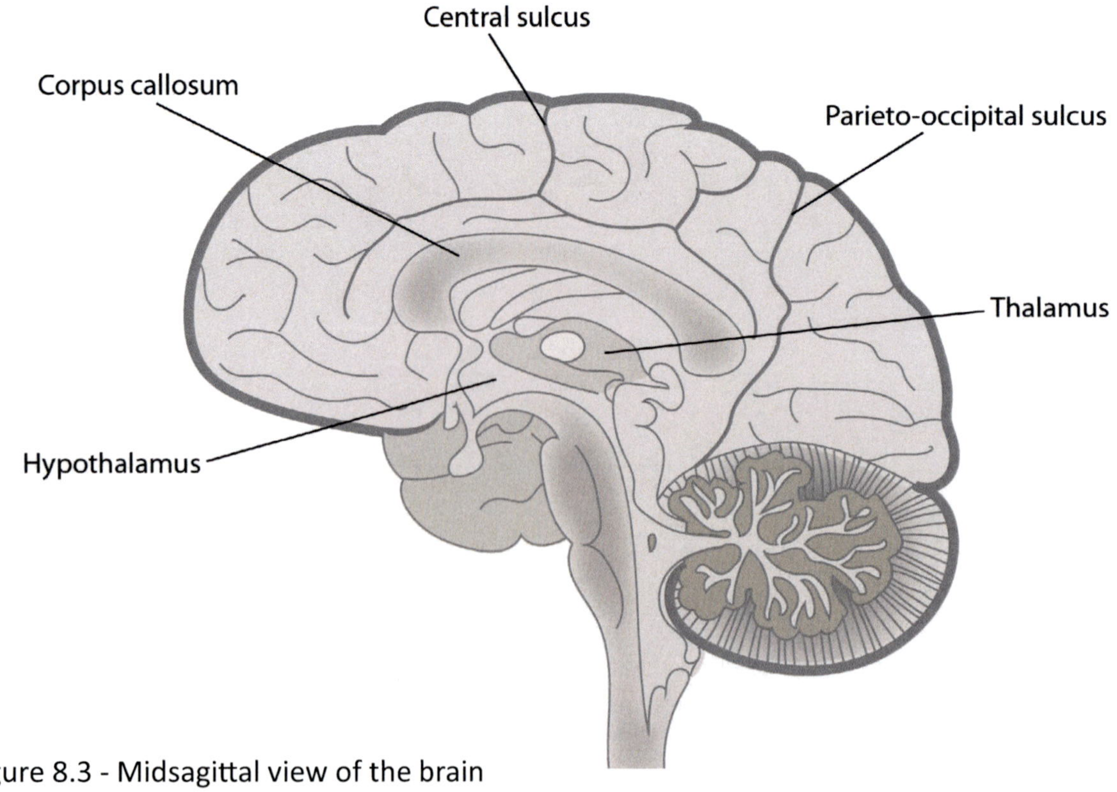

Figure 8.3 - Midsagittal view of the brain

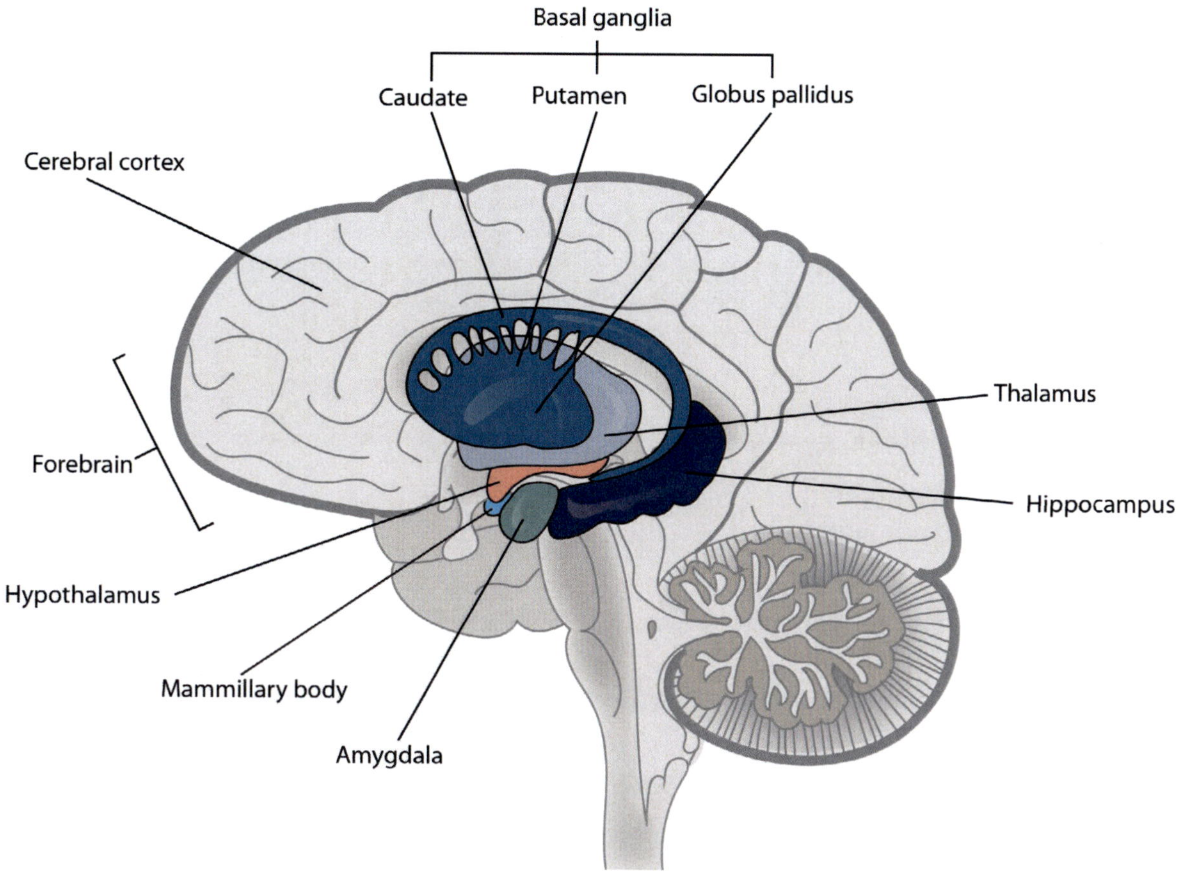

Figure 8.4 - The limbic system and basal ganglia

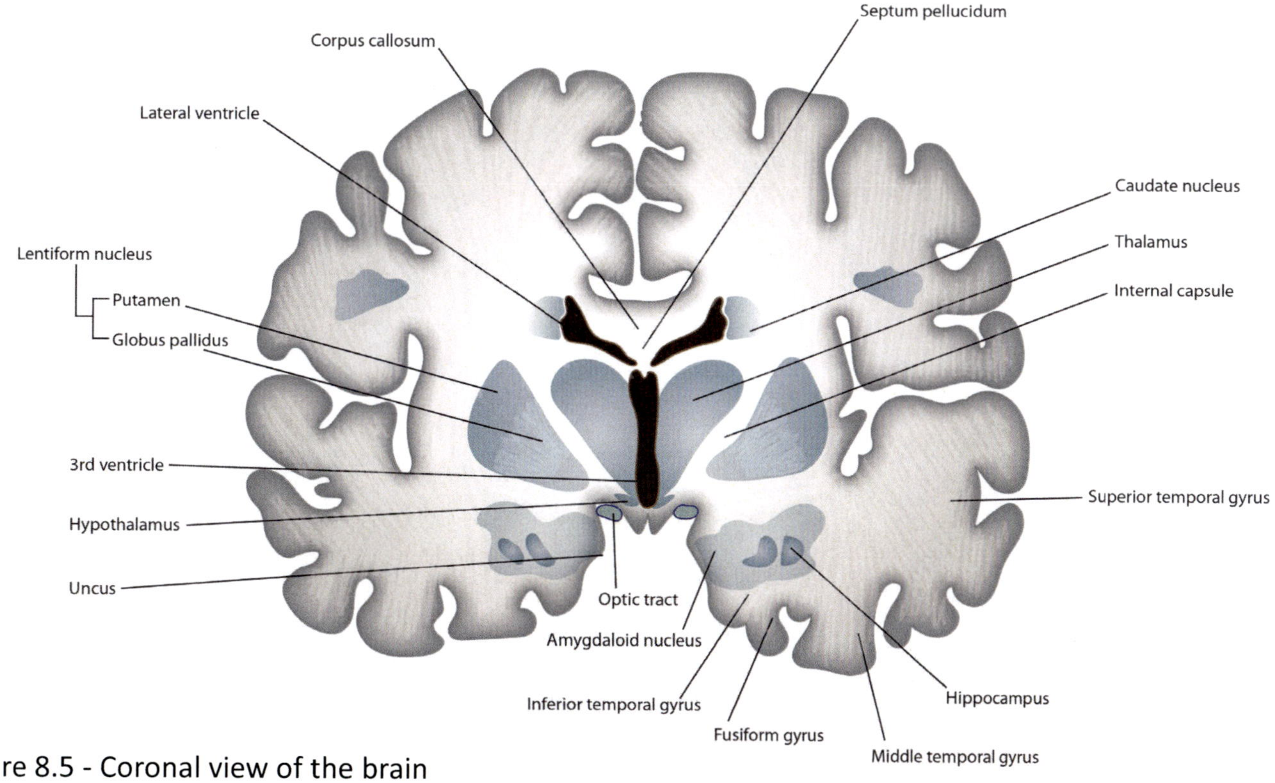

Figure 8.5 - Coronal view of the brain

c) The amygdala is associated with emotions and decision making.

d) The fusiform gyrus is responsible for facial recognition.

e) The uncus is associated with seizures and can compress the third cranial nerve during an uncal herniation.

4. Occipital lobe

a) Primary visual cortex

II. Homunculus (Figure 8.6)

A. A representation of the body superimposed over the precentral and postcentral gyri

1. The precentral gyrus is responsible for movement of the contralateral side.
2. The postcentral gyrus is responsible for tactile sensation of the contralateral side.

III. Internal Capsule (Figure 8.7)

A. Anterior limb

B. Posterior limb

1. The anterior ⅔ of the posterior limb contains motor fibers of the corticospinal tract.
2. The posterior ⅓ of the posterior limb contains sensory fibers of the thalamocortical tract.

C. Genu

1. Contains motor fibers of the corticobulbar tract

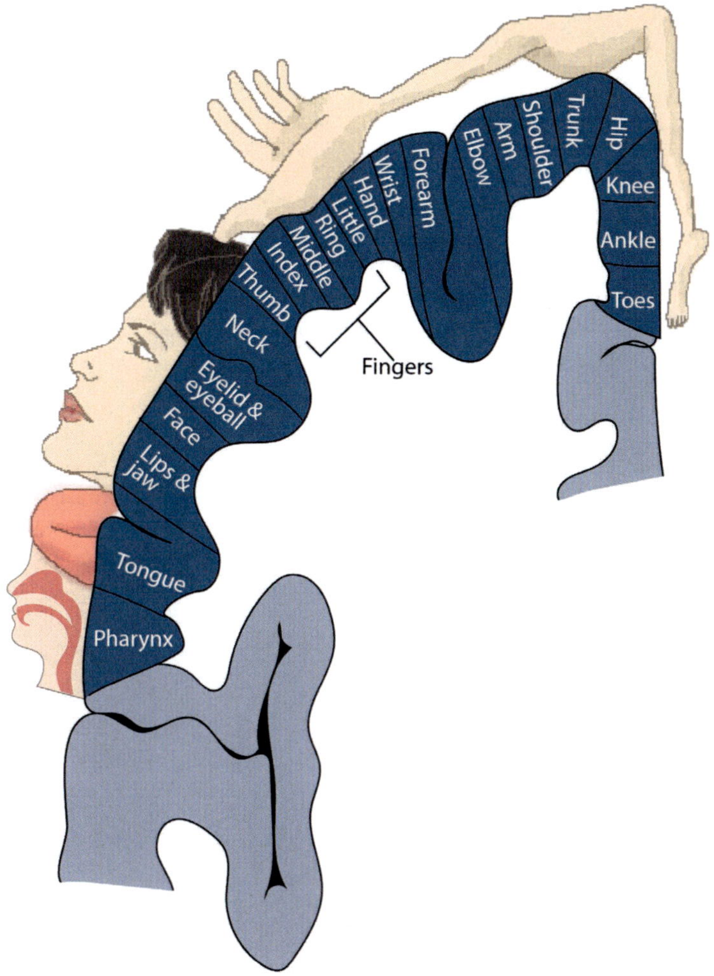

Figure 8.6 - The homunculus

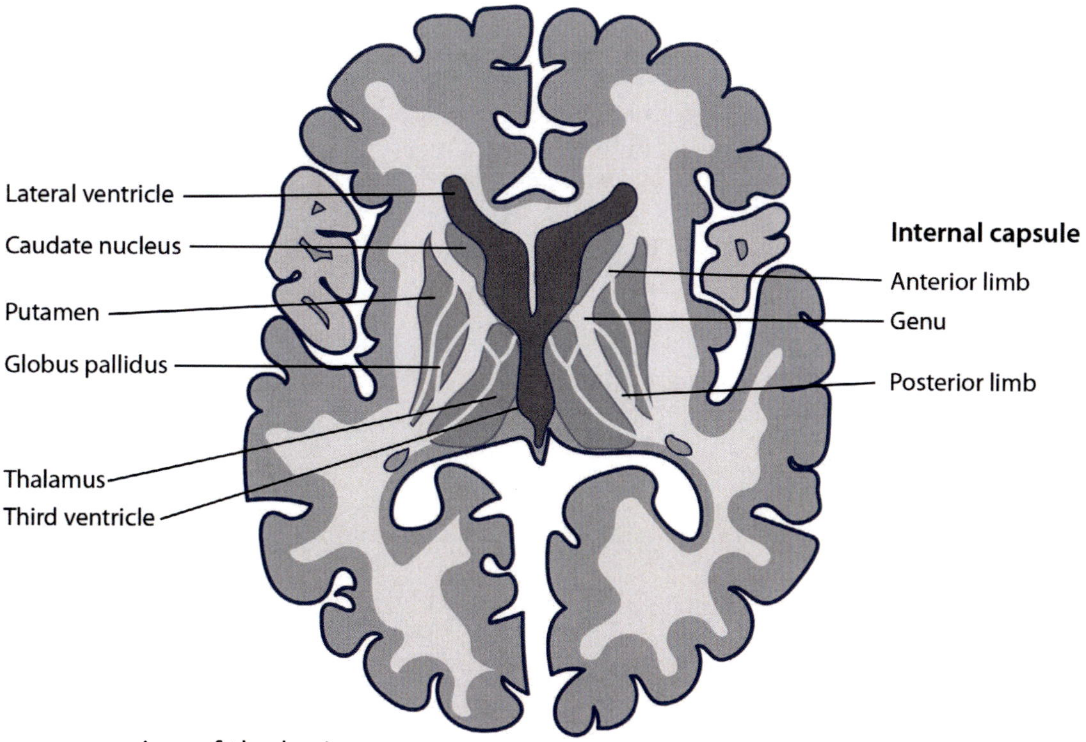

Figure 8.7 - Transverse view of the brain

REVIEW QUESTIONS

1. What symptoms should you suspect in a patient who has damaged the left primary motor cortex?
    - **Right-sided paralysis**
2. How would the left and right eyes be impacted if the left frontal eye field region was damaged?
    - **Left-sided deviation**
3. A 64-year-old right-handed female is brought to the ED after the sudden onset of tingling and burning on the right side of her body. Upon examination there is a complete loss of sensation of the right arm. What region of the brain is damaged?
    - **Left primary sensory cortex (the parietal lobe)**
4. If the entire parietal lobe was involved, what other symptoms would you suspect in this patient (see question above)?
    - **The patient is right-handed → left hemisphere is dominant**
    - **Damage to the angular gyrus of the dominant parietal lobe → Gerstmann syndrome (agraphia, acalculi, finger agnosia, and left-right disorientation)**
5. A 63-year-old male had a stroke one week ago and he no longer recognizes his wife or children when they enter the room. What region of the brain was likely damaged?
    - **The patient has prosopagnosia (can't recognize faces) due to damage to the fusiform gyrus of the temporal lobe**
6. A tumor originating from the medial aspect of the right parieto-occipital sulcus projects anteriorly, compressing the postcentral gyrus. What symptoms would this patient likely experience?
    - **Tumor compresses the medial aspect of the right postcentral gyrus (primary sensory cortex) → sensory abnormalities in the contralateral leg (left leg)**

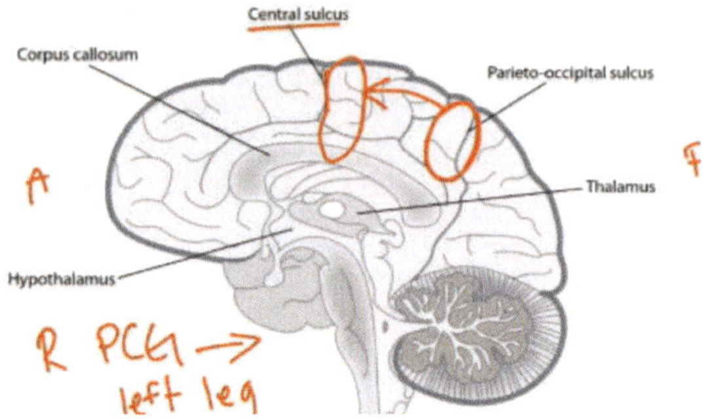

7. A 70-year-old woman presents with paralysis of the right leg. What region of the brain is likely damaged?
    - **The medial aspect of the left precentral gyrus (primary motor cortex)**

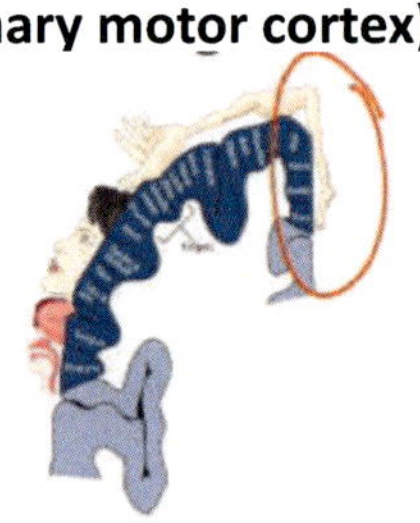

Section II - Spinal Cord, Spinal Tracts, and UMN and LMN

I. Spinal Cord (Figure 8.8)

A. Identification (Figures 8.9 and 8.10)

1. White matter in the spinal cord increases as you move superiorly.
   a) Ascending tracts (dorsal column and spinothalamic tracts) collect as you move up.
   b) Descending tracts (corticospinal tracts) decrease as you move down.
2. The spinal levels T1-L2 are unique because they contain lateral horns.
3. Lumbar and sacral spinal cross sections appear similar. Lumbar is just larger.

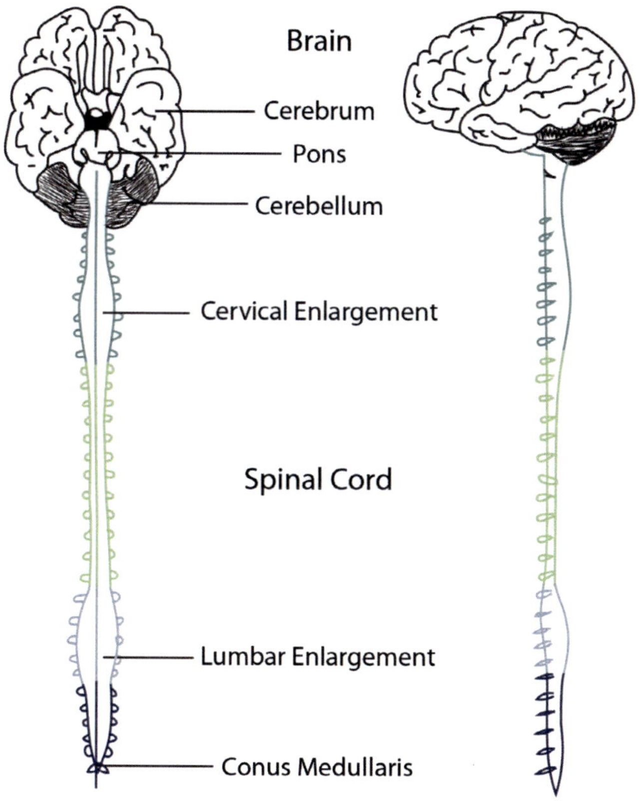

Figure 8.8 - Spinal Cord

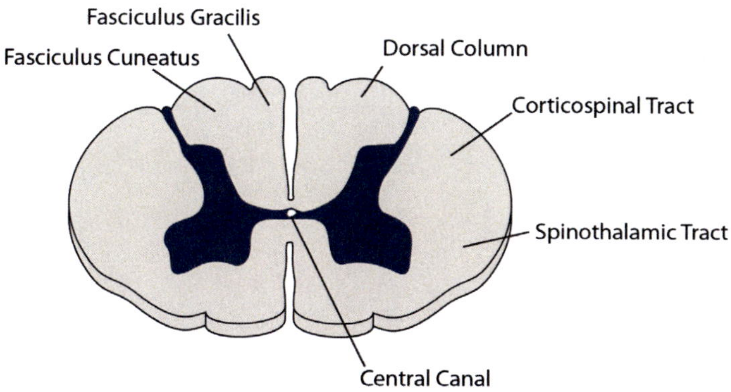

Figure 8.9 - Spinal Cord Cross-Section

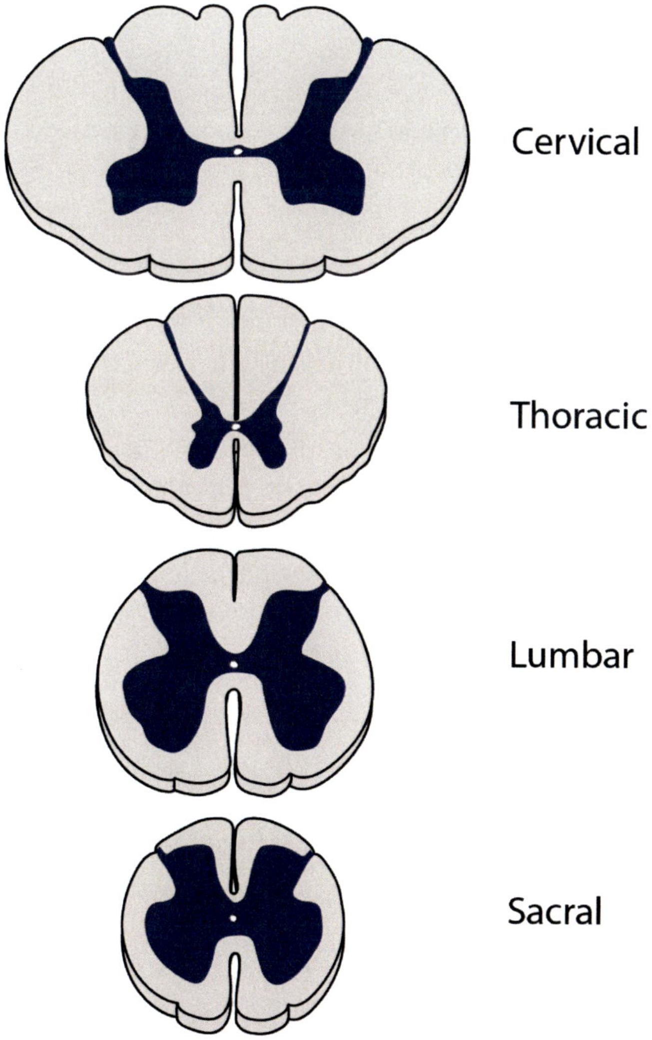

Figure 8.10 - Spinal Cord Levels

B. Spinal nerves (Figure 8.11)

1. All exit above their respective vertebrae from C1 down through C7.
2. C8 exits below C7 and above T1.
3. All exit below their respective vertebrae from T1 down through S5.

C. Lumbar puncture and epidural anesthesia (Figure 8.12)

1. The spinal cord terminates around L1-L2 of the vertebral column but the dura continues until S1-S2.
2. The needle is inserted at L3/L4 or L4/L5 - low enough to avoid the spinal cord and high enough to be within the dural sac.

II. Spinal Tracts

A. Dorsal column (Figure 8.13)

1. Responsible for proprioception and vibration sensation
2. 1st neuron enters DRG → travels up through dorsal column (fasciculus gracilis or fasciculus cuneatus) → synapses in medulla on nucleus gracilis or nucleus cuneatus → 2nd neuron decussates to contralateral medial lemniscus and travels up → synapses on ventroposterolateral (VPL) nucleus in thalamus → 3rd neuron travels to ipsilateral somatosensory cortex
3. Romberg test
    a) Used to identify cause of ataxia (e.g. dorsal column damage v. cerebellar ataxia)
    b) To remain standing, patients require two of the following: proprioception, vision, and vestibular function.
        (1) A patient with absent proprioception (dorsal column damage) will lose balance upon closing their eyes because they are left with only vestibular function.

B. Spinothalamic tracts (Figure 8.14)

1. Responsible for pain and temperature sensation
2. 1st neuron enters DRG → synapses in ipsilateral gray matter posterior horn →

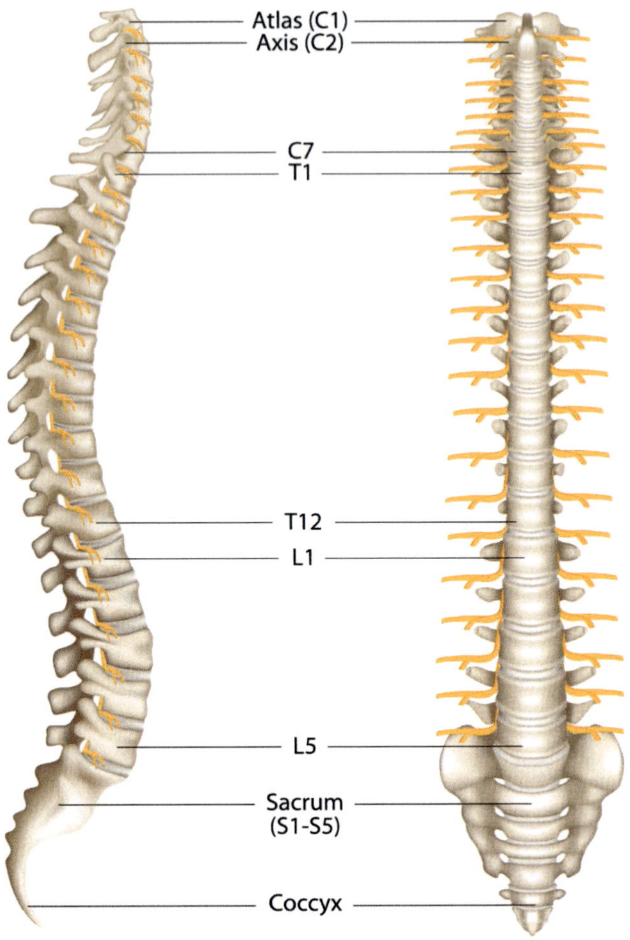

Figure 8.11 - Spinal Nerves

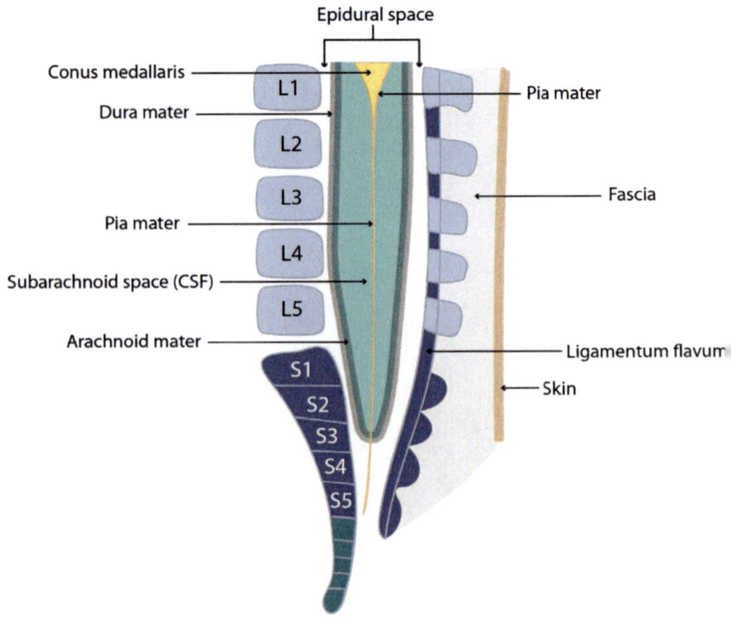

Figure 8.12 - Lumbar Spinal Cord and Layers

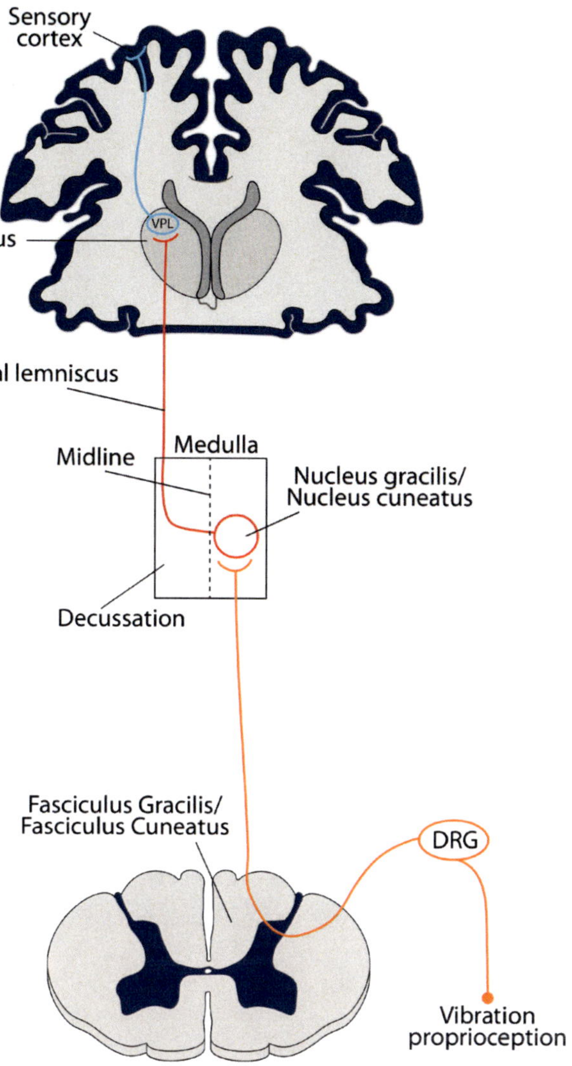

Figure 8.13 - Dorsal Column/Medial Lemniscus Tract

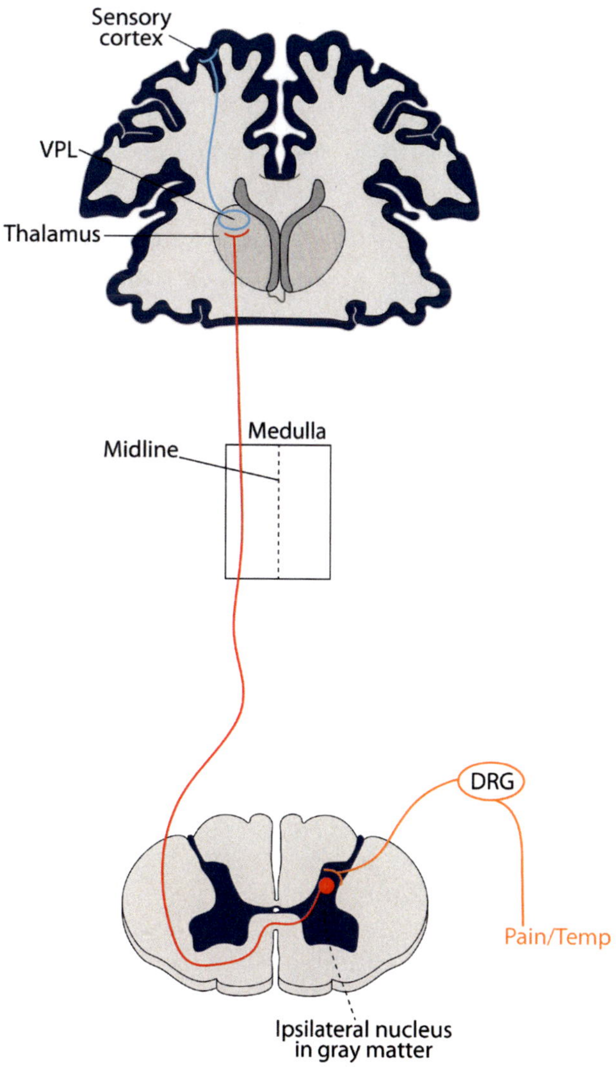

Figure 8.14 - Spinothalamic Tract

2nd neuron decussates through anterior white commissure → ascends through contralateral white matter → synapses on ventroposterolateral (VPL) nucleus in thalamus → 3rd neuron travels to ipsilateral somatosensory cortex

C. Corticospinal tracts (Figure 8.15)

1. Responsible for motor innervation
2. 1st neuron leaves primary motor cortex and travels through internal capsule and reaches the medulla → decussates at medullary pyramids → descends through contralateral posterolateral white matter → synapses in anterior horn of gray matter → 2nd neuron exits spinal cord through anterior root → synapses on neuromuscular junction (NMJ)
3. Upper motor neurons (UMN)
    a) UMNs are the neurons from cortex to the anterior horn within the gray matter of the spinal cord.
    b) Signs of damage include Babinski reflex, spastic paralysis, clasp-knife spasticity, increased tone and reflexes.
4. Lower motor neurons (LMN)
    a) The neuron from the anterior horn gray matter in spinal cord to the NMJ.
    b) Signs of damage include atrophy, fasciculations, decreased tone and reflexes.

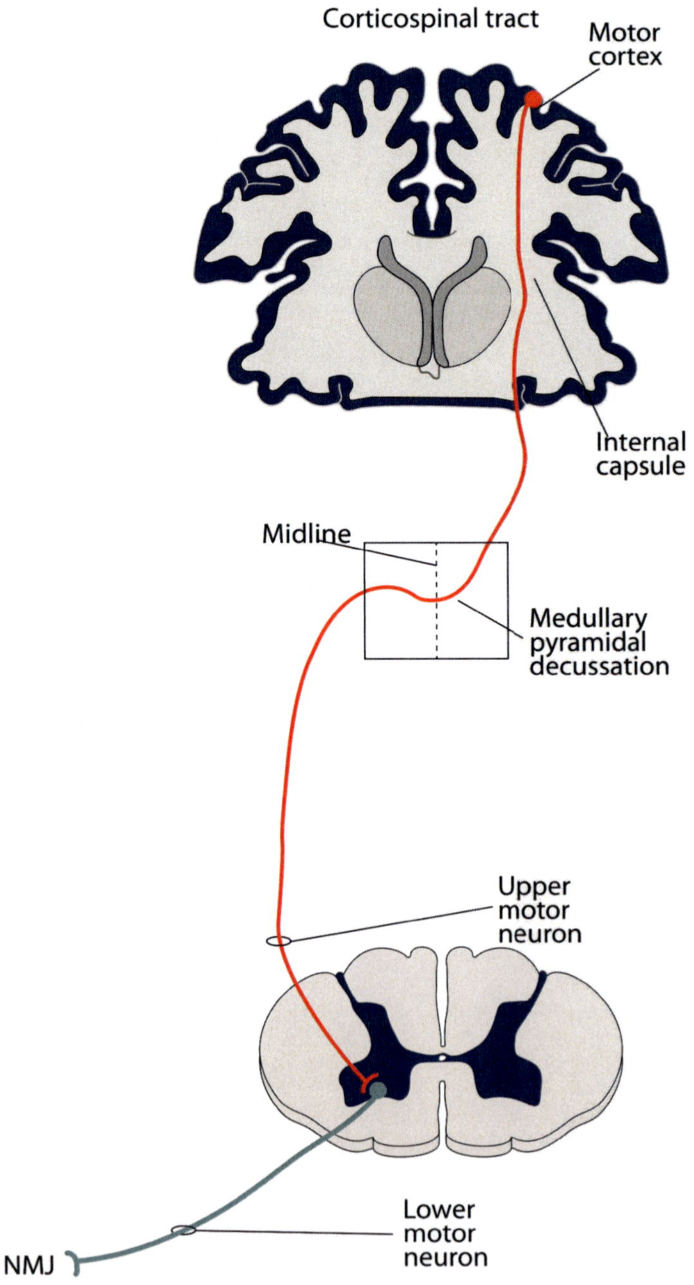

Figure 8.15 - Corticospinal Tract

REVIEW QUESTIONS

1. A patient gets in a car wreck and a radiograph shows that the vertebrae down through C6 have shifted anterior to the vertebrae C7 and below. What spinal nerve is likely damaged?

- **In the cervical spine (C1-C7), each spinal nerve exits above its same-named vertebra**
- **Above C7 vertebra, the C7 spinal nerve would be damaged**

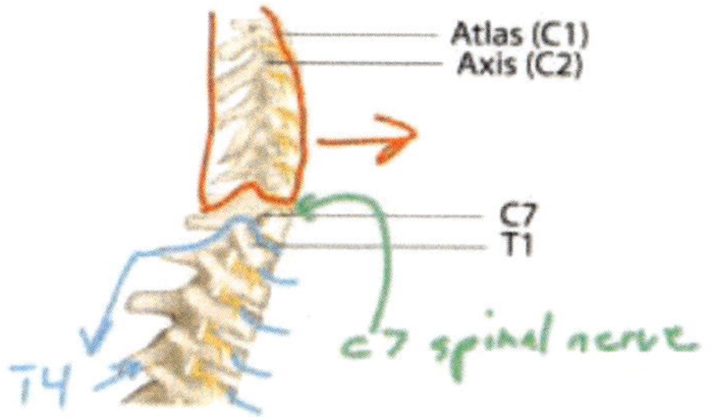

2. A patient is about to receive a lumbar puncture. After puncturing the ligamentum flavum, what layers must the needle penetrate before entering the CSF?

- **Ligamentum flavum → epidural space → dura mater → arachnoid mater → subarachnoid space (CSF)**

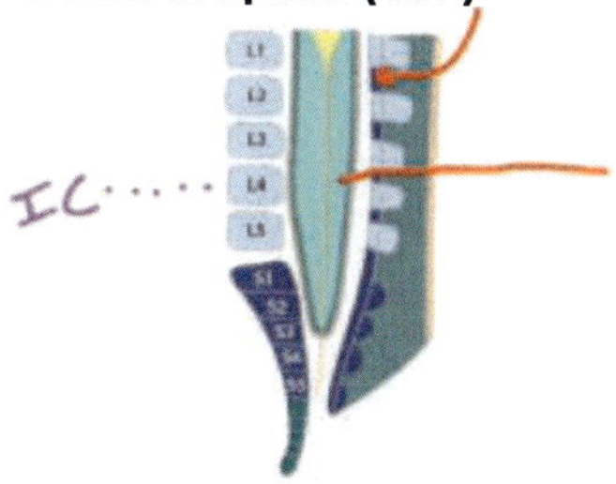

3. A male patient has damaged the left dorsal column at the L1 spinal cord level. What will be his symptoms and where will he experience them?

- **Loss of vibration and proprioception from L1 and below on the ipsilateral side**

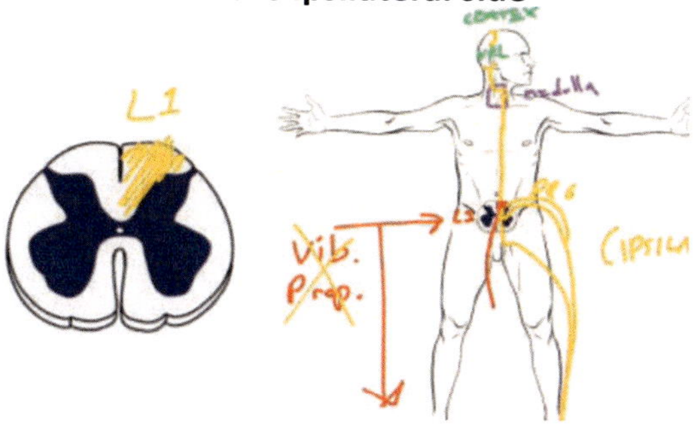

4. What symptoms would a patient experience if only the lateral portion of the right dorsal column was damaged at the C4 spinal cord level?

- **Loss of vibration and proprioception of right arm (fasciculus cuneatus) on the ipsilateral side**

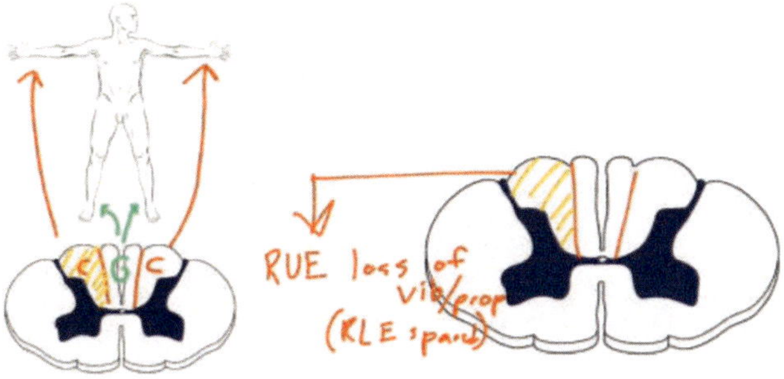

REVIEW QUESTIONS ?

5. A patient is involved in a serious car accident and has lost pain and temperature sensation of the right lower extremity. Where is the lesion likely to be on the spinal cord?

- **Neurologic damage to legs implicates lumbar spinal cord**
- **Loss of pain and temperature implicates spinothalamic damage**
- **Note: If posterior horn of L2 is damaged, L1 and above and L3 and below would still function properly**

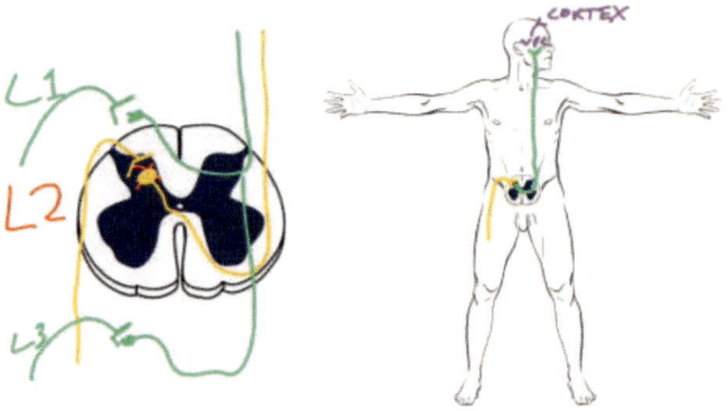

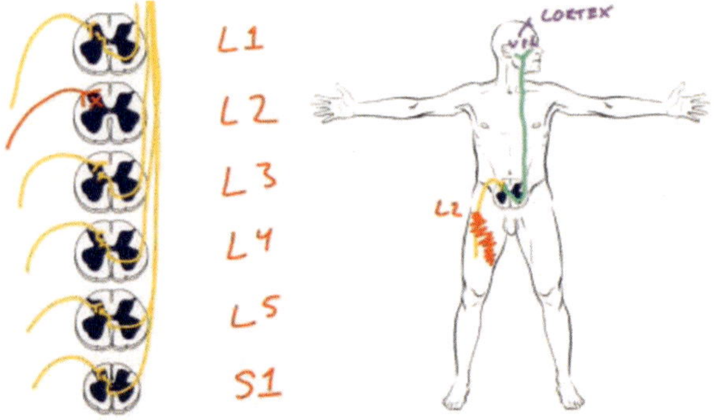

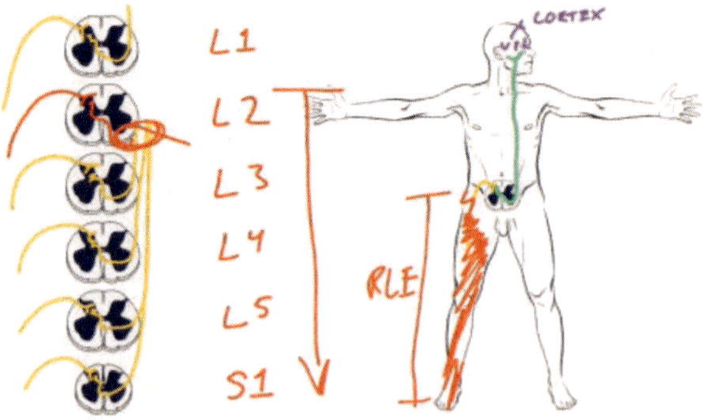

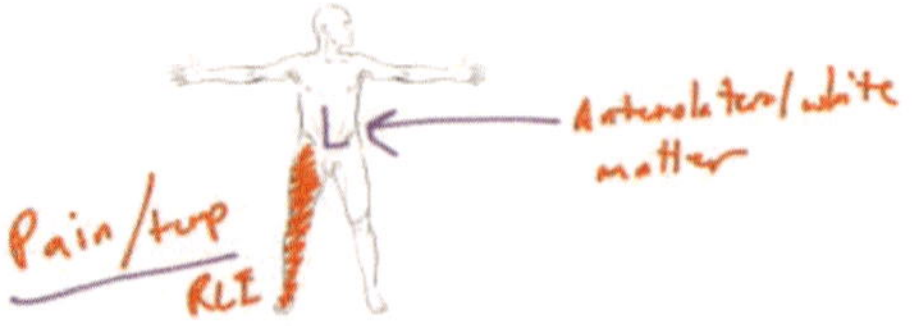

6. A patient has damaged the anterior white commissure of the T1 spinal cord. What symptoms would you expect?

- **Bilateral loss of pain and temperature at the T1 level only**
- **Above and below that level will still decussate and travel as normal**
- **Note: This is classically how syringomyelia presents**

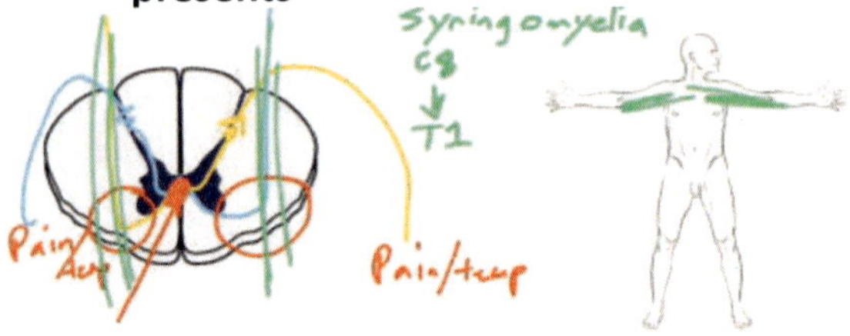

7. A patient has hydrocephalus. What would you expect to have happen to deep tendon reflexes?

- **Hydrocephalus would impact UMN, not LMN**
- **Suspect increased tone, reflexes, Babinski sign, spastic paralysis and clasp-knife spasticity**

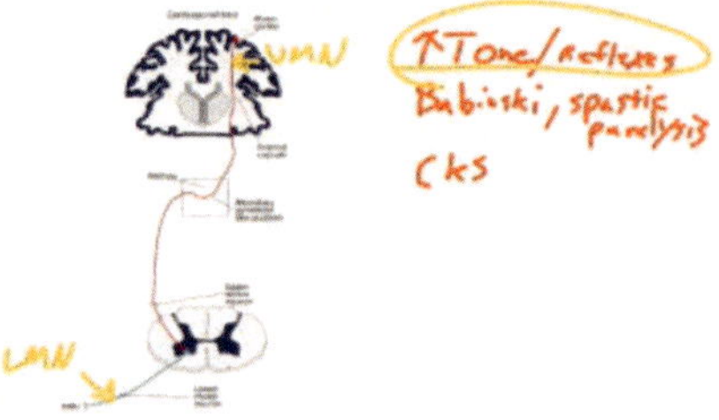

8. An elderly male patient complains of being unable to move his RUE. Upon examination, his RUE is very stiff. Where could the lesion be?

- **This describes spastic paralysis (UMN lesion)**
- **Note: Upon learning there was an MCA stroke, suspect UMN prior to decussation (i.e. left MCA stroke)**

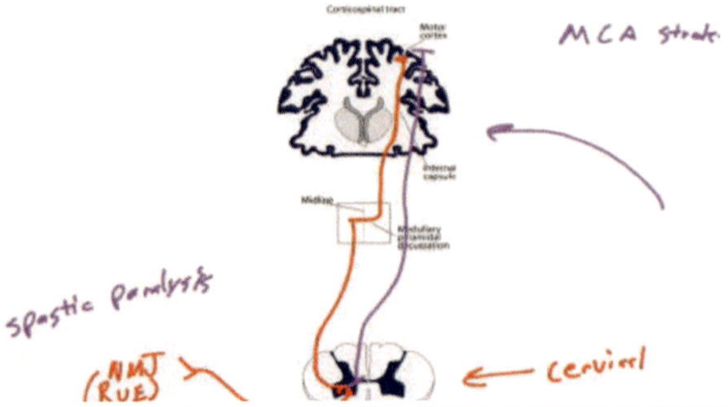

REVIEW QUESTIONS

9. A 5-year-old unvaccinated infant who recently moved to the country has muscle fasciculations of all four limbs. Where is the problem?
   - **Fasciculations indicates LMN lesion**
   - **Poliomyelitis can damage anterior horn cells (LMN nucleus) throughout the spinal cord, causing all limbs to be impacted**

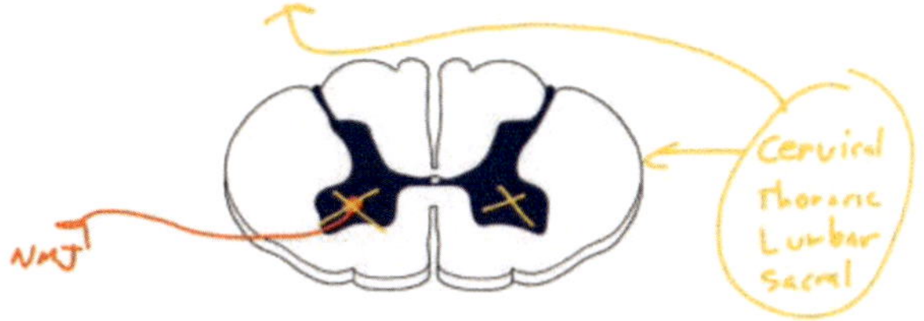

10. A patient has left-sided Brown-Sequard Syndrome at the T9 spinal cord level. What will be the symptoms?
    - **Loss of vibration and proprioception below T9 on ipsilateral side**
    - **Loss of pain and temperature at the T9 level on the ipsilateral side**
    - **Loss of pain and temperature below the T9 level on contralateral side**
    - **Note: Each level of the spinothalamic tract can actually send signals 2 spinal cord levels above each given nerve level (i.e. T9 and T10 levels will have intact pain and temperature sensation with a T9 lesion)**
    - **UMN and LMN lesion signs will be present T9 and below**

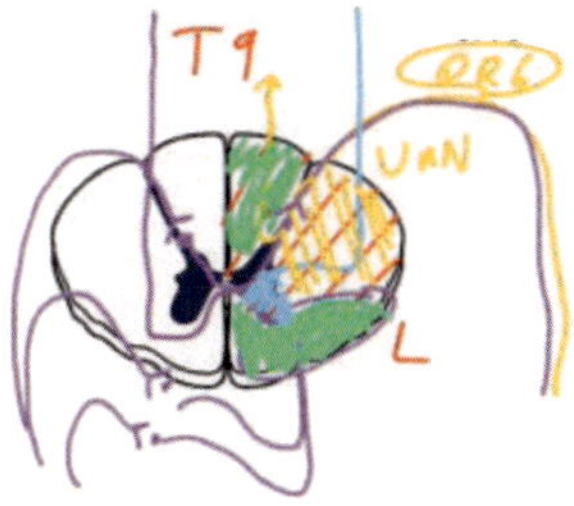

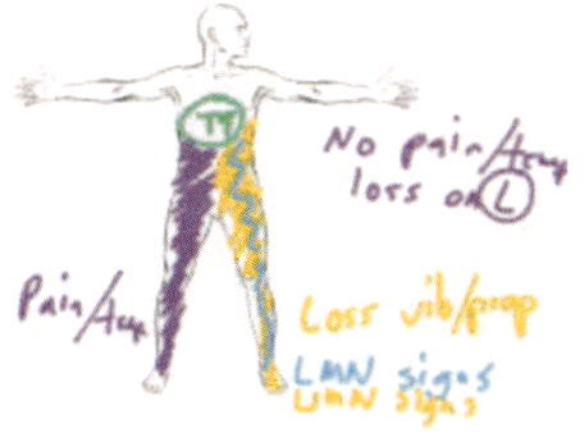

Section III - Cranial Nerves

I. Corticobulbar Tract

A. The neural tract connecting the upper motor neurons and the lower motor neurons of the cranial nerves.

II. Brain Stem

A. Midbrain (Figures 8.16 and 8.17)

1. Contains nuclei for cranial nerves III and IV

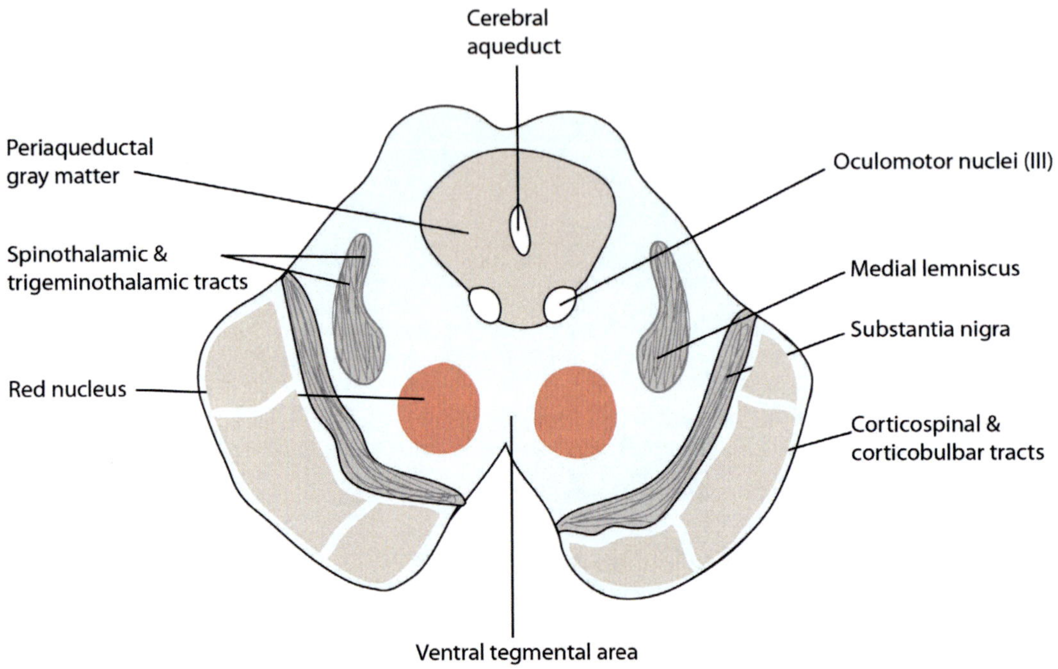

Figure 8.16 - Transverse section of the midbrain

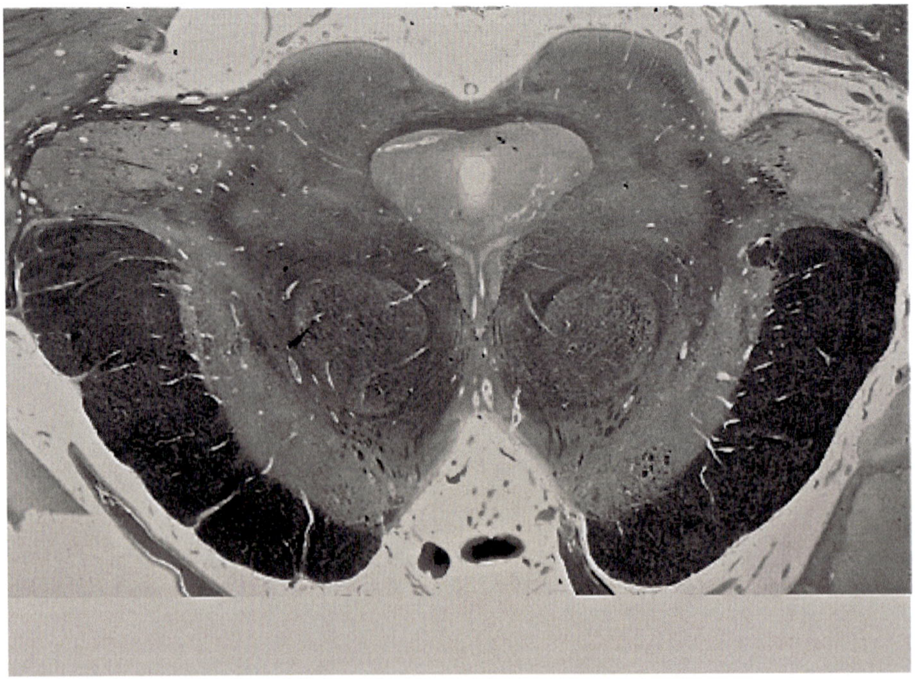

Figure 8.17 - Myelin stain of the midbrain.
(Courtesy of Suzanne Stensaas, Ph.D.; University of Utah School of Medicine)

B. Pons (Figures 8.18 and 8.19)

1. Contains nuclei for cranial nerves V-VIII

C. Medulla (Figures 8.20 and 8.21)

1. Contains nuclei for cranial nerves IX, X, and XII

III. Peripheral Cranial Nerve Branches (Figure 8.22)

A. Most peripheral cranial nerve branches emanate near the region of the cranial nerve nucleus.

1. The peripheral branch of cranial nerve XI emanates from the medulla but the nucleus resides in the cervical spinal cord.

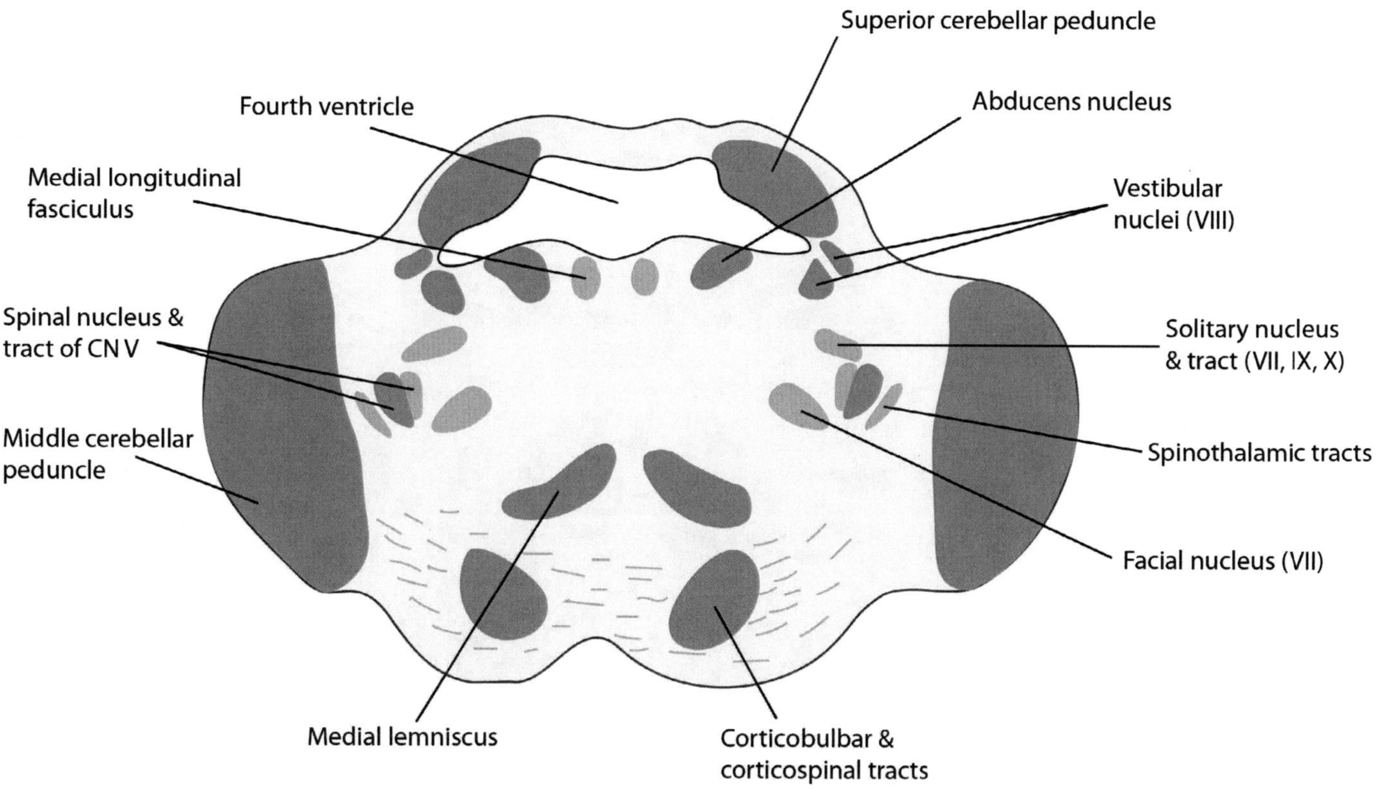

Figure 8.18 - Transverse section of the pons

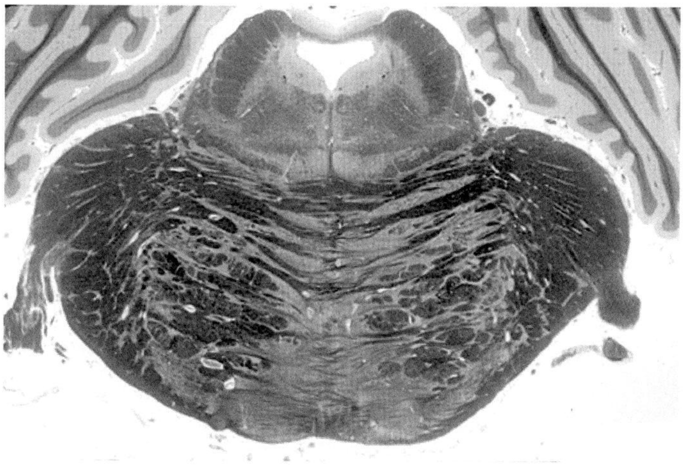

Figure 8.19 - Myelin stain of the pons*

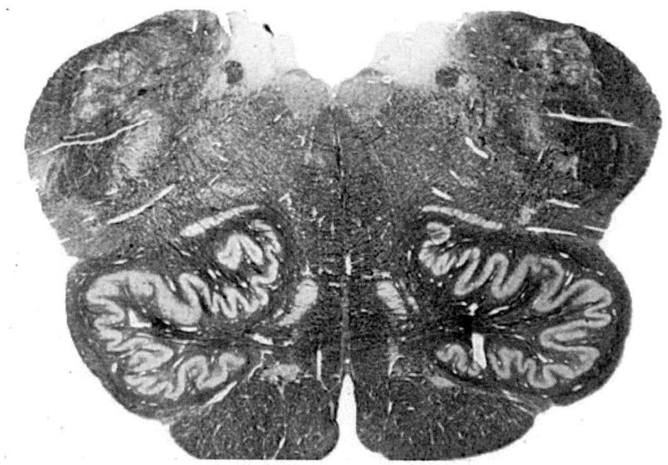

Figure 8.20 - Myelin stain of the medulla*

*Courtesy of Suzanne Stensaas, Ph.D.; University of Utah School of Medicine

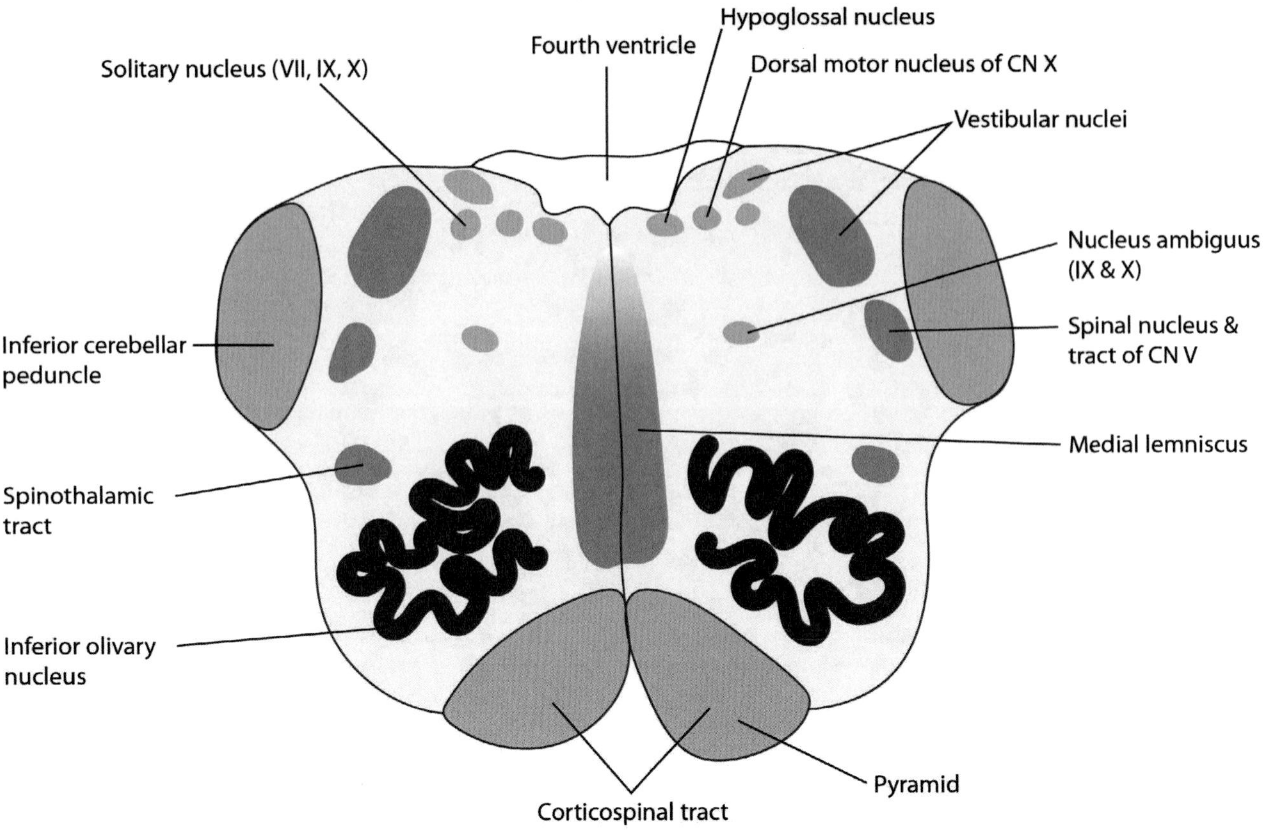

Figure 8.21 - Transverse section of the medulla

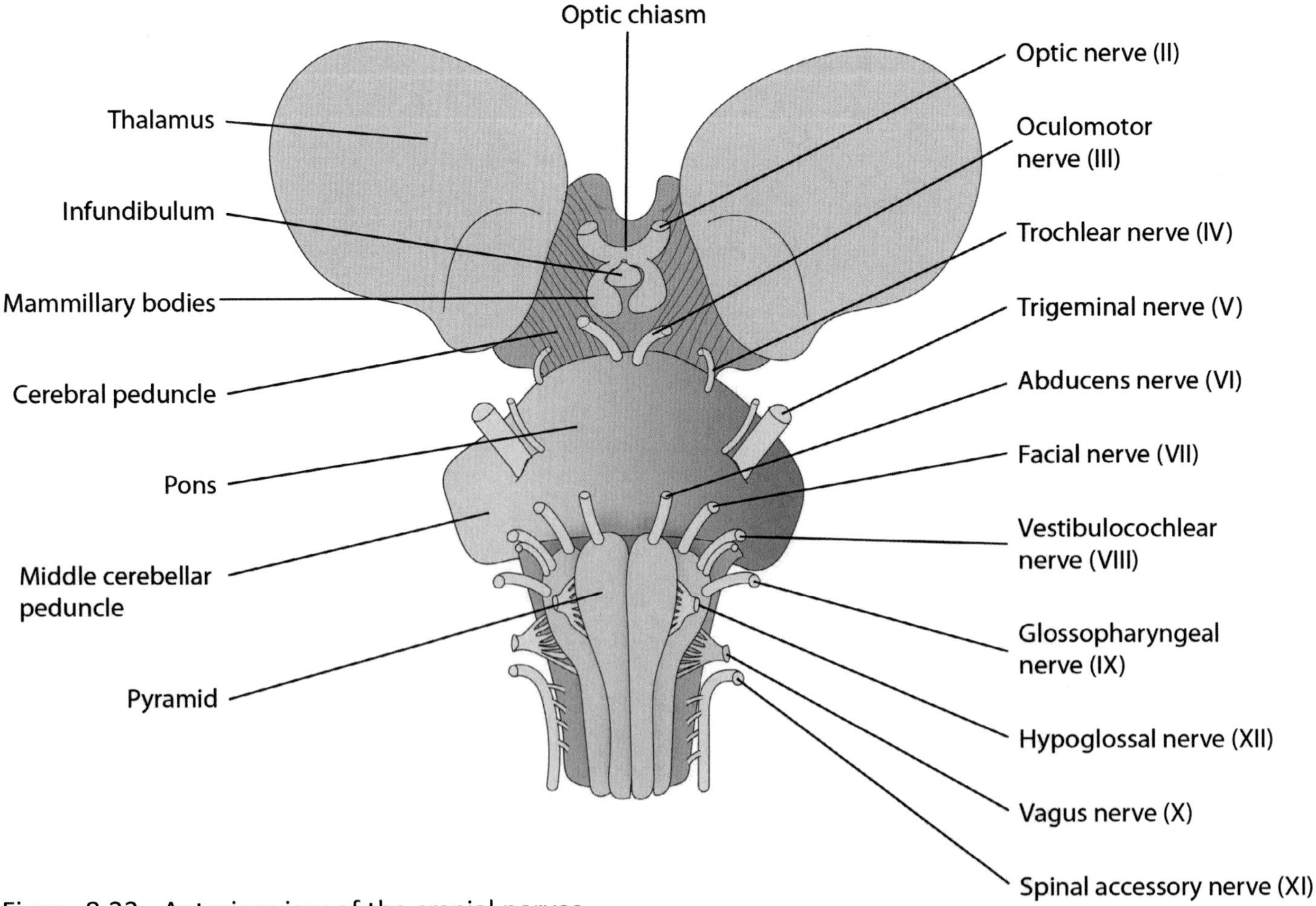

Figure 8.22 - Anterior view of the cranial nerves

B. Each peripheral cranial nerve branch traverses a specific foramen of the skull (Figure 8.23).

C. Cranial nerves II, III, IV, V_1, V_2, and VI pass through the cavernous sinus (Figure 8.24).

IV. See table 8.1 for the names and functions of the cranial nerves.

Table 8.1 - Cranial nerves

Nerve	CN	Function
Olfactory	I	Smell
Optic	II	Vision
Oculomotor	III	Motor output to ocular muscles (superior rectus, medial rectus, inferior rectus, and inferior oblique), eyelid elevation (levator palpebrae superioris), pupillary constriction (pupillary sphincter), and accommodation
Trochlear	IV	Motor output to ocular muscles (superior oblique)
Trigeminal	V	V_1 - ophthalmic: facial sensation of the eyes and forehead V_2 - maxillary: facial sensation around the maxillae V_3 - mandibular: facial sensation around the mandibles, sensation of the anterior ⅔ of the tongue (not taste), and muscles of mastication
Abducens	VI	Motor output to the ocular muscles (lateral rectus)
Facial	VII	Motor output to facial muscles, taste from the anterior ⅔ of the tongue, motor output to the lacrimal glands, closing of the eyelid (orbicularis oculi), motor output to the sublingual and submandibular glands, and auditory modulation (stapedius muscle)
Vestibulocochlear	VIII	Balance and hearing
Glossopharyngeal	IX	Afferent component of the gag reflex, pharyngeal/laryngeal elevation & swallowing (stylopharyngeus), monitor of chemo and baroreceptors of the carotid body and sinus, salivation (parotid gland), and taste and general sensation from the posterior ⅓ of the tongue
Vagus	X	Efferent component of the gag reflex, monitor of the chemo and baroreceptors of the aortic arch, swallowing, soft palate elevation, midline uvula, and parasympathetics to the viscera of the thorax and abdomen
Accessory	XI	Lateral and inferior movements of the head (SCM) and elevation of the shoulders (trapezius)
Hypoglossal	XII	Movement of the tongue

VI. The Trigeminal Cranial Nerve and Tract

A. Information about proprioception and vibration from the right side of the face travels to the right principal nucleus in the pons.

B. Information about pain and temperature from the right side of the face travels to the right spinal trigeminal nucleus in the medulla and cervical spinal cord.

C. After decussating, all sensory information from the principal nucleus and the spinal trigeminal nucleus eventually converges and then ascends up through the brainstem until synapsing on the

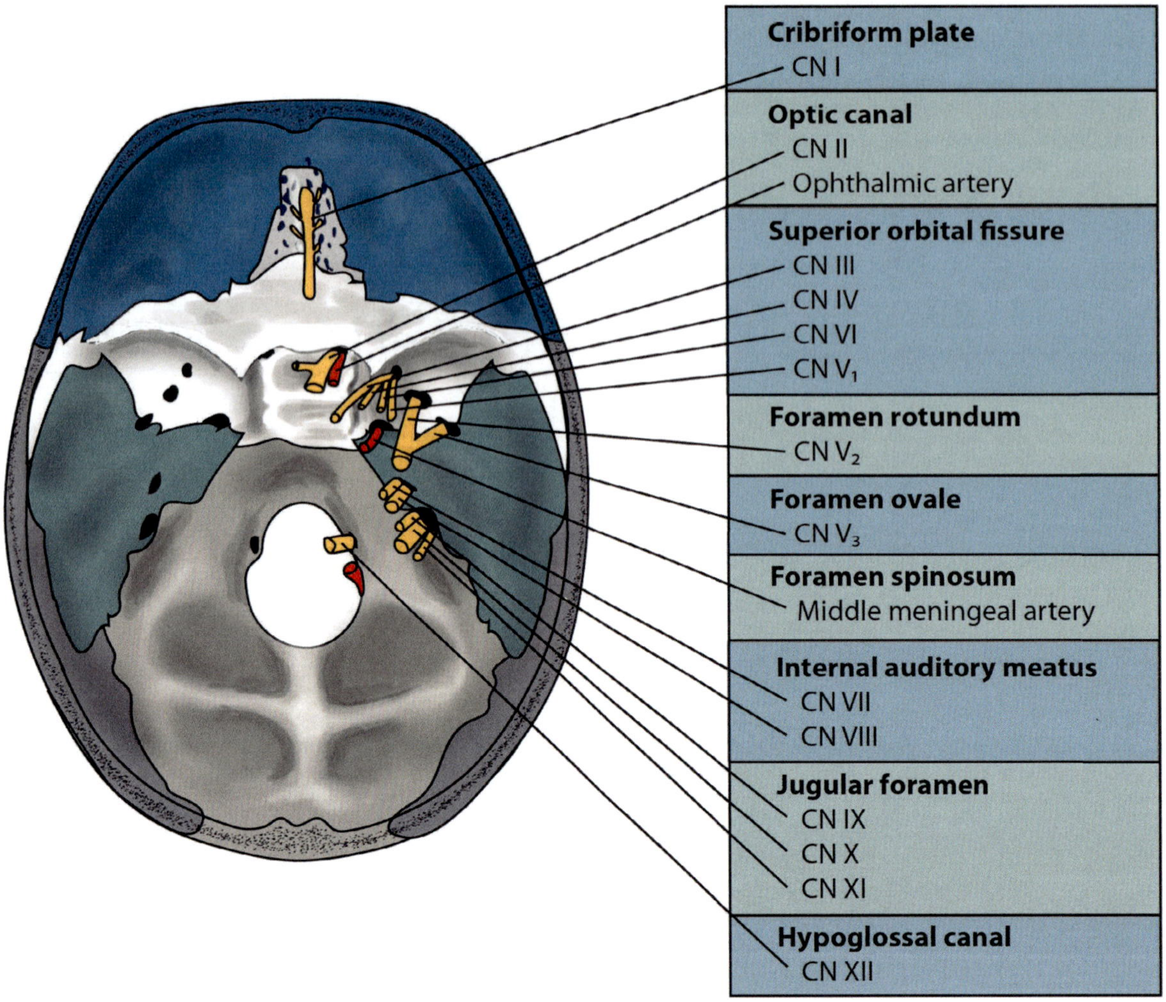

Figure 8.23 - Foramina of the skull

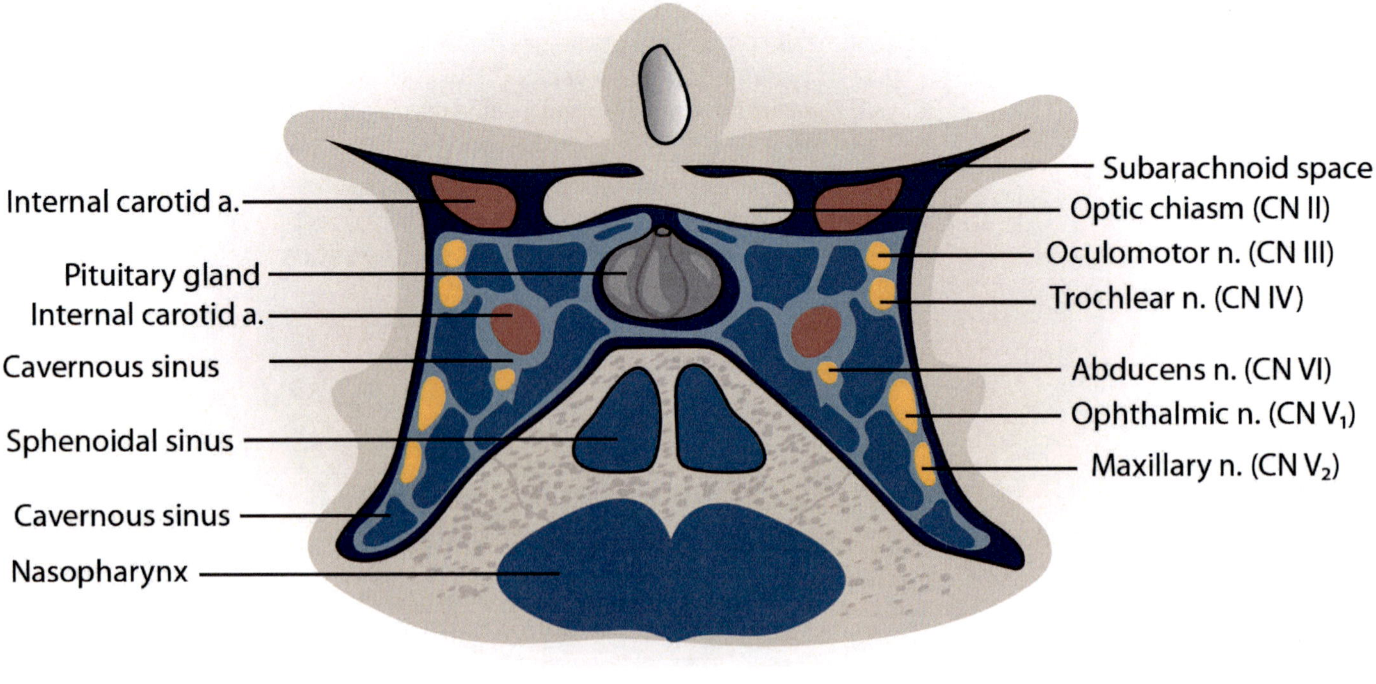

Figure 8.24 - Cavernous sinus

ventral posteromedial nucleus of the thalamus.

D. This information then travels to the primary sensory cortex.

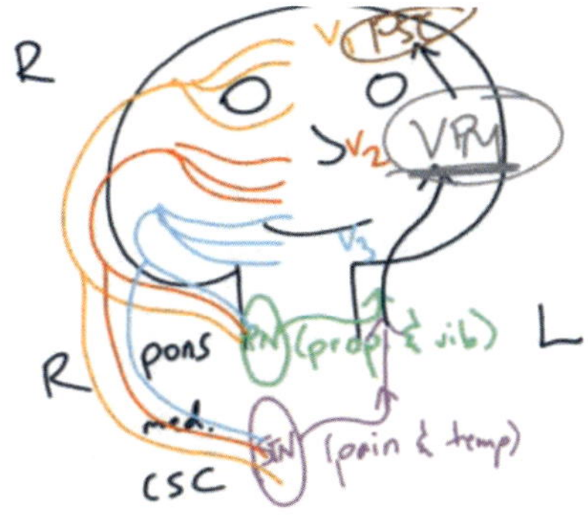

VII. The Facial Nerve

A. The facial nerve is unique because the facial nucleus has an upper and lower component which receives unique innervation from the primary motor cortices (Figure 8.25).

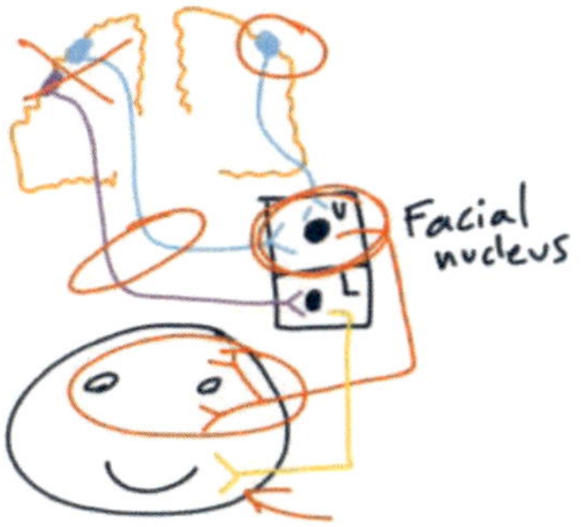

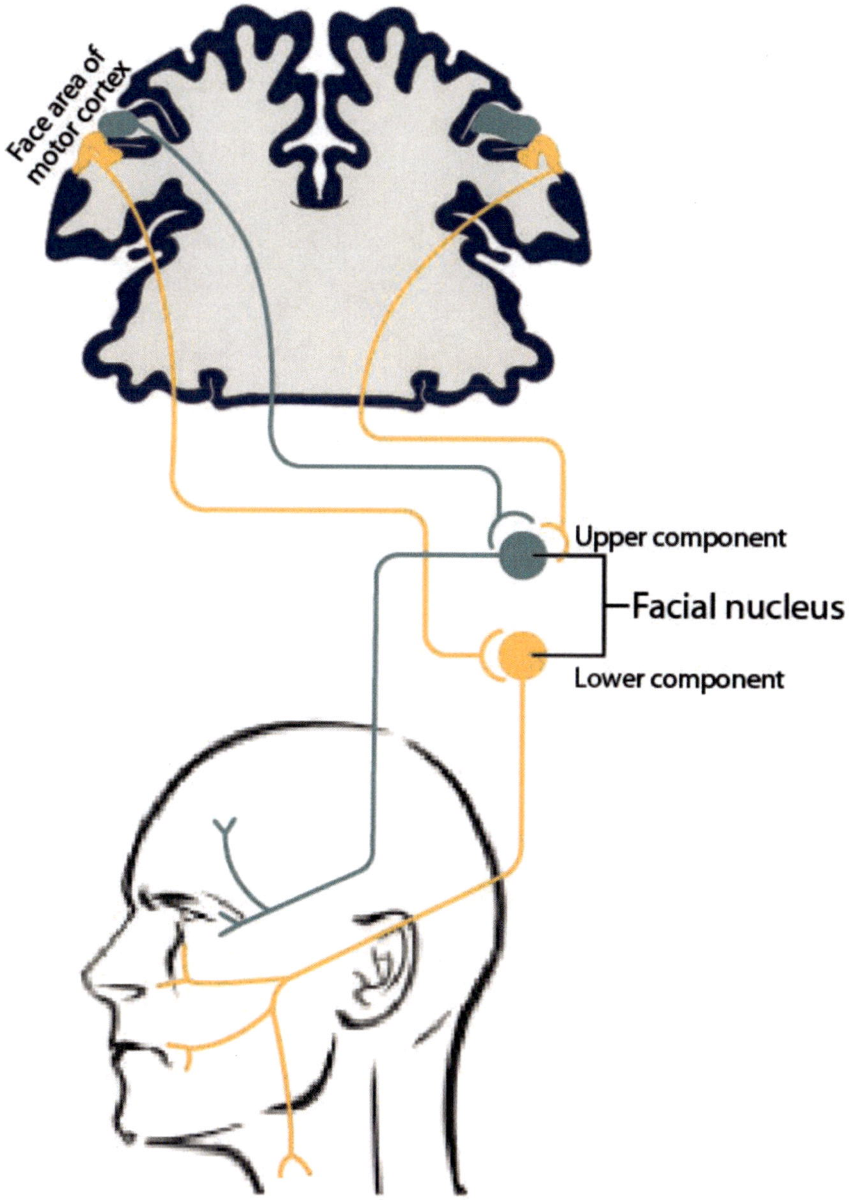

Figure 8.25 - Facial nerve

REVIEW QUESTIONS

1. A patient has an inability to taste on the posterior ⅓ of the right part of her tongue. What part of the brainstem shown below is likely damaged (See figure 8.21)?

    - **Inferior olivary nucleus seen in image → this is the medulla**
    - **The sulcus limitans can distinguish sensory from motor nuclei**
    - **The patient has sensory abnormalities → damaged region must be lateral to the sulcus limitans on the right side of the medulla (this is where the glossopharyngeal nerve nucleus would be)**

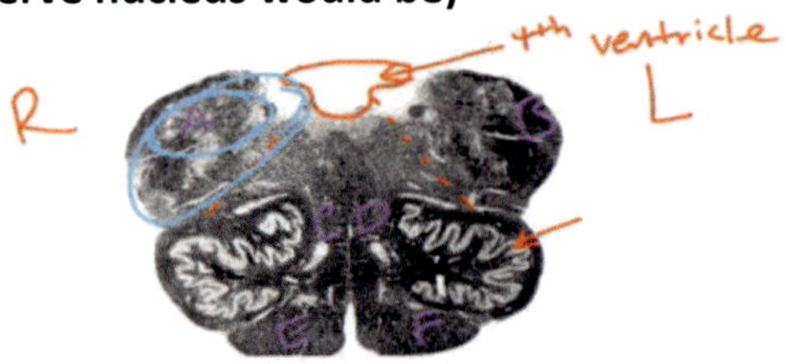

2. What symptoms should you suspect in a patient with a fractured right jugular foramen?

    - **Cranial nerves 9-11 traverse the jugular foramen → see table 8.1 for possible symptoms**

Nerve	CN	Function
Olfactory	I	Smell
Optic	II	Vision
Oculomotor	III	Motor output to ocular muscles (superior rectus, medial rectus, inferior rectus, and inferior oblique), eyelid elevation (levator palpebrae superioris), pupillary constriction (pupillary sphincter), and accommodation
Trochlear	IV	Motor output to ocular muscles (superior oblique)
Trigeminal	V	V_1 - ophthalmic: facial sensation of the eyes and forehead V_2 - maxillary: facial sensation around the maxillae V_3 - mandibular: facial sensation around the mandibles, sensation of the anterior ⅔ of the tongue (not taste), and muscles of mastication
Abducens	VI	Motor output to the ocular muscles (lateral rectus)
Facial	VII	Motor output to facial muscles, taste from the anterior ⅔ of the tongue, motor output to the lacrimal glands, closing of the eyelid (orbicularis oculi), motor output to the sublingual and submandibular glands, and auditory modulation (stapedius muscle)
Vestibulocochlear	VIII	Balance and hearing
Glossopharyngeal	IX	Afferent component of the gag reflex, pharyngeal/laryngeal elevation & swallowing (stylopharyngeus), monitor of chemo and baroreceptors of the carotid body and sinus, salivation (parotid gland), and taste and general sensation from the posterior ⅓ of the tongue
Vagus	X	Efferent component of the gag reflex, monitor of the chemo and baroreceptors of the aortic arch, swallowing, soft palate elevation, midline uvula, and parasympathetics to the viscera of the thorax and abdomen
Accessory	XI	Lateral and inferior movements of the head (SCM) and elevation of the shoulders (trapezius)
Hypoglossal	XII	Movement of the tongue

3. A 32-year-old woman with uncontrolled type one diabetes presents with sinus pain and tachypnea. Upon further examination you suspect involvement of the cavernous sinus. What other symptoms would this patient likely have due to involvement of the cavernous sinus?

    - **This patient is in diabetic ketoacidosis → ↑ risk for mucor and rhizopus infection → thrombosis of the cavernous sinus → damage to cranial nerves III, IV, V_1, V_2, and VI → see table 8.1 for possible symptoms**

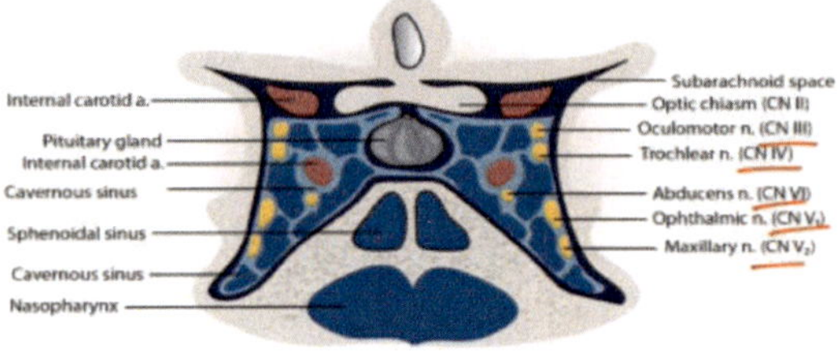

Nerve	CN	Function
Olfactory	I	Smell
Optic	II	Vision
Oculomotor	III	Motor output to ocular muscles (superior rectus, medial rectus, inferior rectus, and inferior oblique), eyelid elevation (levator palpebrae superioris), pupillary constriction (pupillary sphincter), and accommodation
Trochlear	IV	Motor output to ocular muscles (superior oblique)
Trigeminal	V	V_1 - ophthalmic: facial sensation of the eyes and forehead V_2 - maxillary: facial sensation around the maxillae V_3 - mandibular: facial sensation around the mandibles, sensation of the anterior ⅔ of the tongue (not taste), and muscles of mastication
Abducens	VI	Motor output to the ocular muscles (lateral rectus)
Facial	VII	Motor output to facial muscles, taste from the anterior ⅔ of the tongue, motor output to the lacrimal glands, closing of the eyelid (orbicularis oculi), motor output to the sublingual and submandibular glands, and auditory modulation (stapedius muscle)
Vestibulocochlear	VIII	Balance and hearing
Glossopharyngeal	IX	Afferent component of the gag reflex, pharyngeal/laryngeal elevation & swallowing (stylopharyngeus), monitor of chemo and baroreceptors of the carotid body and sinus, salivation (parotid gland), and taste and general sensation from the posterior ⅓ of the tongue
Vagus	X	Efferent component of the gag reflex, monitor of the chemo and baroreceptors of the aortic arch, swallowing, soft palate elevation, midline uvula, and parasympathetics to the viscera of the thorax and abdomen
Accessory	XI	Lateral and inferior movements of the head (SCM) and elevation of the shoulders (trapezius)
Hypoglossal	XII	Movement of the tongue

4. A plastic surgeon accidentally cuts the nerve that passes through the left parotid gland. What symptoms will the patient likely experience as a result of the mistake?

    - **The facial nerve (CN VII) passes through the parotid gland → damage to peripheral aspect of left facial nerve → complete left-sided facial paralysis**

left facial nerve
1) UMN
2) LMN
3) peripheral → complete paralysis

REVIEW QUESTIONS

5. When the patient is asked to say, “ah” in attempt to elevate the palate, the uvula deviates to the right. What cranial nerve shown below is likely damaged (see figure 8.22)?

- **Cranial nerve X is responsible for keeping the uvula midline**
- **Damage to CN X → contralateral deviation.**
- **The left vagus nerve is damaged**

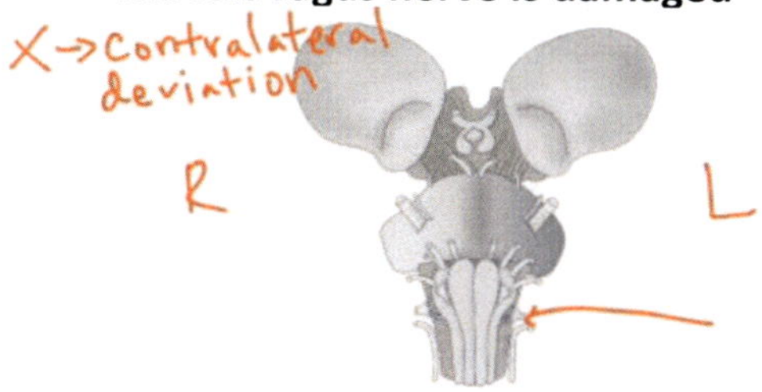

6. A 65-year-old female presents to the neurologist with numbness of the anterior tongue with taste intact and difficulty chewing food. The damaged nerve passes through which foramen of the skull?

- **V_3**
- **Mandibular branch of the trigeminal nerve is damaged → passes through the foramen ovale.**

Nerve	CN	Function
Olfactory	I	Smell
Optic	II	Vision
Oculomotor	III	Motor output to ocular muscles (superior rectus, medial rectus, inferior rectus, and inferior oblique), eyelid elevation (levator palpebrae superioris), pupillary constriction (pupillary sphincter), and accommodation
Trochlear	IV	Motor output to ocular muscles (superior oblique)
Trigeminal	V	V_1 - ophthalmic: facial sensation of the eyes and forehead V_2 - maxillary: facial sensation around the maxillae V_3 - mandibular: facial sensation around the mandibles, sensation of the anterior ⅔ of the tongue (not taste), and muscles of mastication
Abducens	VI	Motor output to the ocular muscles (lateral rectus)
Facial	VII	Motor output to facial muscles, taste from the anterior ⅔ of the tongue, motor output to the lacrimal glands, closing of the eyelid (orbicularis oculi), motor output to the sublingual and submandibular glands, and auditory modulation (stapedius muscle)
Vestibulocochlear	VIII	Balance and hearing
Glossopharyngeal	IX	Afferent component of the gag reflex, pharyngeal/laryngeal elevation & swallowing (stylopharyngeus), monitor of chemo and baroreceptors of the carotid body and sinus, salivation (parotid gland), and taste and general sensation from the posterior ⅓ of the tongue
Vagus	X	Efferent component of the gag reflex, monitor of the chemo and baroreceptors of the aortic arch, swallowing, soft palate elevation, midline uvula, and parasympathetics to the viscera of the thorax and abdomen
Accessory	XI	Lateral and inferior movements of the head (SCM) and elevation of the shoulders (trapezius)
Hypoglossal	XII	Movement of the tongue

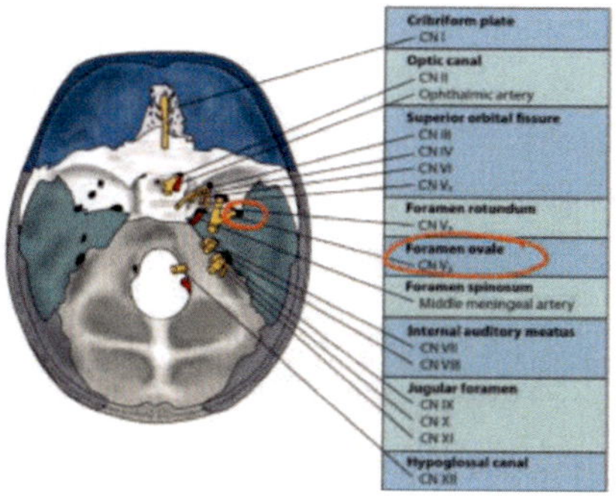

7. A patient presents with deviation of the left eye toward the midline when asked to look straight ahead. The neurologist suspects a tumor compressing which region of the brain?

- **The abducens nerve (CN VI) innervates the lateral rectus muscle (responsible for lateral movement of the eye)**
- **Damage to CN VI → unopposed medial force → medial deviation of the left eye**
- **The nucleus of CN VI is located in the pons**

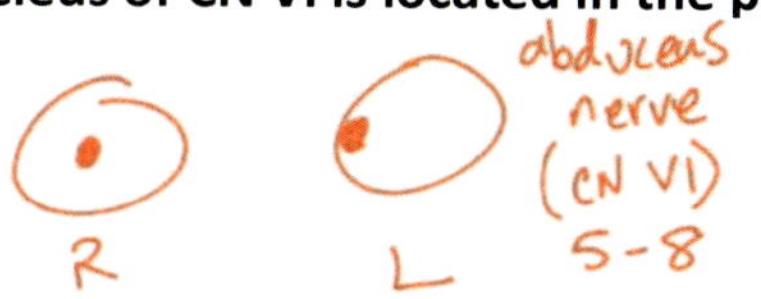

8. A newborn has a cleft upper lip secondary to Patau syndrome. The nerve that innervates this region passes through which foramen of the skull?

- **The upper lip is innervated by the maxillary branch of the trigeminal nerve (V_2)**
- **V_2 passes through the foramen rotundum**

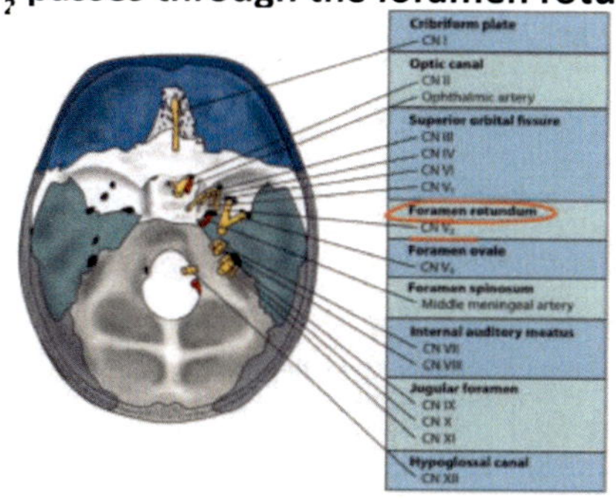

9. When a patient is asked to look to the left the left eye moves laterally and the right eye moves medially and slightly superior. What part of the brainstem is likely involved?

- **The trochlear nerve (CN IV) innervates the superior oblique muscle (responsible for downward movement and intorsion)**
- **Damage to the right CN IV → excessive upward pull on the eye → upward deviation of the right eye**
- **CN IV is located in the midbrain**

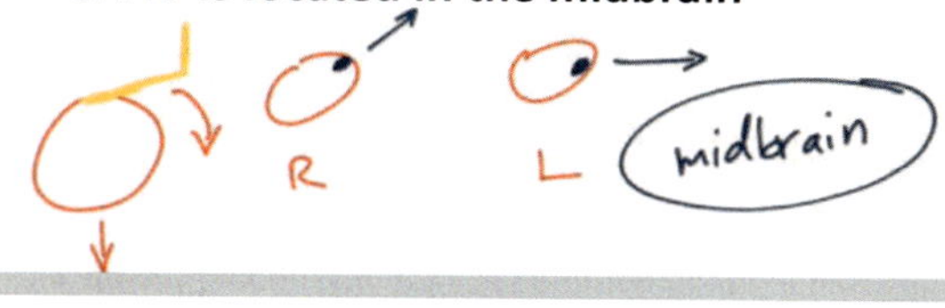

REVIEW QUESTIONS

10. How would damage to the facial nerve alter hearing?

- **The facial nerve (CN VII) innervates the stapedius muscle which normally dampens sound.**
- **Damage to CN VII → hyperacusis**

11. An MRI shows a fracture of the right hypoglossal canal. What symptoms would be present in the patient?

- **The hypoglossal nerve (CN XII) traverses the hypoglossal canal.**
- **Damage to the hypoglossal nerve (CN XII) results in ipsilateral tongue deviation.**
- **Right-sided damage → right-sided tongue deviation**

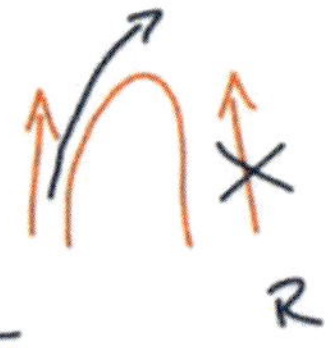

12. One month ago a 23-year-old male developed a ring-like rash after hiking in the Appalachian Mountains. He presents to the ED today due to complete paralysis of the right side of his face. What region of the brain is likely involved?

- **This patient has Lyme disease due to infection from the microorganism borrelia burgdorferi.**
- **Stage II of Lyme disease → facial nerve palsy due to damage to the lower motor neuron → complete paralysis of the ipsilateral face.**
- **The facial nerve nucleus is located in the pons.**

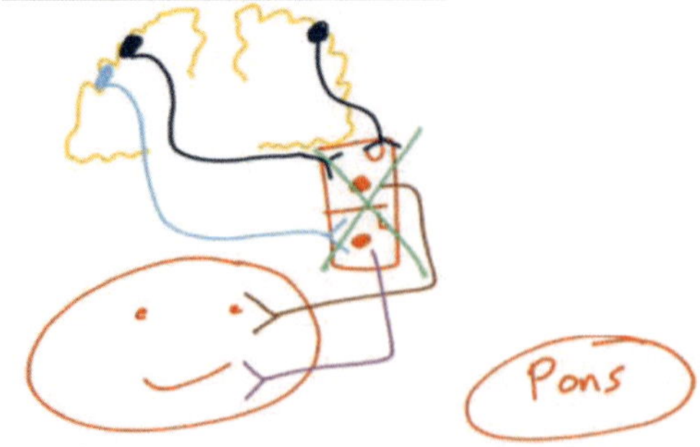

13. A 26-year-old male presents to the ED after an automobile accident. Upon examination the physician notices several abnormalities of the right eye including ptosis, mydriasis, and an inability to look to the left. What foramen of the skull was likely fractured?

- **The oculomotor nerve (CN III) is damaged.**
- **This traverses the superior orbital fissure.**

CN III

Nerve	CN	Function
Olfactory	I	Smell
Optic	II	Vision
Oculomotor	III	Motor output to ocular muscles (superior rectus, medial rectus, inferior rectus, and inferior oblique), eyelid elevation (levator palpebrae superioris), pupillary constriction (pupillary sphincter), and accommodation
Trochlear	IV	Motor output to ocular muscles (superior oblique)
Trigeminal	V	V_1 - ophthalmic: facial sensation of the eyes and forehead V_2 - maxillary: facial sensation around the maxillae V_3 - mandibular: facial sensation around the mandibles, sensation of the anterior ⅔ of the tongue (not taste), and muscles of mastication
Abducens	VI	Motor output to the ocular muscles (lateral rectus)
Facial	VII	Motor output to facial muscles, taste from the anterior ⅔ of the tongue, motor output to the lacrimal glands, closing of the eyelid (orbicularis oculi), motor output to the sublingual and submandibular glands, and auditory modulation (stapedius muscle)
Vestibulocochlear	VIII	Balance and hearing
Glossopharyngeal	IX	Afferent component of the gag reflex, pharyngeal/laryngeal elevation & swallowing (stylopharyngeus), monitor of chemo and baroreceptors of the carotid body and sinus, salivation (parotid gland), and taste and general sensation from the posterior ⅓ of the tongue
Vagus	X	Efferent component of the gag reflex, monitor of the chemo and baroreceptors of the aortic arch, swallowing, soft palate elevation, midline uvula, and parasympathetics to the viscera of the thorax and abdomen
Accessory	XI	Lateral and inferior movements of the head (SCM) and elevation of the shoulders (trapezius)
Hypoglossal	XII	Movement of the tongue

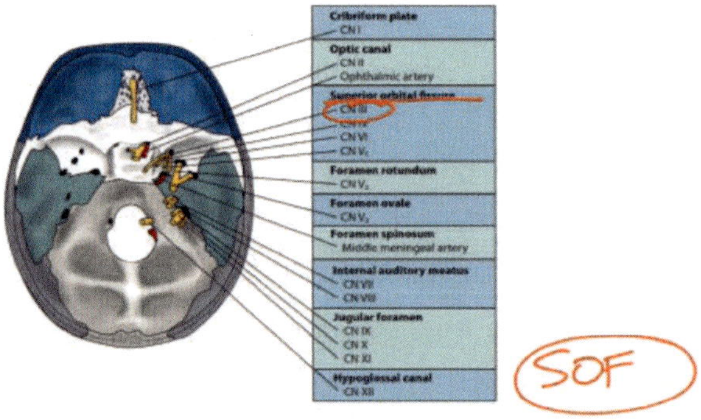

Section IV - Thalamus, Hypothalamus, and Limbic System

I. Thalamus, Hypothalamus, and Limbic System

A. Thalamus (Figure 8.3)

1. See Table 8.2 for important nuclei, inputs & outputs, and the processed sensation.

Table 8.2 - The thalamus

Nuclei	Input	Processed Sensation	Output
Lateral geniculate nucleus	Optic nerve	Sight	Occipital lobe (calcarine sulcus)
Medial geniculate nucleus	Auditory pathway (inferior colliculus)	Hearing	Auditory cortex
Ventral posterolateral nucleus	Spinothalamic and dorsal column	Pain, temperature, proprioception and vibration	Primary sensory cortex
Ventral posteromedial nucleus	Taste and trigeminal pathways	Taste and sensation from the face	Primary sensory cortex
Ventral lateral nucleus	Cerebellum and basal ganglia	Motor information	Motor cortex

II. Hypothalamus (Figure 8.3)

A. See Table 8.3 for important nuclei and corresponding function.

Table 8.3 - The hypothalamus

Hypothalamic nuclei	Functions
Anterior	Decreases body temperature during states of hyperthermia
Posterior	Increases body temperature during states of hypothermia
Lateral	Mediates hunger
Ventromedial	Mediates satiety
Supraoptic	Synthesizes and secretes ADH
Suprachiasmatic	Regulation of circadian rhythm
Arcuate	Secretion of hormones (dopamine, GNRH, and GH)
Paraventricular	Synthesizes and secretes oxytocin

III. Limbic System (Figure 8.4 and 8.5)

A. The mammillary bodies and the hippocampus are associated with memory.

1. Thiamine deficiency can result in damage to the mammillary bodies.
2. The hippocampus is highly susceptible to damage under hypoxic conditions.

B. The amygdala is associated with emotions and decision making.

1. Bilateral damage to this region results in hyperorality, hyperphagia, and hypersexuality (Klüver-Bucy syndrome).

REVIEW QUESTIONS

1. Researchers are studying a hypothalamic nucleus that may be damaged in patients with Prader-Willi syndrome. What nucleus are the researchers most likely studying?

- **Patients with Prader-Willi syndrome have hyperphagia**
- **The ventromedial nucleus (VMN) of the hypothalamus is responsible for satiety**
- **Damage to the VMN → hyperphagia**
- **Researches are most likely studying the VMN**

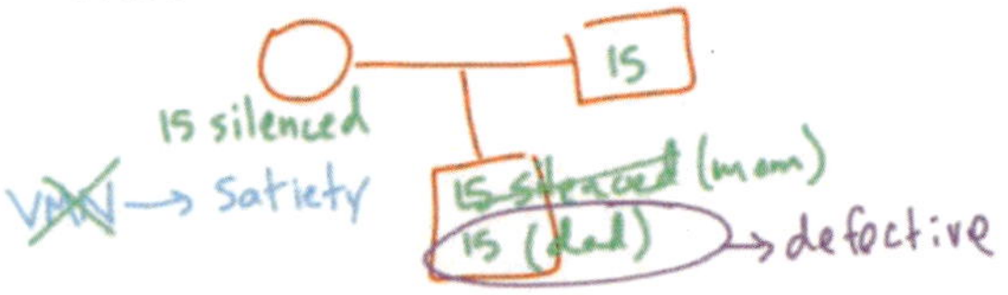

2. A 72-year-old female presents with loss of proprioception, vibration, temperature, and pain on the left side of her body. What thalamic nucleus is likely damaged?

- **The spinothalamic tract conveys information about pain and temperature**
- **The dorsal columns convey information about proprioception and vibration**
- **Both tracts synapse on the ventroposterolateral (VPL) nucleus of the thalamus**
- **Right VPL is likely damaged**

d? Right VPL

ST → pain & temp → VPL
DC → prop & vib →

3. A 28-year-old homeless man presents to the ED after being mugged. He repeatedly asks where he is and seems confused. Upon exam you notice complete paralysis of the eyes. What region of the brain is likely damaged?

- **This patient has Wernicke-Korsakoff syndrome due to vitamin B1 (thiamine) deficiency → mammillary bodies are damaged**

Wernicke-Korsakoff syndrome

mammillary bodies

4. A 24-year-old man recently returned from his first trip to Mount Everest. During his ascent he became injured and lost several liters of blood. Since returning he has had difficulty forming new memories. What region of the brain was likely damaged?

- **This patient experienced severe hypoxia**
- **The hippocampus is highly sensitive to hypoxia**
- **Damaged hippocampus → inability to form new memories**

Section V - Cerebellum

I. Cerebellar Anatomy (Figure 8.26)

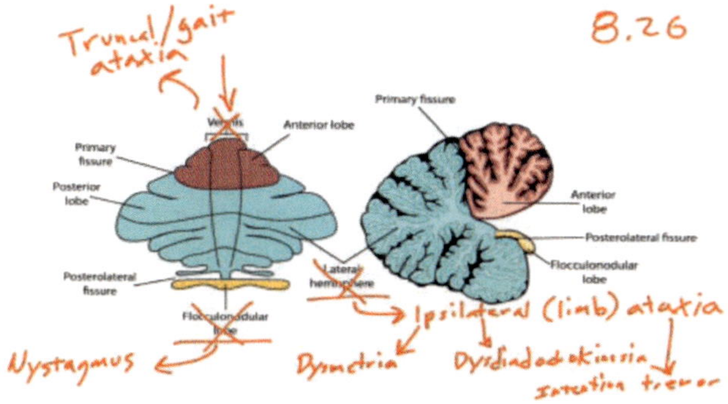

A. Hemispheres (cerebrocerebellum): coordination of limbs (lateral corticospinal tract)

1. Lesions cause limb ataxia

a) Intention tremor: trembling when making a movement

b) Dysmetria: undershoot or overshoot with finger

c) Dysdiadochokinesia: cannot perform rapid alternating movements

B. Vermis (spinocerebellum) colon coordination of axial muscles (anterior corticospinal tract)

1. Lesions cause truncal ataxia

a) Lack of coordination while walking (gait ataxia), maintaining posture while seated

b) Maintaining posture while walking or seated (postural ataxia)

C. Flocculonodular lobe (vestibulocerebellum): involved with coordination of eye movements

1. Lesions cause truncal ataxia:

a) Lack of coordination while walking (gait ataxia), maintaining posture while seated

b) Maintaining posture while walking or seated (postural ataxia)

c) Nystagmus: repetitive, uncontrollable eye movements

II. Layers and fibers (Figure 8.27)

A. White matter: signal (action potentials) enters and exits the cerebellar cortex through this

B. Molecular layer: signal processing

C. Granule layer: signal input to molecular layer

D. Purkinje layer: sends outgoing fibers to deep nuclei; releases GABA

III. Deep Nuclei of Cerebellum (Figure 8.28)

A. Dentate (lateral)

B. Emboliform

C. Globose

D. Fastigial (medial)

E. Each nuclei corresponds to a specific location of the cerebellum

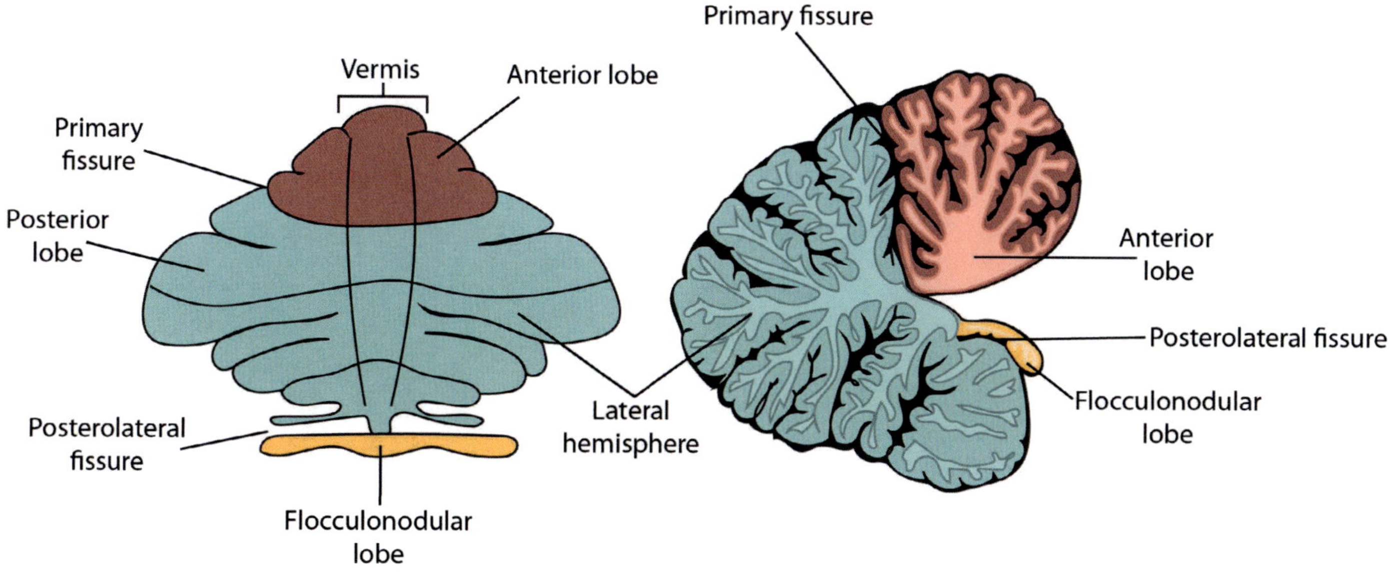

Figure 8.26 - Cerebellum Anatomy

1. Medial nuclei interact with medial cerebellar cortex
2. Lateral nuclei with lateral cerebellar cortex

F. All receive inhibitory (GABA) input from Purkinje neurons

G. All send axons out of the cerebellum via cerebellar peduncles

IV. Peduncles and Tracts (Figure 8.29)

A. Superior peduncle

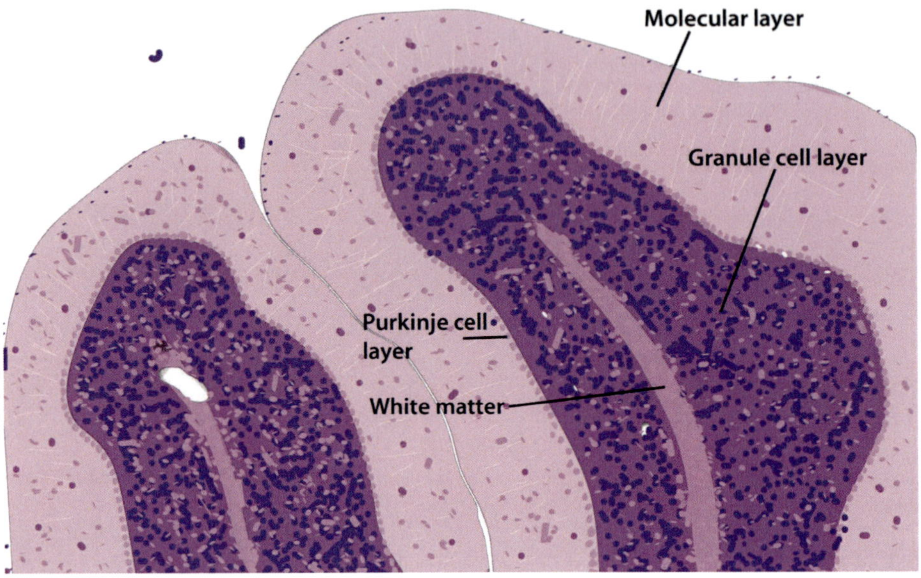

Figure 8.27 - Cerebellum Layers

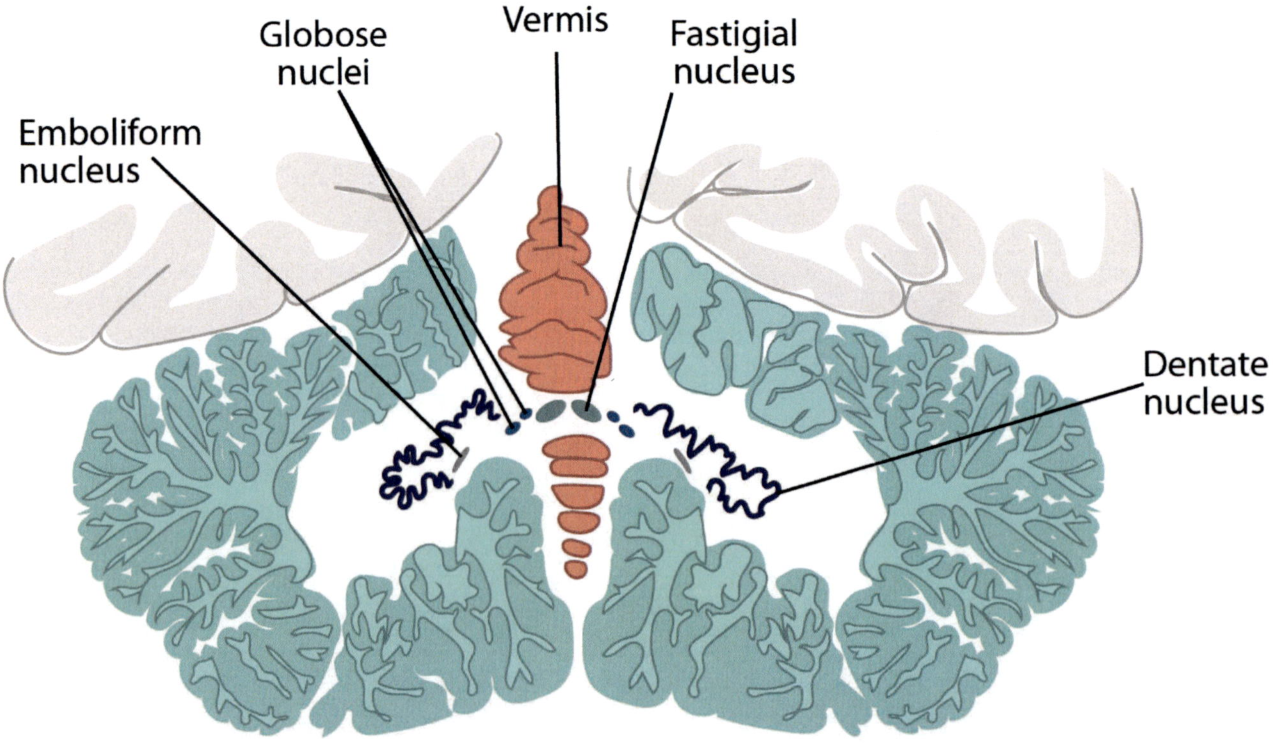

Figure 8.28 - Deep Nuclei of the Cerebellum

1. Proprioceptive *out to* contralateral VL nucleus of thalamus → motor cortex (cerebellothalamic tract)

B. Middle peduncle

1. "Intention" *in from* contralateral cerebral motor cortex (corticopontocerebellar tract)

C. Inferior peduncle

1. Proprioceptive *in from* spinal cord (spinocerebellar tract)

V. Vestibulocerebellar Tract (Figure 8.30)

A. Vestibular nuclei (VN) → flocculonodular lobe → back to VN → CN VI, III, and IV

B. Pathway remains ipsilateral

C. Damage → nystagmus

VI. Dominating Cerebellum Questions

A. Hemisphere lesions cause limb ataxia (intention tremor, dysmetria, dysdiadochokinesia) on the ipsilateral side.

B. Vermis lesions cause gait/truncal ataxia.

C. Flocculonodular lobe lesions cause gait/truncal ataxia and nystagmus.

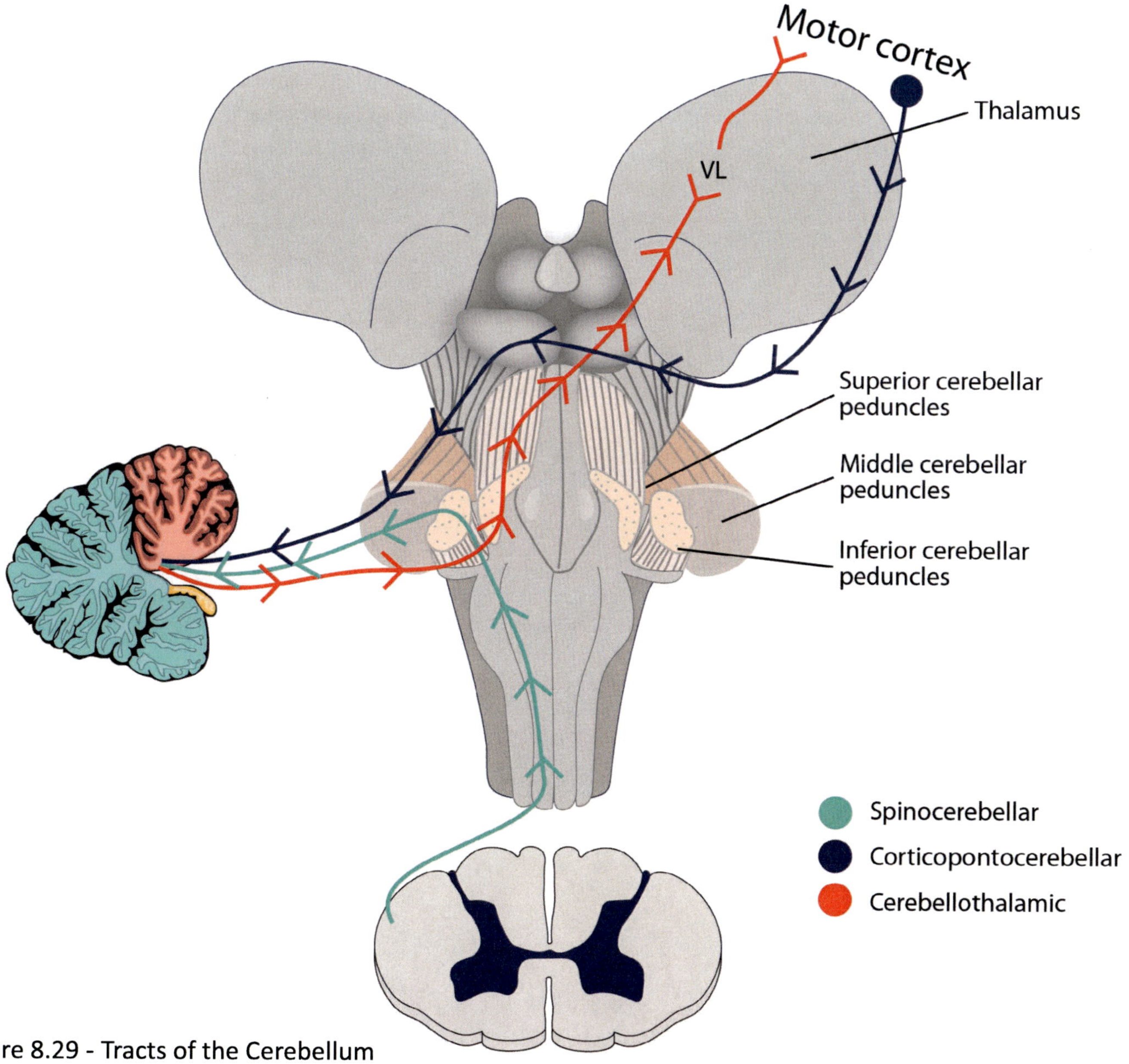

Figure 8.29 - Tracts of the Cerebellum

REVIEW QUESTIONS

1. During a neurological exam, a patient is unable to touch the clinician's finger with his right finger. However, he is able to touch the clinician's finger with his left finger. A CT scan reveals a tumor in the cerebellum. Where in the cerebellum would you expect to find the tumor?

   - **Dysmetria (right-sided)**
     ↓
     Hemisphere lesion (right)

2. A patient seems to have uncoordinated movements while walking. If cerebellar damage is the cause of this presentation, where is the damage likely to be?

   - **Truncal ataxia implicates vermis or flocculonodular lobe (will also have nystagmus)**

   gait/truncal ataxia
   Vermis
   FN Lobe
   No nystagmus

How to approach Cerebellum Questions:

- **Hemisphere lesions cause limb ataxia (intention tremor, dysmetria, dysdiadochokinesia) on the ipsilateral side**
- **Vermis lesions cause gait/truncal ataxia**
- **Flocculonodular lobe lesions cause gait/ truncal ataxia and nystagmus**

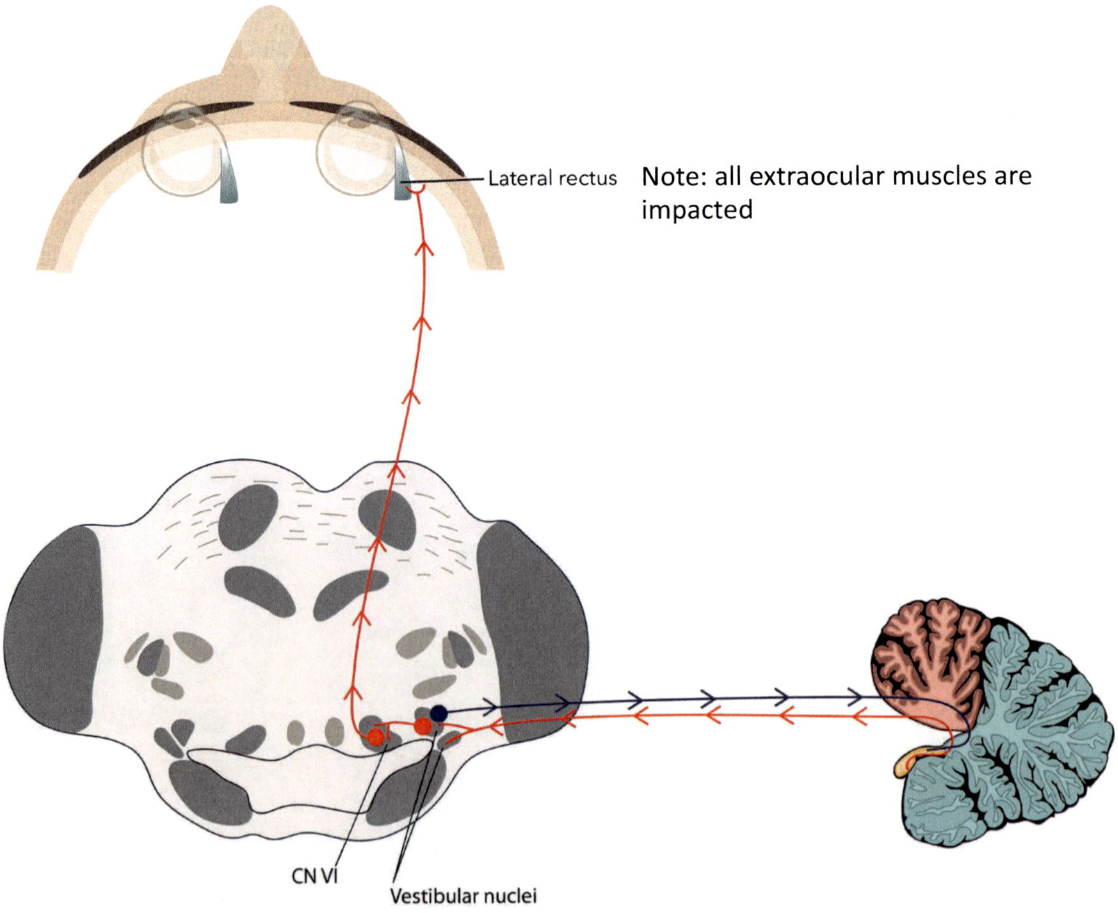

Note: all extraocular muscles are impacted

Figure 8.30 - Flocculonodular Lobe and Cranial Nerve VI

Section VI - Basal Ganglia and Dopaminergic Pathways

I. Basal Ganglia (Figure 8.31)

A. Plays a role in voluntary movements and maintaining posture

B. Composed of the striatum and lentiform

C. Striatum (aka: dorsal striatum)

1. Caudate

a) Just lateral to the lateral ventricles

2. Putamen (just lateral to the internal capsule)

D. Lentiform

1. Globus pallidus (medial to the putamen)

2. Putamen

E. Subthalamic nucleus

1. Normally increases activation of the globus pallidus internus (GPi). The GPi normally inhibits the thalamus which results in decreased activation of the motor cortex and decreased movement.

F. Substantia Nigra pars compacta (SNc)

1. See Nigrostriatal Pathway below

II. Direct (excitatory) Pathway

A. Increase movement

B. Motor cortex → stimulation of striatum (caudate and putamen) → GABA released → increased inhibition of globus pallidus internus → decreased inhibition of thalamus (ventrolateral nucleus) → increased excitement of the motor cortex → increased movement

III. Dopaminergic pathway (Figure 8.32)

A. Project axons to various locations in the brain to deliver dopamine

1. There are four major pathways

2. Nigrostriatal (destruction → Parkinson's)

3. b) Mesolimbic (hyperactivity → positive symptoms)

4. c) Mesocortical (hypoactivity → negative symptoms)

B. Nigrostriatal pathway

1. Cell bodies in the substantia nigra pars compacta (SNc)

2. Axons project to the striatum (caudate and putamen) and release dopamine.

3. Dopamine stimulates the D1 and D2 receptors in the putamen.

4. D1 receptor stimulation → excitatory pathway stimulation → increased movement

5. D2 receptor stimulation → inhibitory pathway inhibition → increased movement

6. Hypoactivity of the pathway → Parkinson-like symptoms (rigidity, bradykinesia, tremors)

C. Mesolimbic pathway

1. Cell bodies reside in the ventral tegmental area (VTA).

2. Regulates behavior and cognition

3. Ventral tegmental area (VTA) releases dopamine → travels to nucleus accumbens.

4. Ventral tegmental area

a) Major production site for dopamine

5. Nucleus accumbens

a) Reward center of the brain. Associated with drugs/addiction, food, sex, etc.

6. Increased activity of the pathway results in the positive symptoms associated with schizophrenia (delusions and hallucinations).

D. Mesocortical pathway

1. Cell bodies reside in the ventral tegmental area (VTA).

2. Axons project to the prefrontal cortex

3. The prefrontal cortex is responsible for motor planning, personality expression, and decision making.

4. Decreased activity of the pathway results in the negative symptoms associated with schizophrenia (limited speech and flat affect).

E. Tuberoinfundibular pathway

1. Cell bodies reside in the hypothalamus.
2. Axons project to the anterior pituitary.
3. Dopamine release at the anterior pituitary causes inhibition of prolactin secretion.

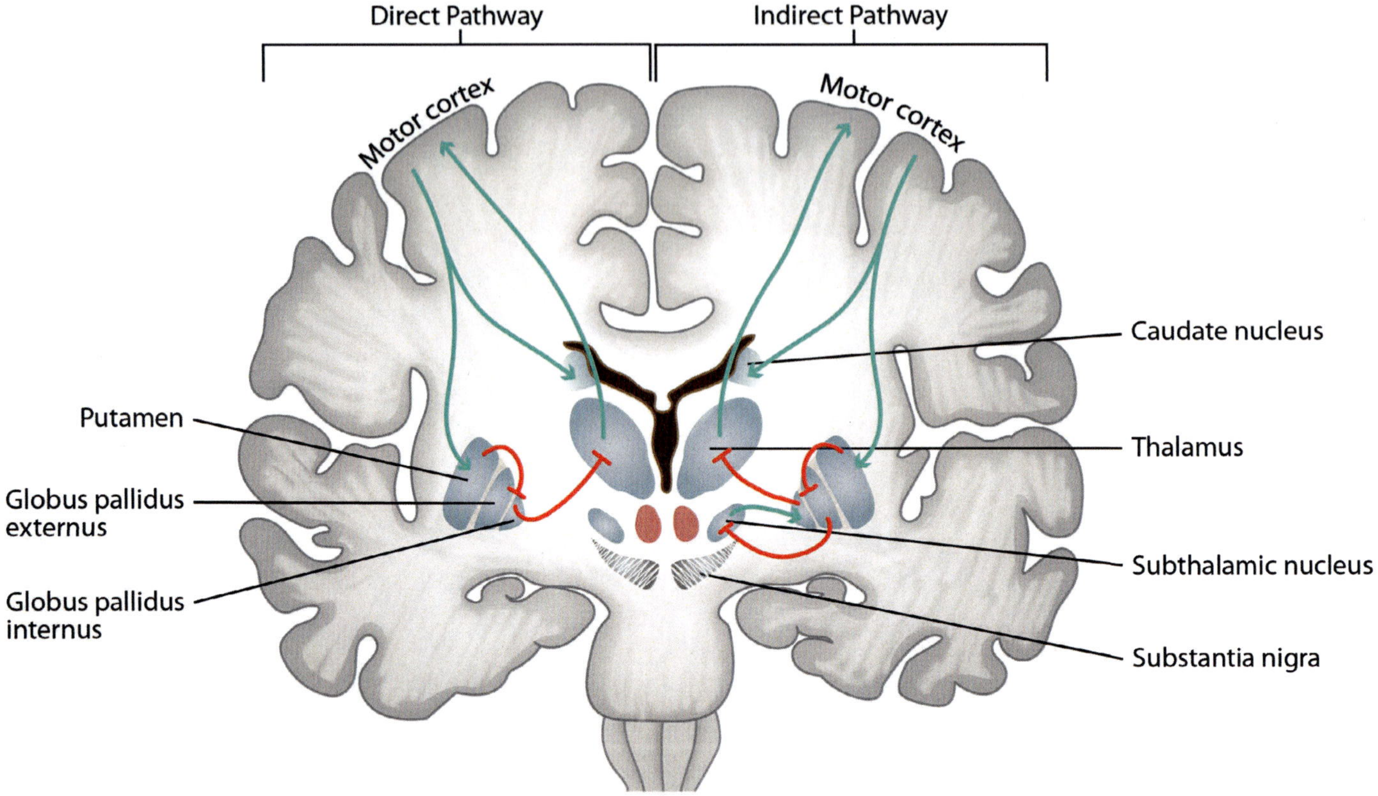

Figure 8.31 - Basal Ganglia

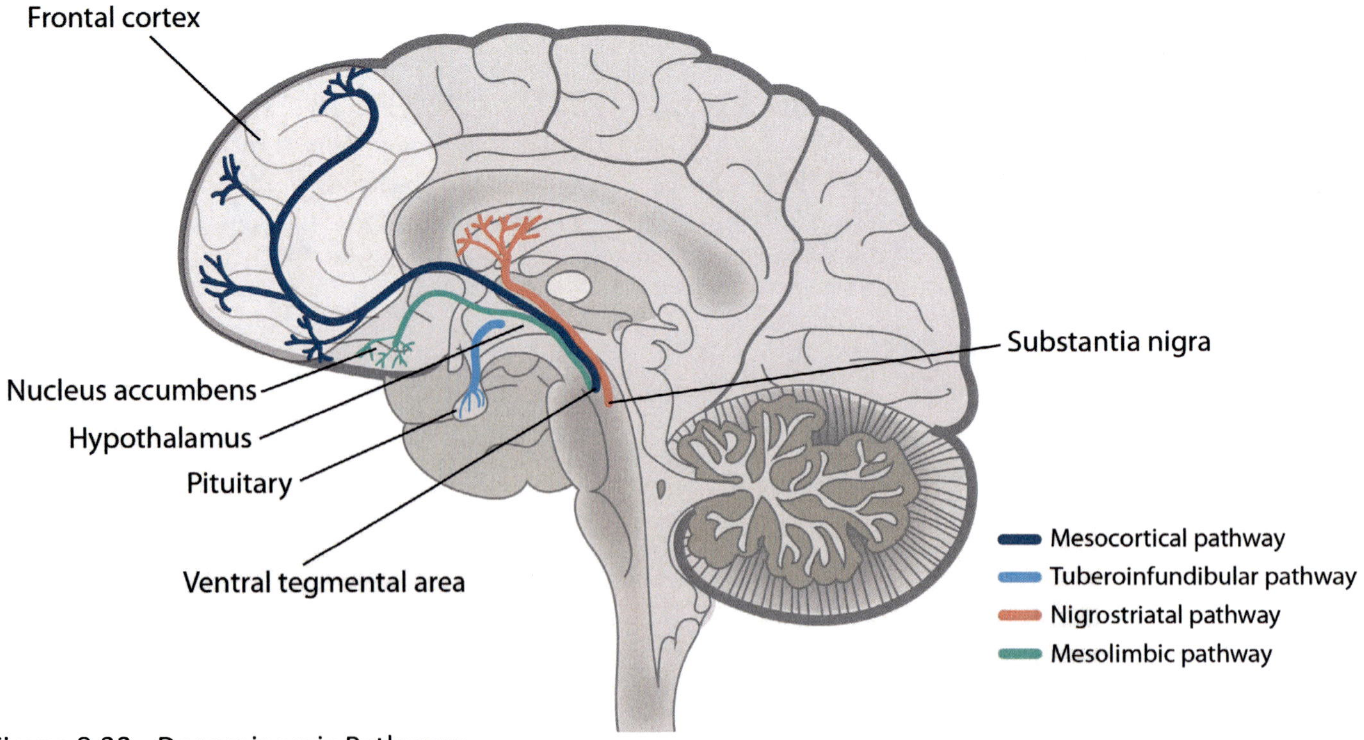

Figure 8.32 - Dopaminergic Pathways

REVIEW QUESTIONS

1. A 27-year-old female presents with rapid, involuntary movements in both arms. She was adopted and is unable to provide an adequate family history. From the image below, what region of the brain is likely damaged?

   - **This describes chorea (Huntington's disease striatum damage), whereas hemiballismus (STN) is unilateral, wild flailing**

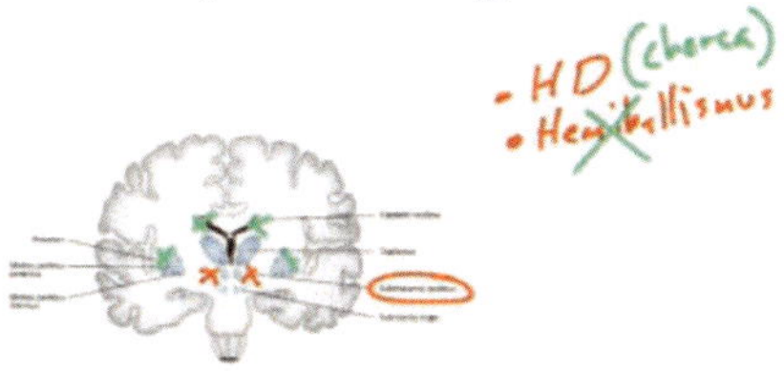

2. What symptoms would you expect with damage to the substantia nigra?

   - **Loss of D1 and D2 receptor stimulation, leading to decreased stimulation of basal ganglia and the motor cortex (decreased movement)**

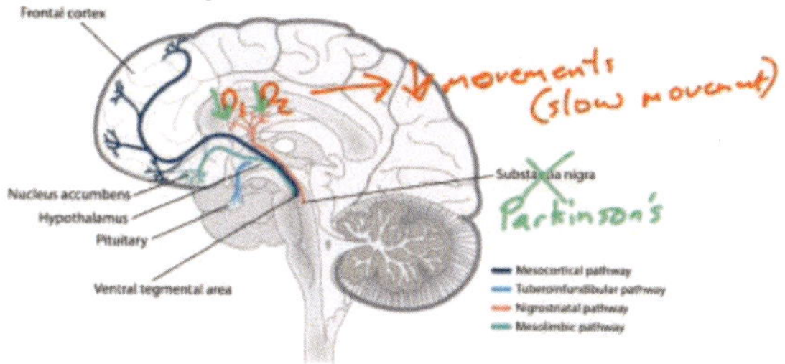

3. What pathway is affected causing a flat affect in a schizophrenic patient?

   - **The prefrontal cortex is responsible for emotion and motivation**
   - **Note: Mesolimbic pathway (nucleus accumbens) stimulation provides positive symptoms in schizophrenia**

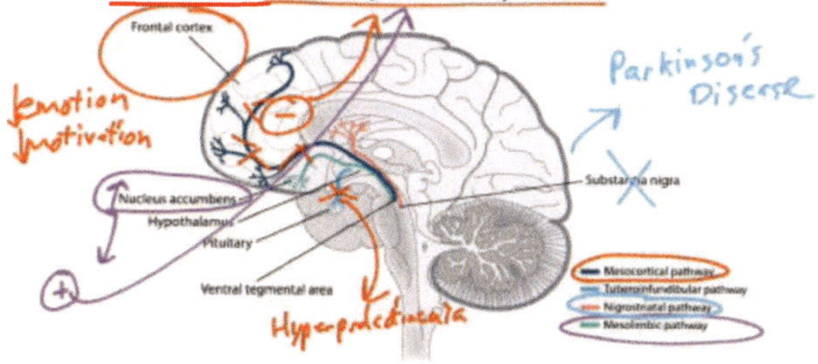

I. Auditory Pathway (Figures 8.33, 8.34, and 8.35)

A. Auditory canal of outer ear → tympanic membrane of middle ear → auditory ossicles (malleus, incus, stapes) → oval window → fluid displacement within cochlea → basilar membrane vibrates → hair cells within basilar membrane press against tectorial membrane → oscillating potential generated → firing of CN VIII in the midbrain → fibers ascend through lateral lemniscus to ipsilateral + contralateral superior olivary nucleus and ipsilateral + contralateral inferior colliculus

II. Tonotopy and Hearing Loss (Figure 8.36)

A. Sounds produce vibrations of a certain frequency.

B. Each frequency is associated with a specific part along the cochlea.

C. Base of cochlea = high frequency

1. Lost in noise-induced and presbycusis

D. Helicotrema of cochlea = low frequency

III. Rinne Test

A. Tuning fork placed near, but not touching the ear (air)

B. Tuning fork placed on bony area surrounding ear (bone)

C. Air > bone = normal hearing

1. Or sensorineural hearing loss (inner ear)

D. Bone > air = conductive hearing loss (outer to middle ear)

IV. Weber Test

A. Tuning fork placed on top of skull

B. Localizes hearing loss to affected ear in conductive hearing loss

1. Right = left (normal)
2. Right > left (left-sided hearing loss)
3. Right < left (right-sided hearing loss)

C. Localizes to the unaffected ear in sensorineural hearing loss

V. Vestibular System (Figure 8.37)

A. Maintains balance

B. Composed of 3 semicircular canals and the utricle and saccule

C. Semicircular canals are filled with endolymph.

D. Hair cells with cilia are within the endolymph.

E. Vestibular transduction occurs when cilia of hair cells move against the endolymph → vestibular fibers to vestibular nerve in pons.

1. Alteration to endolymph (i.e. BBPV or Meniere's disease) will cause vertigo.

VI. Vestibular-Ocular Reflex (Figure 8.38)

A. Maintains image in center

B. Head turn to the left:

1. Cortical stimulation → fast phase (nystagmus) eye movement left
2. Increased firing of left vestibular system → vestibular-ocular reflex stimulation → slow phase eye movement right

C. If unconscious → no cortical input → no fast phase, no nystagmus

D. If damaged brainstem/vestibular function → no VOR → no slow phase

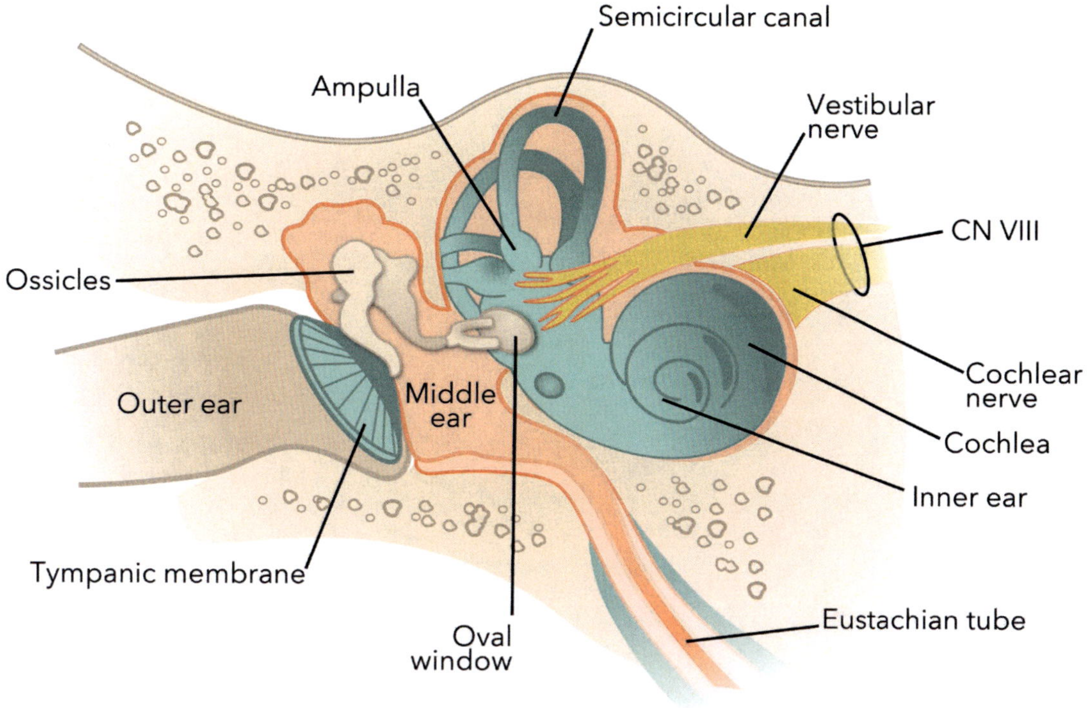

Figure 8.33 - Auditory Anatomy

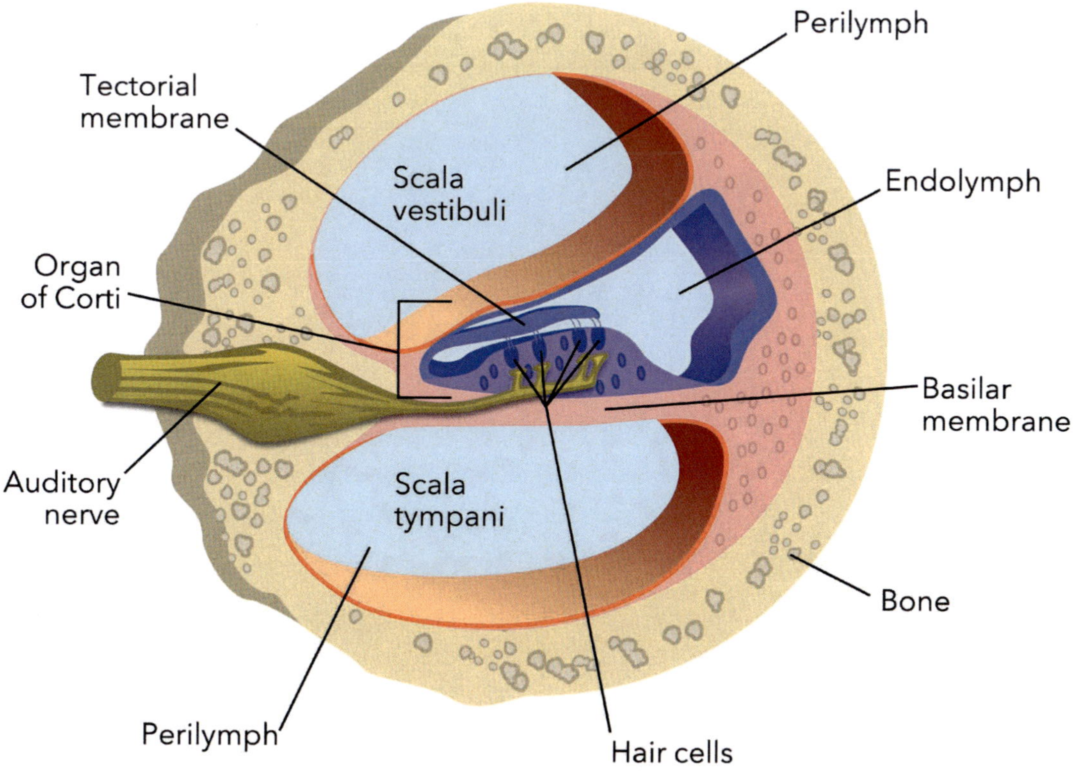

Figure 8.34 - Cross-Section of the Cochlea

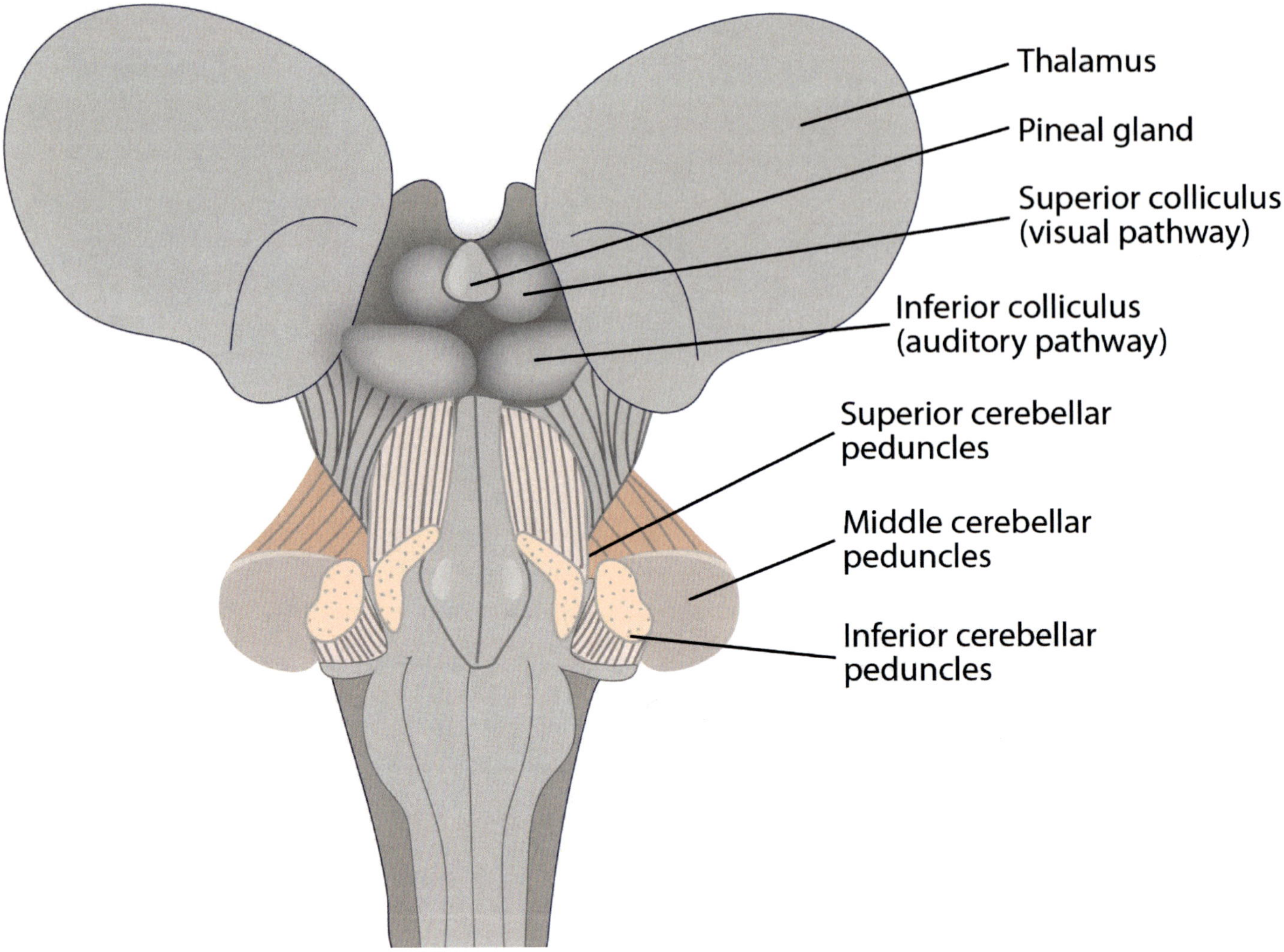

Figure 8.35 - Auditory Anatomy (Brainstem)

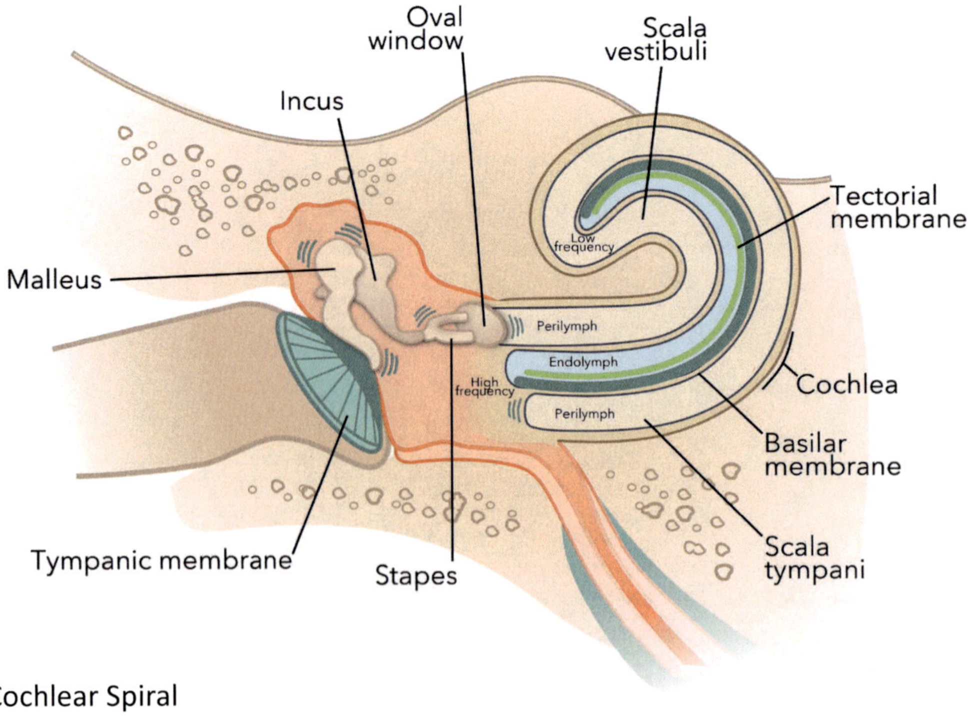

Figure 8.36 - Cochlear Spiral

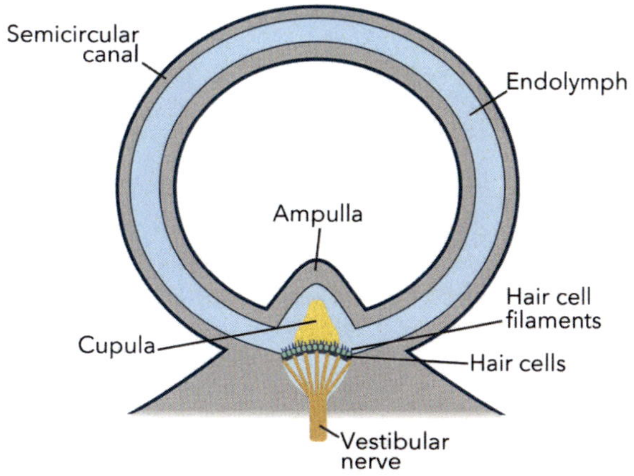

Figure 8.37 - Semicircular Canal

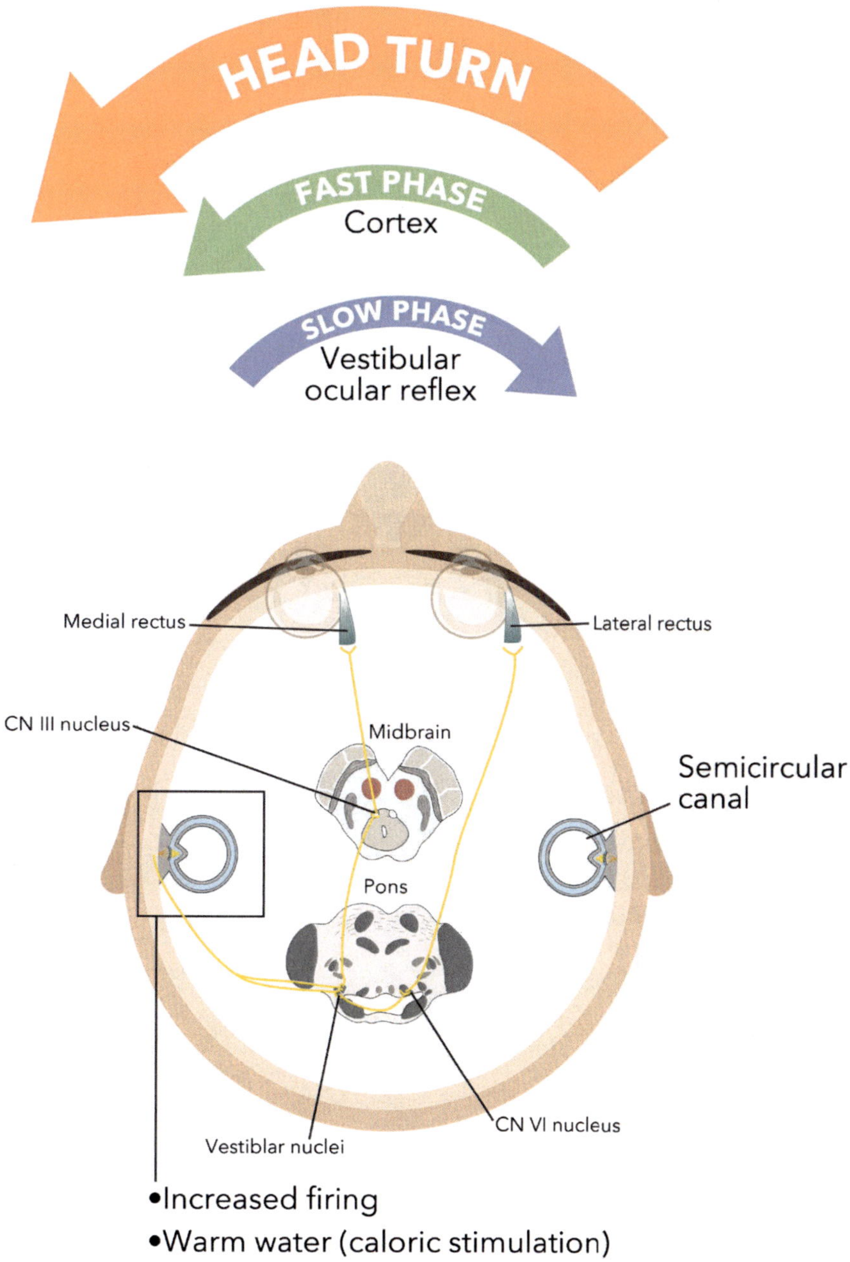

Figure 8.38 - Vestibular-Ocular Reflex

REVIEW QUESTIONS

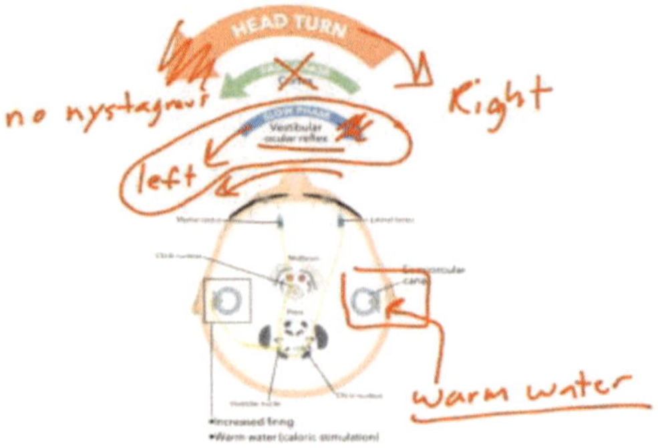

1. A 70-year-old male factory worker complains of hearing loss. What part of the cochlea is likely responsible for this loss, the base or the apex?

    - **This describes noise-induced hearing loss, resulting in damage to the base (high frequency)**

noise-induced HL → base of cochlea damaged

low frequency HL or High frequency HL

2. A patient describes a muffling of sound in the right ear following a boating trip. Upon physical exam, there appears to be water lateral to the ear drum. What would be the results of the Rinne hearing test?

    - **Based on the description of the trauma, suspect conductive hearing loss**
    - **Rinne test would reveal bone conduction would be louder than air conduction**

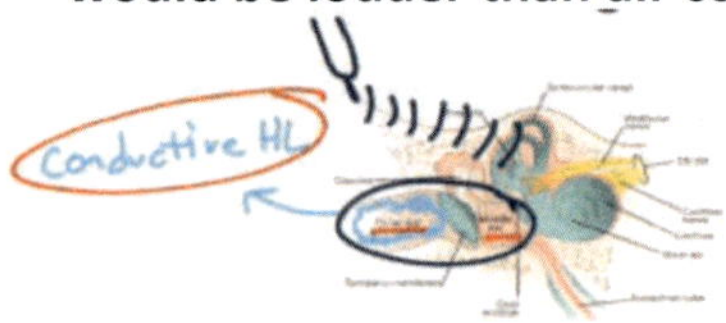

Bone > air

3. A female patient is unconscious following a car wreck. The medics on site are able to elicit a normal pupillary light reflex, indicating proper brainstem function. If caloric stimulation with warm water was performed in the right ear, how would the patient's eyes respond?

    - **Warm water in right ear makes the brain think the head is turning to the right**
    - **Since the patient is unconscious, don't expect the fast phase (motor cortex) or nystagmus**
    - **The eyes should drift to the left (slow phase) since the brainstem is functional**

Section VIII - Ophthalmology

I. Visual Pathway (Figure 8.39)

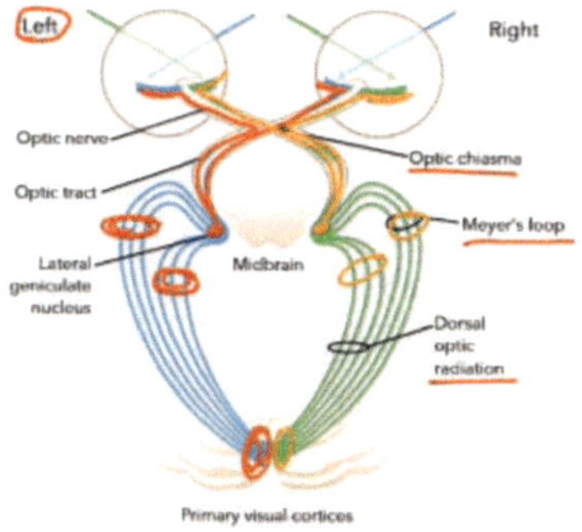

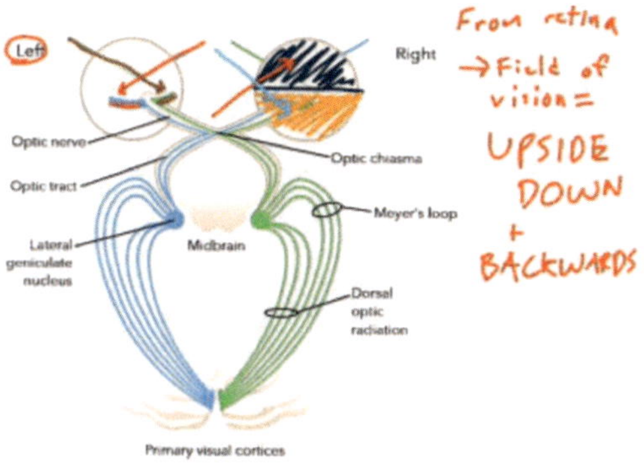

A. Temporal hemiretina → optic nerve → ipsilateral optic chiasm and optic tract → ipsilateral lateral geniculate body → ipsilateral optic radiations (dorsal optic radiation and Meyer's loop) → ipsilateral primary visual cortex

B. Nasal hemiretina → optic nerve → contralateral optic chiasm and optic tract → contralateral lateral geniculate body → contralateral optic radiations (dorsal optic radiation and Meyer's loop) → contralateral primary visual cortex

C. Dorsal optic radiations traverse the parietal lobe → synapse on the upper occipital cortex

D. Meyer loop (lateral optic radiations) traverse the temporal lobe → synapse on the lower occipital cortex

E. Lesion locations and the resulting visual field can be seen on figure 8.40.

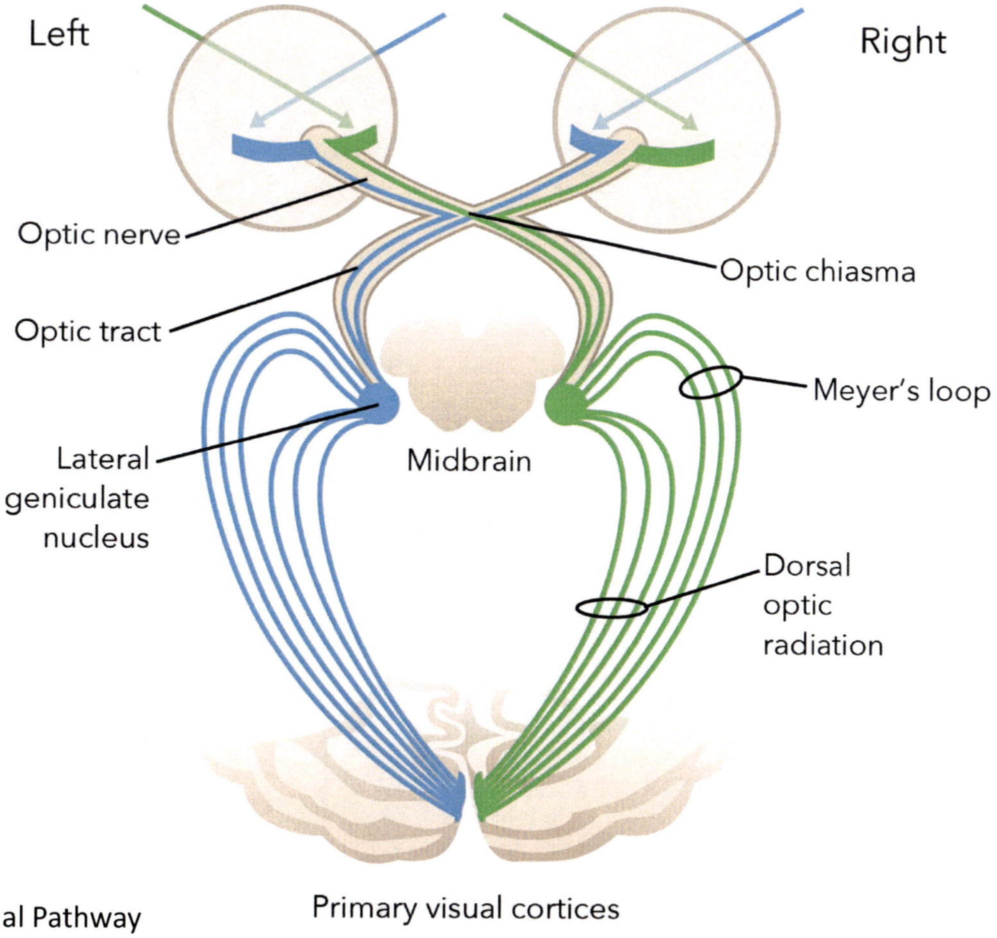

Figure 8.39 - Visual Pathway

F. Rocking visual field questions
   1. Determine the location of lesion in the visual pathway
   2. Determine what part of the retina will be dysfunctional
   3. Determine the field of vision deficit

II. Macula
   A. The macula is a part of the retina.
   B. The PCA supplies blood to the occipital cortex but the region responsible for macular vision receives blood from the MCA. PCA stroke → contralateral homonymous hemianopia with macular sparing

III. Blood Supply to the Visual Pathway (Figure 8.41)
   A. Retina → ophthalmic artery (internal carotid)
   B. Optic nerve and chiasm → branches of the ACA
   C. Optic tract → anterior choroidal (MCA) and posterior communicating

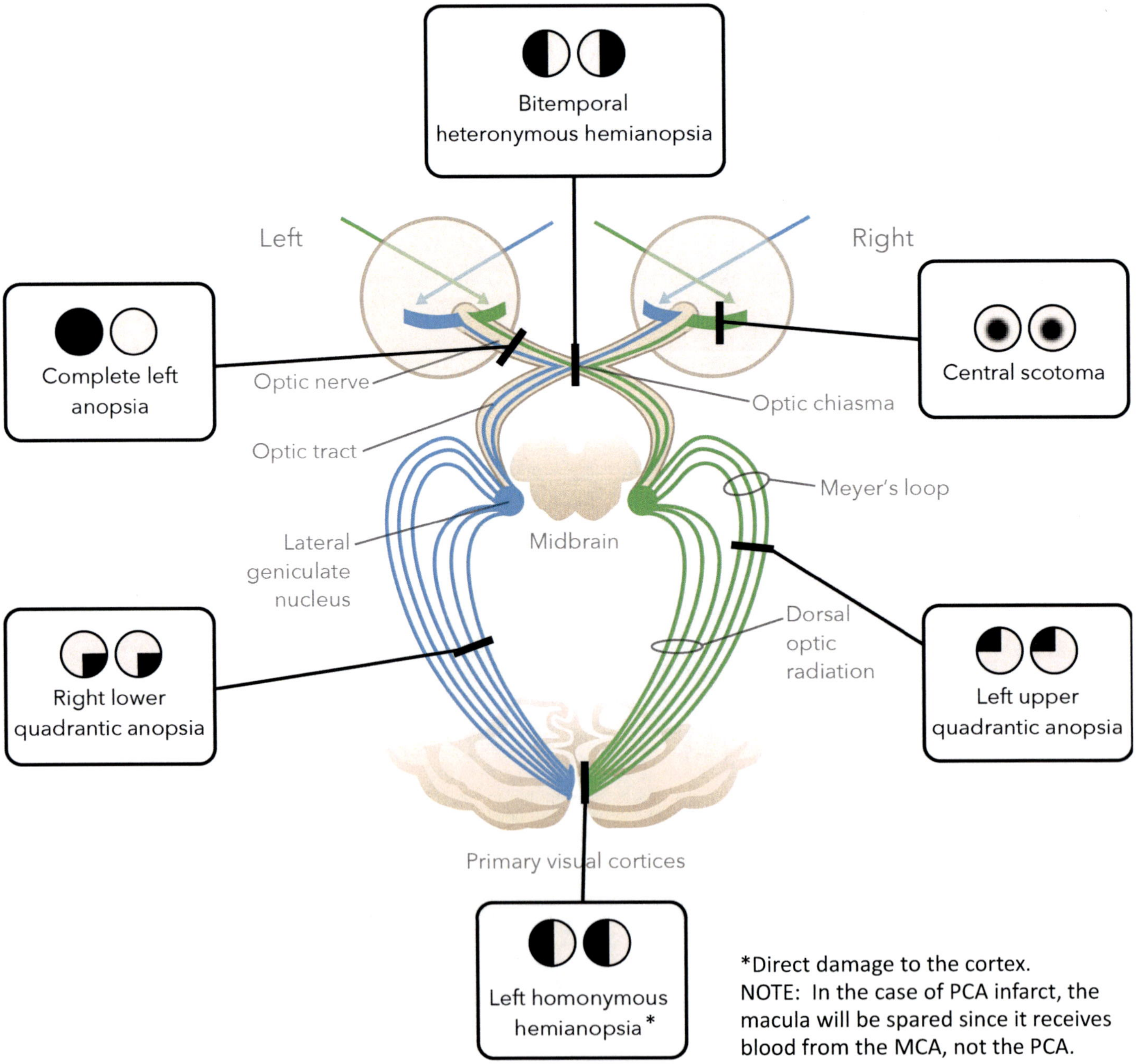

Figure 8.40 - Visual Pathway Lesions

D. Lateral geniculate nucleus → anterior choroidal (MCA) and posterior choroidal (ACA) arteries

E. Optic radiations → MCA and PCA

F. Occipital cortex → PCA (macular area supplied by MCA)

IV. Parasympathetic Innervation (Figure 8.42)

A. Mediated by CN III

B. Edinger-Westphal nucleus → ciliary ganglion → short ciliary nerve → pupillary sphincter muscle → miosis

C. Edinger-Westphal nucleus → ciliary ganglion → short ciliary nerve → ciliary muscle → accommodation of lens

D. Pupillary light reflex (Figure 8.43)

1. Retina receives light stimulus → CN II to pretectal nucleus in midbrain → fibers travel to ipsilateral and contralateral Edinger-Westphal nucleus → CN III to ciliary ganglion bilaterally → short ciliary nerve → pupillary sphincter muscle → miosis

V. Sympathetic Innervation (Figure 8.44)

A. Hypothalamus → lateral tegmentum → lateral horn gray matter of C8-T2 → exits at T1 to enter sympathetic chain → superior cervical ganglion at C2 → long ciliary nerve → pupillary dilator muscle → mydriasis

B. Superior cervical ganglion → superior tarsal muscle → lid retraction

C. The superior cervical ganglion also sends fibers to the sweat glands (sweating) and blood vessels (constriction) of the face and forehead

1. Horner's syndrome

a) Loss of long ciliary nerve innervation → miosis

b) Loss of superior tarsal muscle innervation → ptosis

c) Loss of sweat gland innervation → anhidrosis

d) Loss of vasoconstriction → vasodilation

Vascular Supply

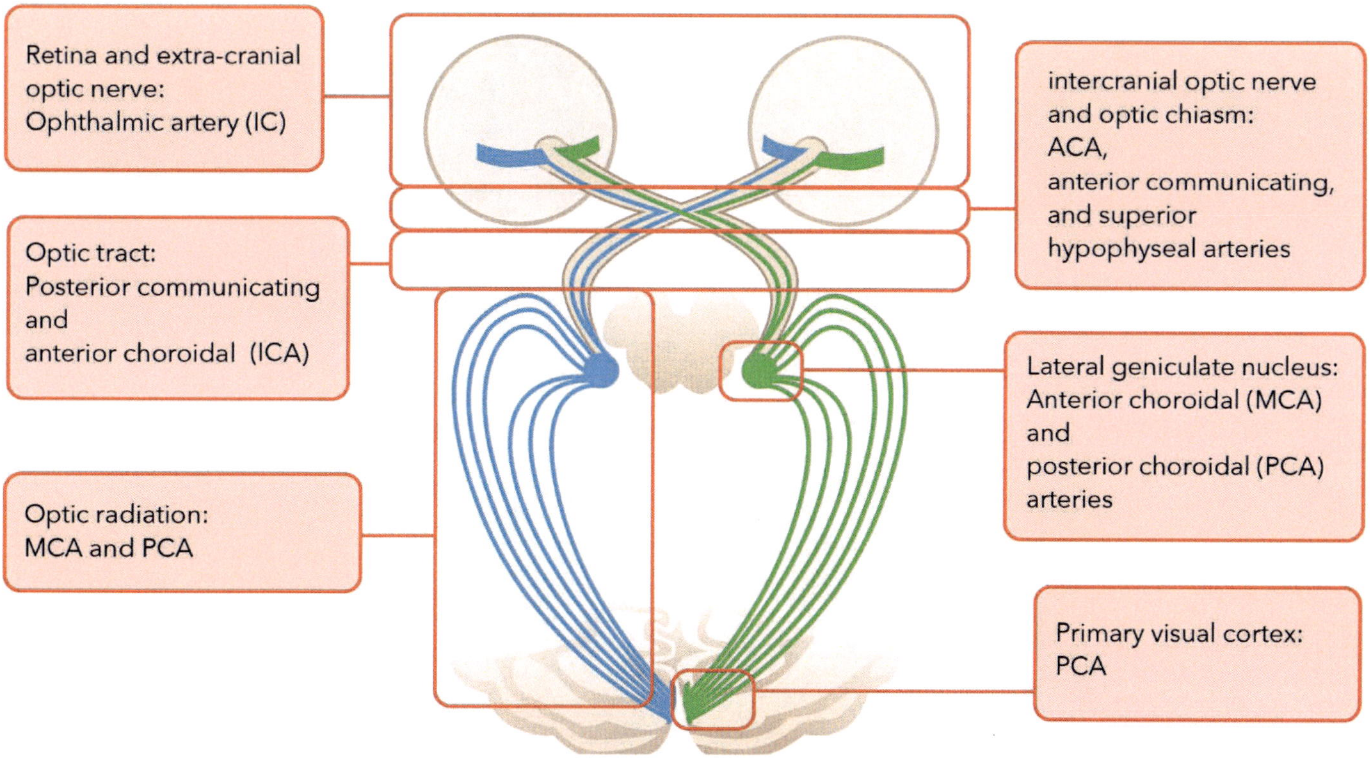

Figure 8.41 - Vascular Supply of the Visual Pathway

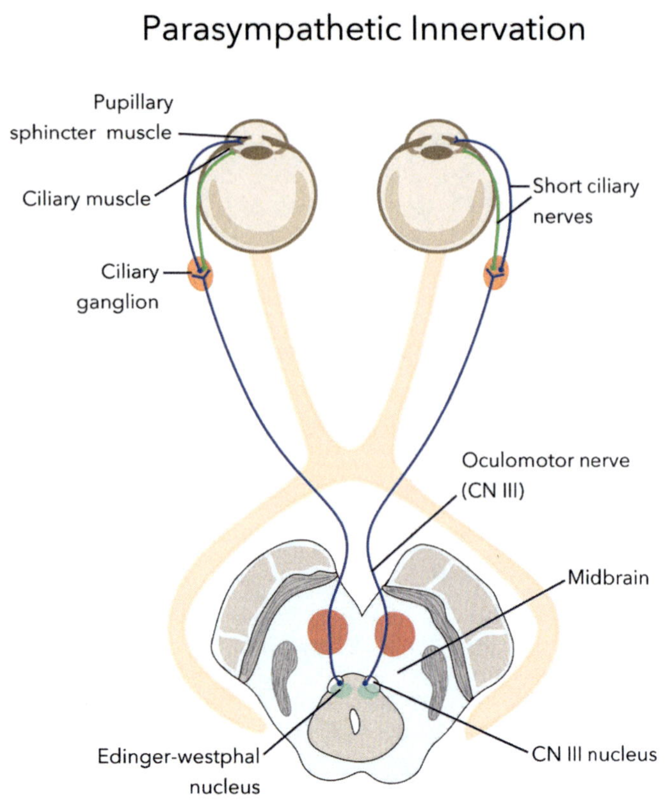

Figure 8.42 - Parasympathetic Innervation of the Visual Pathway

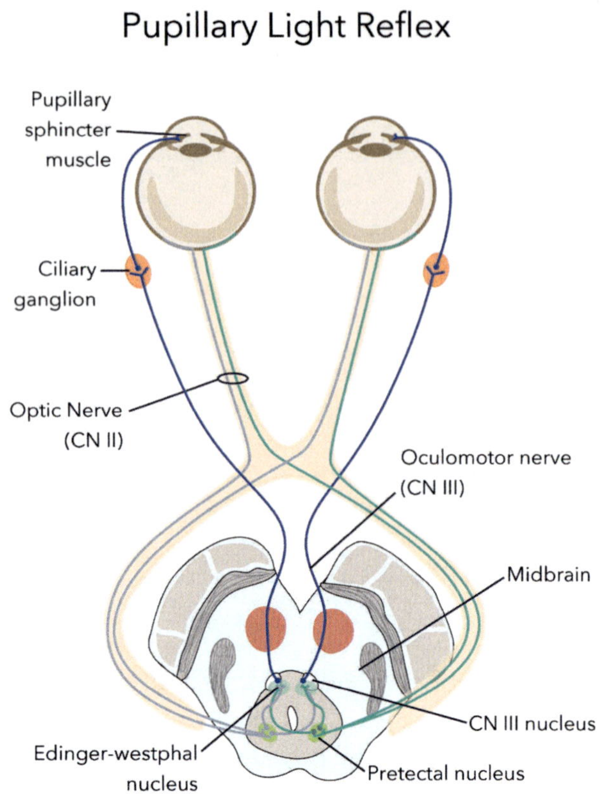

Figure 8.43 - Pupillary Light Reflex

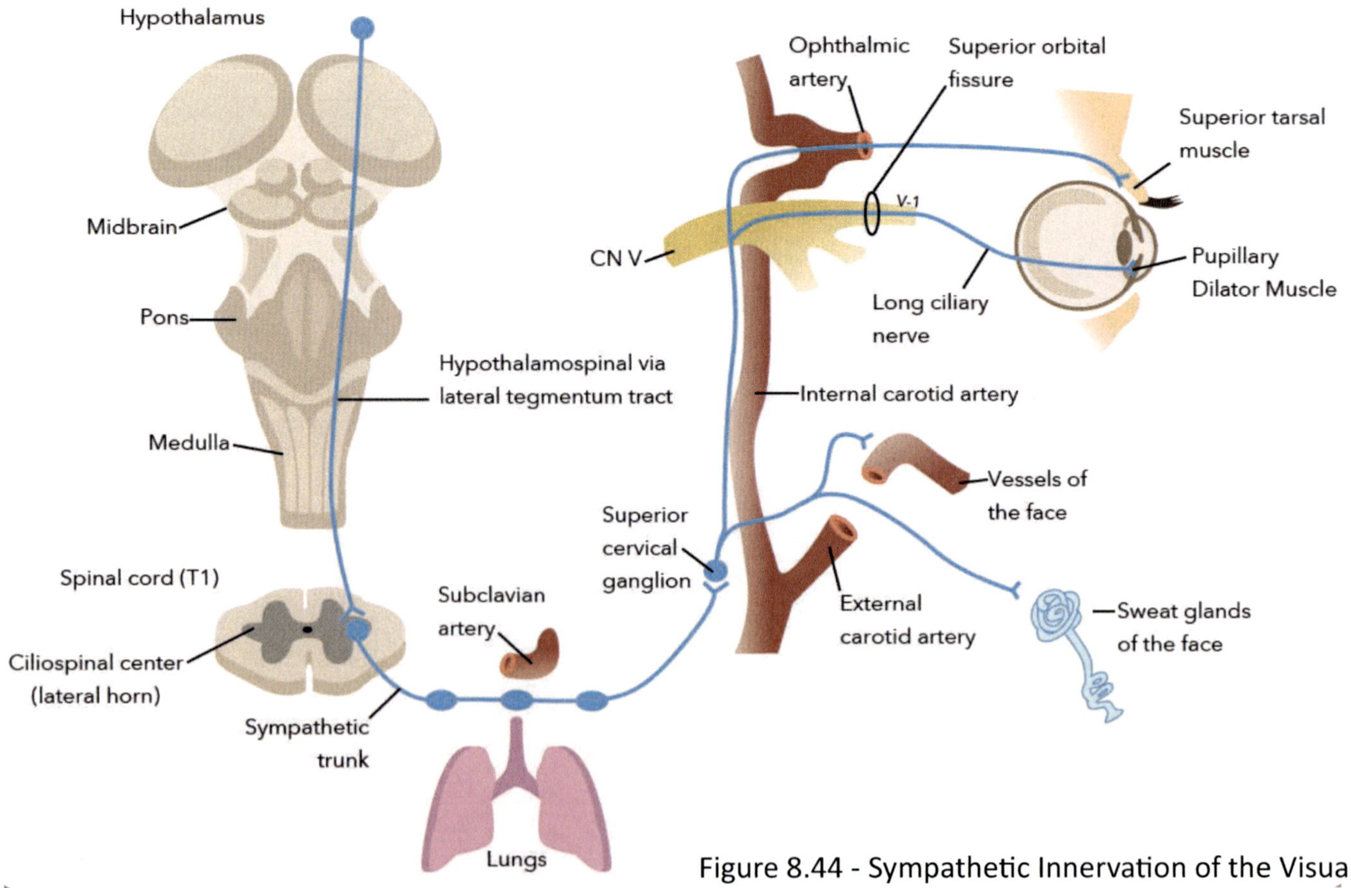

Figure 8.44 - Sympathetic Innervation of the Visual Pathway and Horner's Syndrome

VI. Horizontal Gaze Pathway (Figure 8.45)

A. Right frontal eye field → left paramedian pontine reticular formation (PPRF) in pons → left abducens nucleus (CN VI) in pons → right medial longitudinal fasciculus (MLF) → right medial rectus subnucleus (CN III) in midbrain

B. Net effect: Left lateral rectus muscle and the right medial rectus muscle stimulated at the same time → eyes look left

C. Internuclear Ophthalmoplegia (INO)

1. Right INO = right MLF damage = double vision when looking left = nystagmus of left eye
2. Left INO = left MLF damage = double vision when looking right = nystagmus of right eye
3. MLF and CN VI are located in medial pons
4. CN III is located in medial midbrain

VII. Vertical Gaze Pathway (Figures 8.3 and 8.16)

A. Superior colliculus is responsible for ensuring both eyes move up and down together (conjugate gaze)

B. The superior colliculus located on the dorsal midbrain

C. Can be damaged by pineal gland tumor

VIII. Ocular Muscles

A. Medial rectus → adduct

B. Lateral rectus → abduct

C. Superior rectus → elevate

D. Inferior rectus → depress

E. Superior oblique → abduct, depress, internally rotate

F. Inferior oblique → abduct, elevate, externally rotate

G. $LR_6SO_4R_3$

1. Lateral rectus via CN VI (lesion → medial deviation)
2. Superior oblique via CN IV (lesion → medial/upward deviation)
3. The rest via CN III (lesion → lateral/downward deviation, mydriasis)

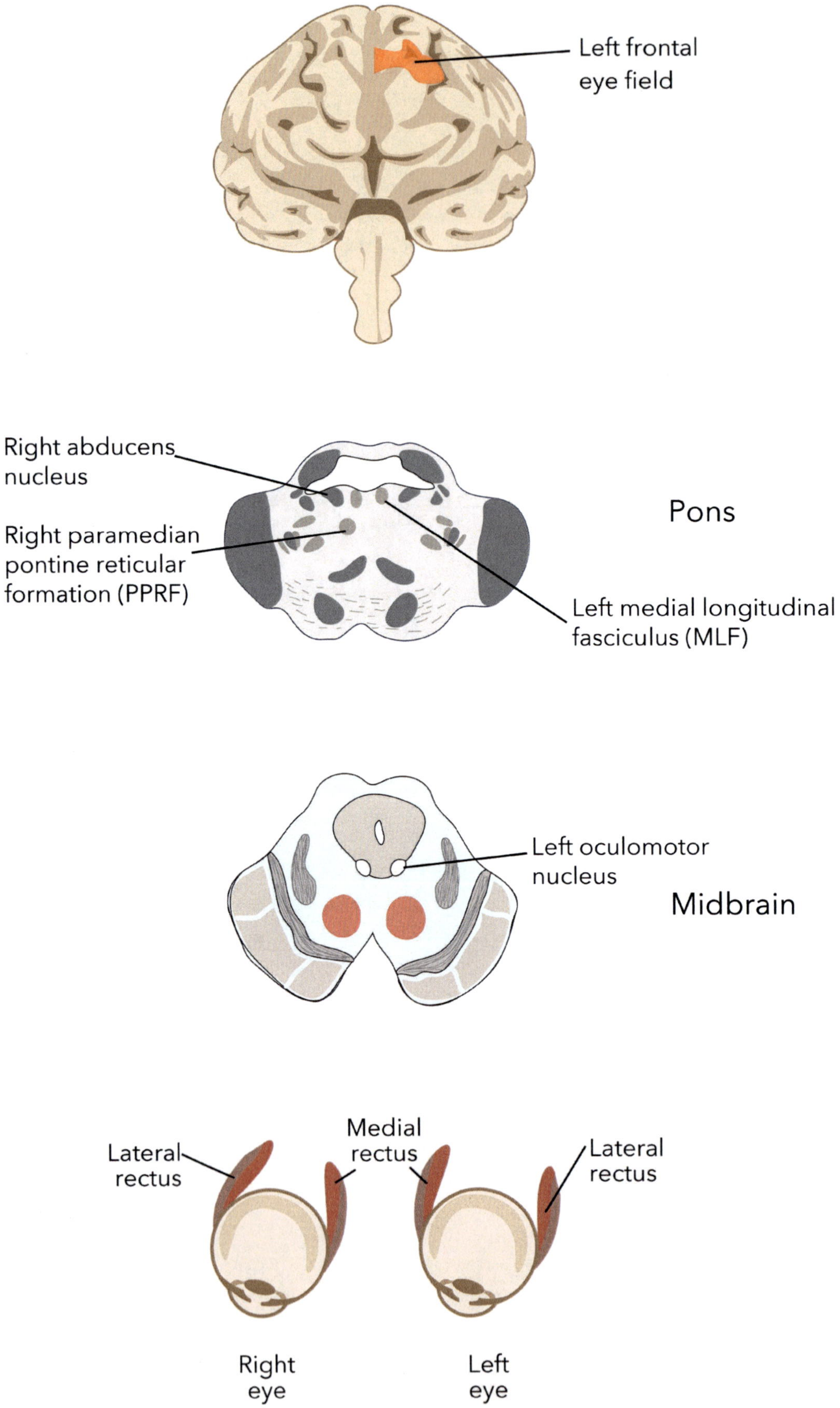

Figure 8.45 - Horizontal Gaze Pathway and Internuclear Ophthalmoplegia

REVIEW QUESTIONS

1. A patient is unable to visualize anything on her left. What part of the visual pathway is likely damaged?

   - **Left visual field is absent (left homonymous hemianopsia)**
   - **Remember the upside down and backwards rule: Pathway from right hemiretina (bilaterally) and back to the occipital cortex could be damaged**

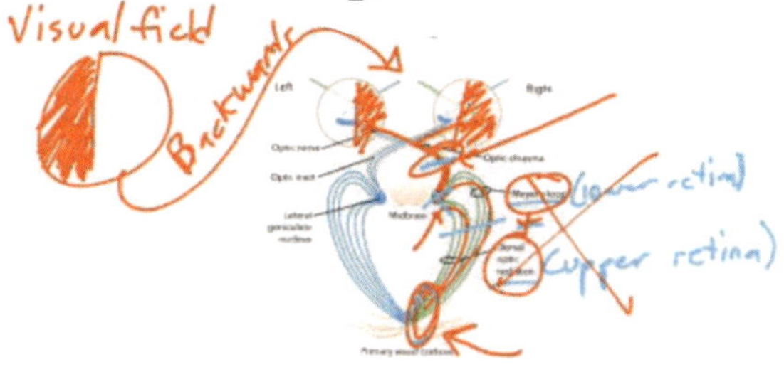

2. An elderly female patient has a tumor in the left temporal lobe. What visual field defect might she have as a result of the tumor?

   - **The Meyer's loop traverses the temporal lobe and is responsible for the lower retina (left lower quadrant damage)**
   - **Remember upside and backwards rule: right upper quadrantic field defect**

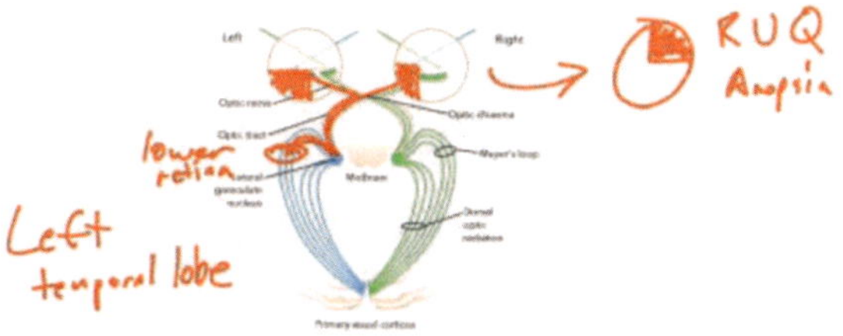

3. A 64-year-old female patient complains of a blurry spot in the middle of her vision. Where is there damage likely to be?

   - **This describes central loss of vision which could be due to MCA damage or central retina damage**

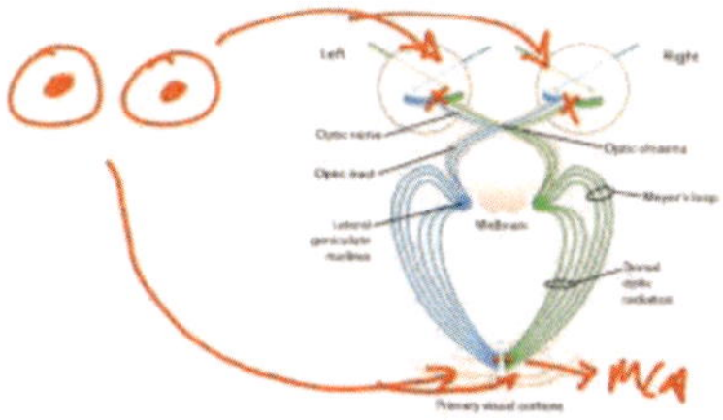

4. A 73-year-old male patient is found unconscious on his living room floor. After regaining consciousness he complains of loss of vision on the left side with full vision in the center. Neurologic imaging indicates a stroke. Where was the stroke likely to be?

   - **This describes left homonymous hemianopsia**
   - **Remember upside and backwards rule: Right hemiretina pathway and back could be damaged**
   - **Macular sparing indicates PCA infarct (MCA supplies central vision)**

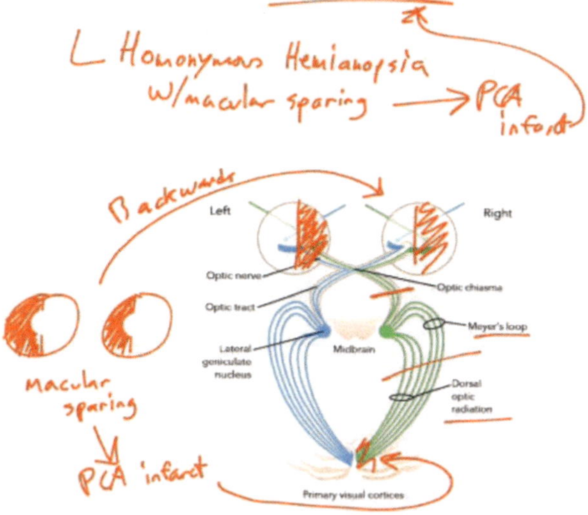

5. A patient has a severe retinal detachment in the left eye. How will the right eye respond when light is shone through the left eye?

   - **Left retinal detachment implies left afferent (optic nerve) damage, resulting in no signal reaching the brainstem and no constriction of either pupil**

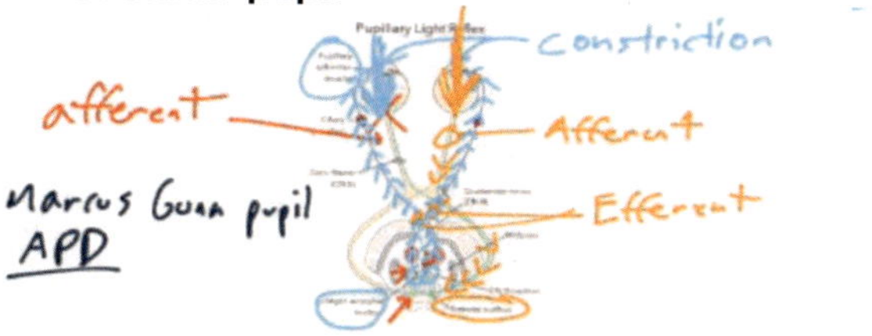

REVIEW QUESTIONS

6. A patient is unconscious following a car crash. The medic shines a light in both eyes without any constriction of either pupil. If brain damage caused the failed pupillary light reflex, what structure would be implicated?

- **Midbrain**

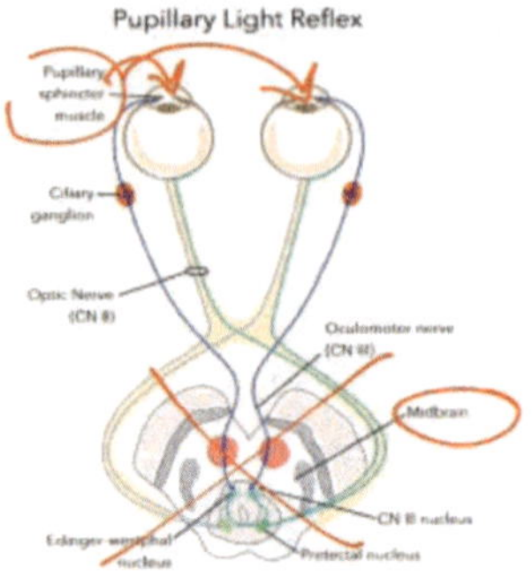

7. The left MLF is damaged. What will happen when the patient looks to the left?

- **When looking right: The left medial rectus muscle will not be stimulated, resulting in nystagmus from right eye and left eye remaining straight**
- **When looking left: Normal gaze because the left MLF was not needed**

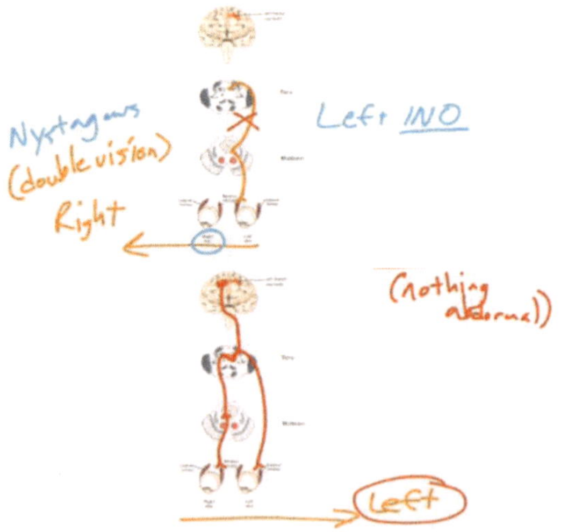

8. A patient demonstrates right-sided INO. When will she likely experience double vision?

- **Right INO indicates right MLF damage**
- **Double vision will occur when looking left because the right eye will remain forward**

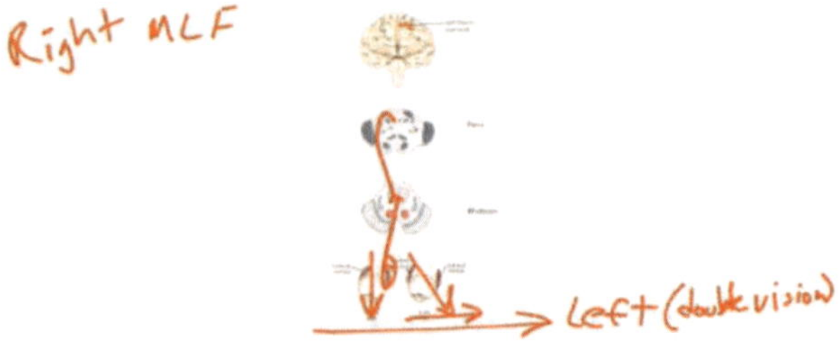

9. A patient demonstrates right-sided INO and experiences double vision when looking left. Convergence is intact. Where in the brain is the lesion?

- **Pons: Near the fourth ventricle on the medial side (motor nuclei are found medial to the sulcus limitans)**
- **Medulla: Not an testable/identifiable location**

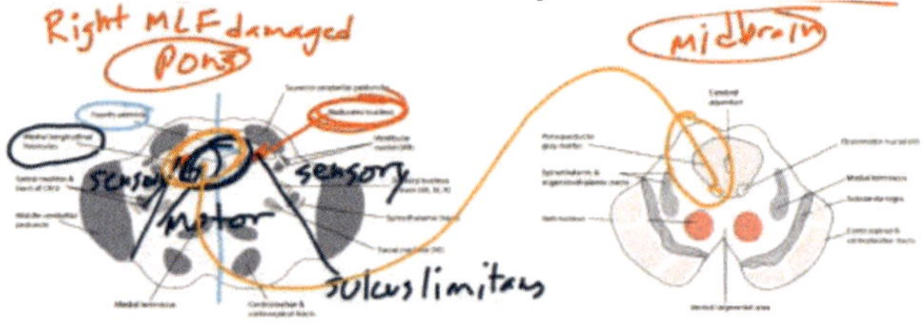

10. A patient develops right-sided ptosis and miosis secondary to Brown-Sequard syndrome. What was damaged, the post-ganglionic or pre-ganglionic sympathetic fibers?

- **Brown-Sequard syndrome damages the spinal cord (preganglionic fibers)**

The Oculosympathetic Pathway

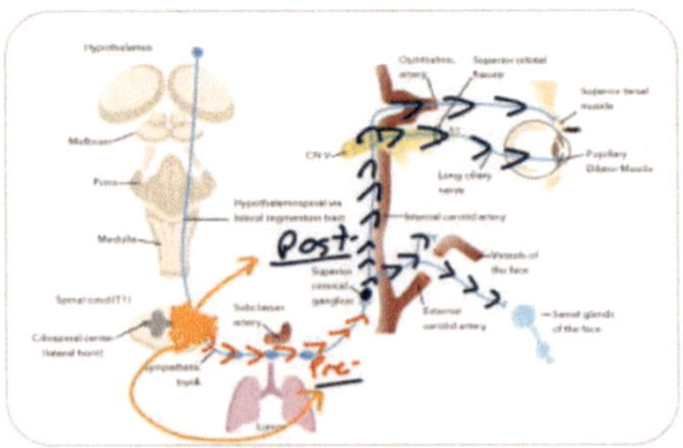

The Oculosympathetic Pathway

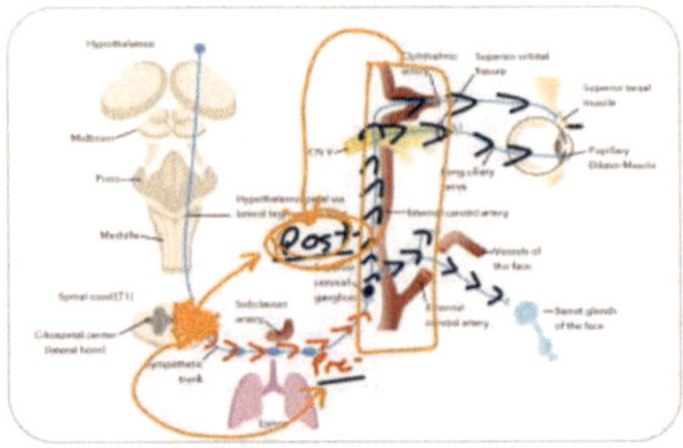

Section IX - Neurovasculature

I. Vasculature

A. Blood brain barrier

1. Composed of endothelial cells, astrocytes, and pericytes.

B. Figure 8.46 provides a general overview of the neurovascular anatomy.

C. Figure 8.47 shows an inferior view of the Circle of Willis.

D. Figure 8.48 shows the important neurovascular territories supplied by the cerebral circulation.

E. Figure 8.49 provides a coronal view of the lenticulostriate arteries.

F. Table 8.4 provides an overview of the effects of strokes.

Table 8.4 - Strokes

Artery	Lesioned Area & Symptoms
Anterior cerebral artery	1. Medial aspect of primary sensory and motor cortices → contralateral motor and sensory deficits of the leg
Middle cerebral artery	1. Lateral aspect of primary sensory and motor cortices → contralateral motor and sensory deficits of the face and arm
Lenticulostriate artery	1. Basal ganglia → movement abnormalities (highly variable depending on the region damaged) 2. Internal capsule → contralateral paralysis and sensory deficits of the entire body
Posterior cerebral artery	1. Visual cortex → contralateral hemianopia with sparing of the macula
Basilar artery	1. Midbrain, pons, and medulla are all damaged. The structures below are spared: 1. CN III → vertical eye movement and blinking intact 2. Reticular activating system (reticular formation and tegmentum) → preserved consciousness
Anterior inferior cerebellar artery (lateral pontine syndrome)	1. Lateral pons a) Facial nucleus → ipsilateral facial paralysis b) Solitary nucleus → taste deficit from the anterior ⅔ of the tongue c) Vestibular nuclei → vertigo and nystagmus d) Spinal nucleus and tract of CN V → ipsilateral facial deficits of pain and temperature e) Spinothalamic tract → contralateral deficits of pain and temperature f) Inferior cerebellar peduncle → ataxia, dysmetria, and falls toward lesioned side g) Lateral tegmentum → interruption of the hypothalamospinal tract (sympathetic innervation of the face)
Posterior inferior cerebellar artery / vertebral artery (lateral medullary syndrome)	1. Lateral medulla a) Nucleus ambiguous → dysphagia and dysphonia b) Vestibular nuclei → vertigo and nystagmus c) Spinal nucleus and tract of CN V → ipsilateral facial deficits of pain and temperature d) Spinothalamic tract → contralateral deficits of pain and temperature e) Inferior cerebellar peduncle → ataxia, dysmetria, and falls toward lesioned side f) Lateral tegmentum → interruption of the hypothalamospinal tract (sympathetic innervation of the face)
Anterior spinal artery (paramedian branches)	1. Corticospinal tract → contralateral hemiparesis 2. Medial lemniscus → contralateral loss of vibration and proprioception 3. Hypoglossal nuclei → ipsilateral tongue deviation

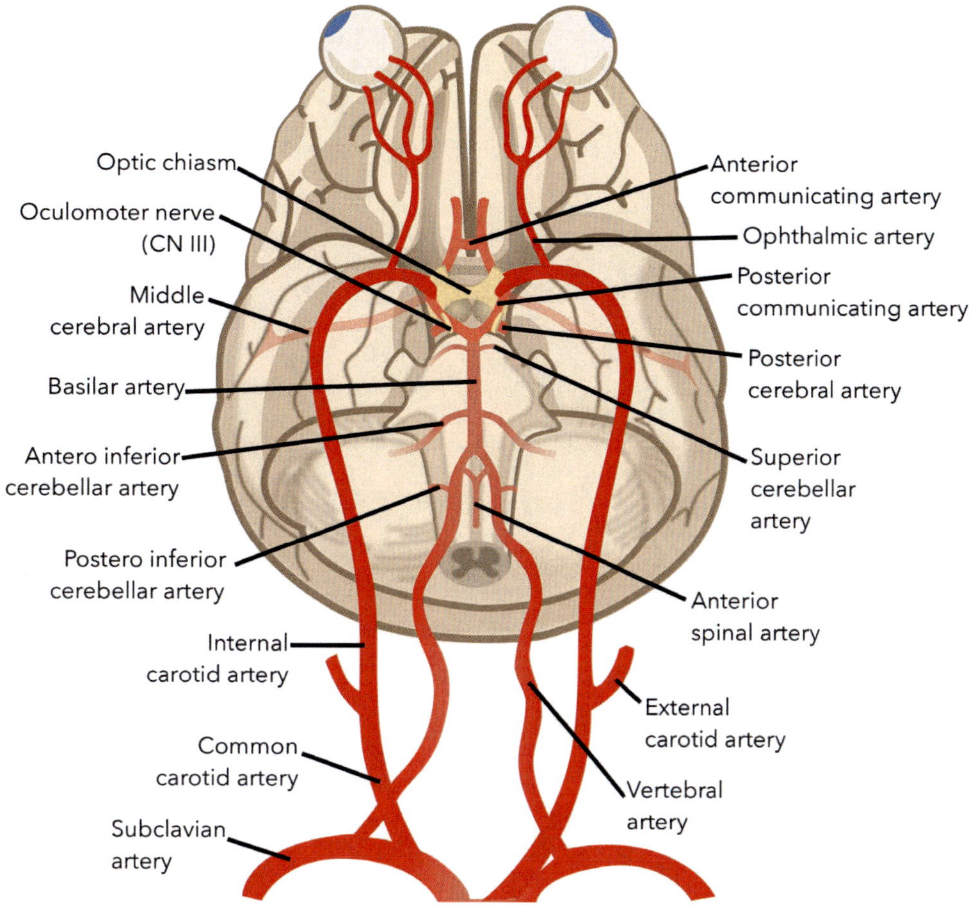

Figure 8.46 - Neurovascular anatomy overview

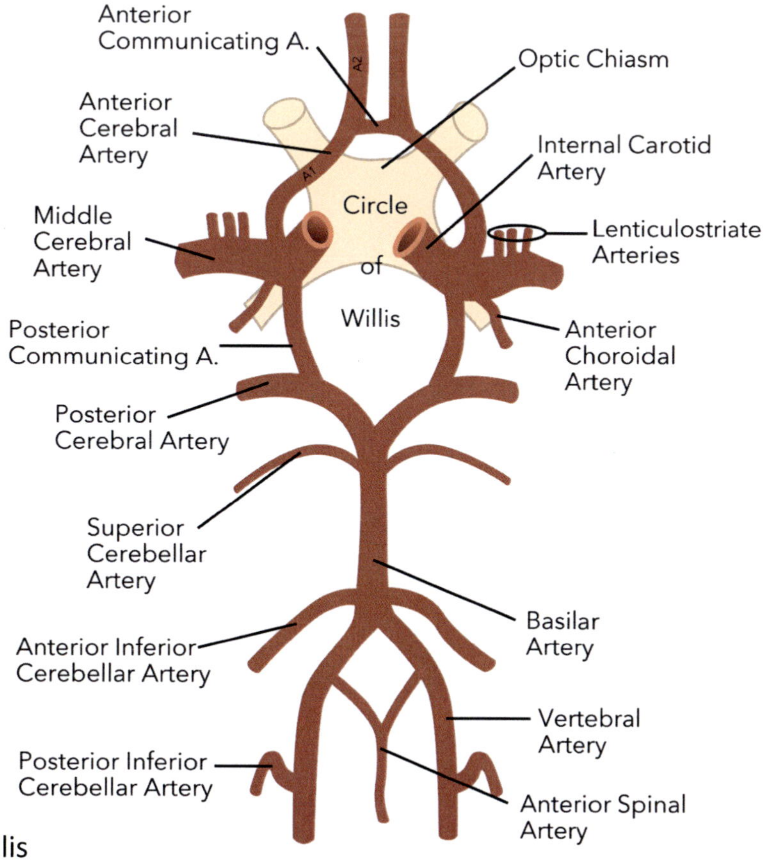

Figure 8.47 - Circle of Willis

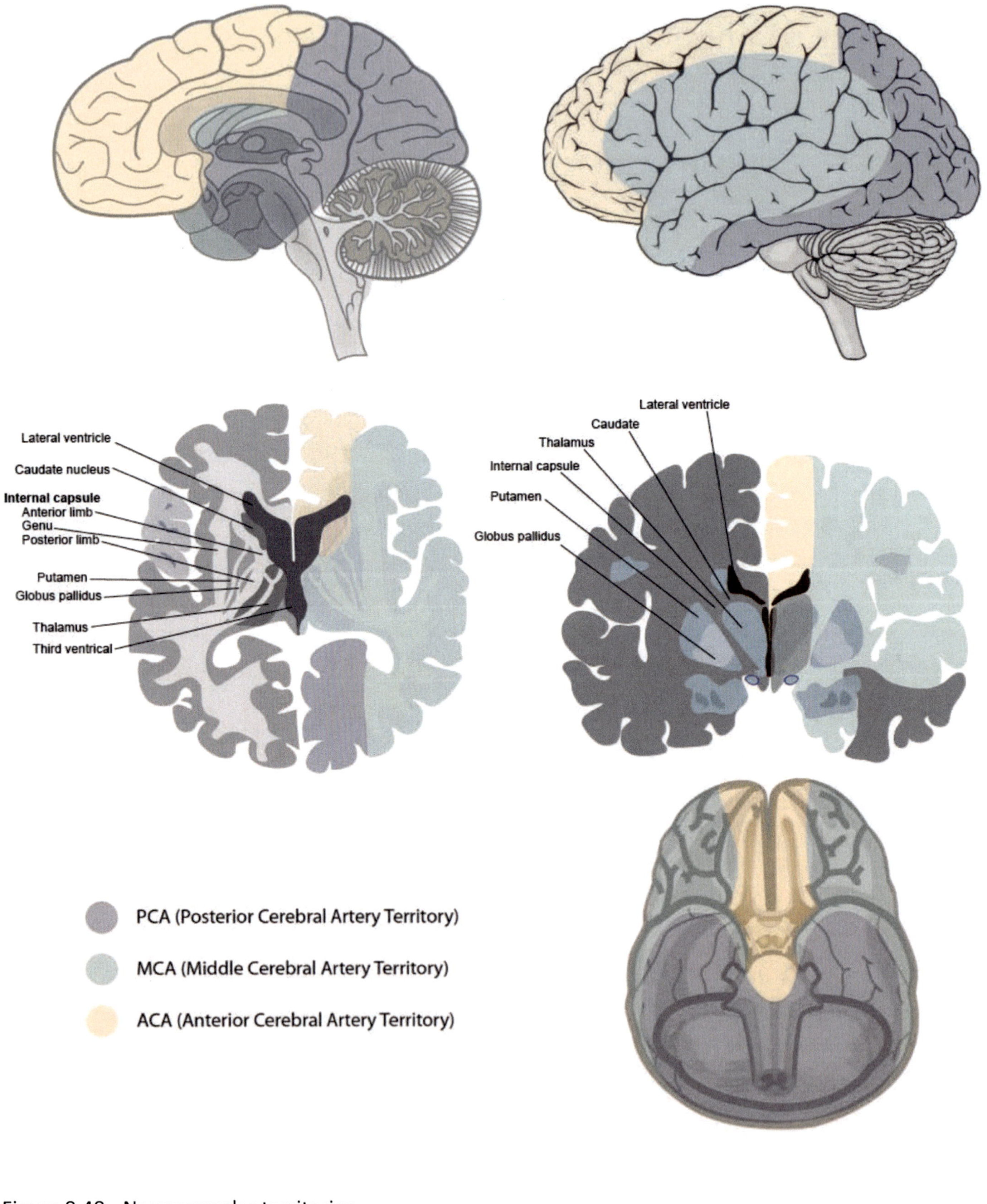

Figure 8.48 - Neurovascular territories

II. Aneurysms (Table 8.5)

Table 8.5 - Aneurysms

Aneurysm	Lesioned Area & Symptoms
Middle cerebral artery	1. Rupture results in a stroke of the MCA distribution, resulting in identical symptoms to that of an MCA stroke (contralateral paralysis and sensory deficits of the face and upper limb)
Lenticulostriate artery	1. Rupture commonly results in damage to the striatum and internal capsule → contralateral paralysis and sensory deficits of the entire body
Anterior communicating artery	1. Rupture results in a stroke of the ACA distribution, resulting in identical symptoms to that of an ACA stroke (contralateral paralysis and sensory deficits of the lower limb) 2. Can compress the optic chiasm, resulting in bitemporal hemianopia
Posterior communicating artery	1. Compression of the superficial parasympathetic fibers of CN III results in mydriasis and ptosis 2. Compression of the deep somatic fibers of CN III can result in paralysis of the corresponding ocular muscles (superior rectus, medial rectus, inferior rectus, and inferior oblique)

A. Balloon-like dilation of an artery.

1. Saccular (berry) aneurysm
   a) Most commonly associated with connective tissue disorders (i.e. Ehlers-Danlos syndrome), smoking, and age.
   b) An aneurysm can rupture resulting in a subarachnoid hemorrhage and/or ischemia, or can compress nearby structures.
2. Charcot-Bouchard microaneurysm
   a) Highly associated with chronic hypertension.
   b) Most commonly seen in the lenticulostriate arteries.

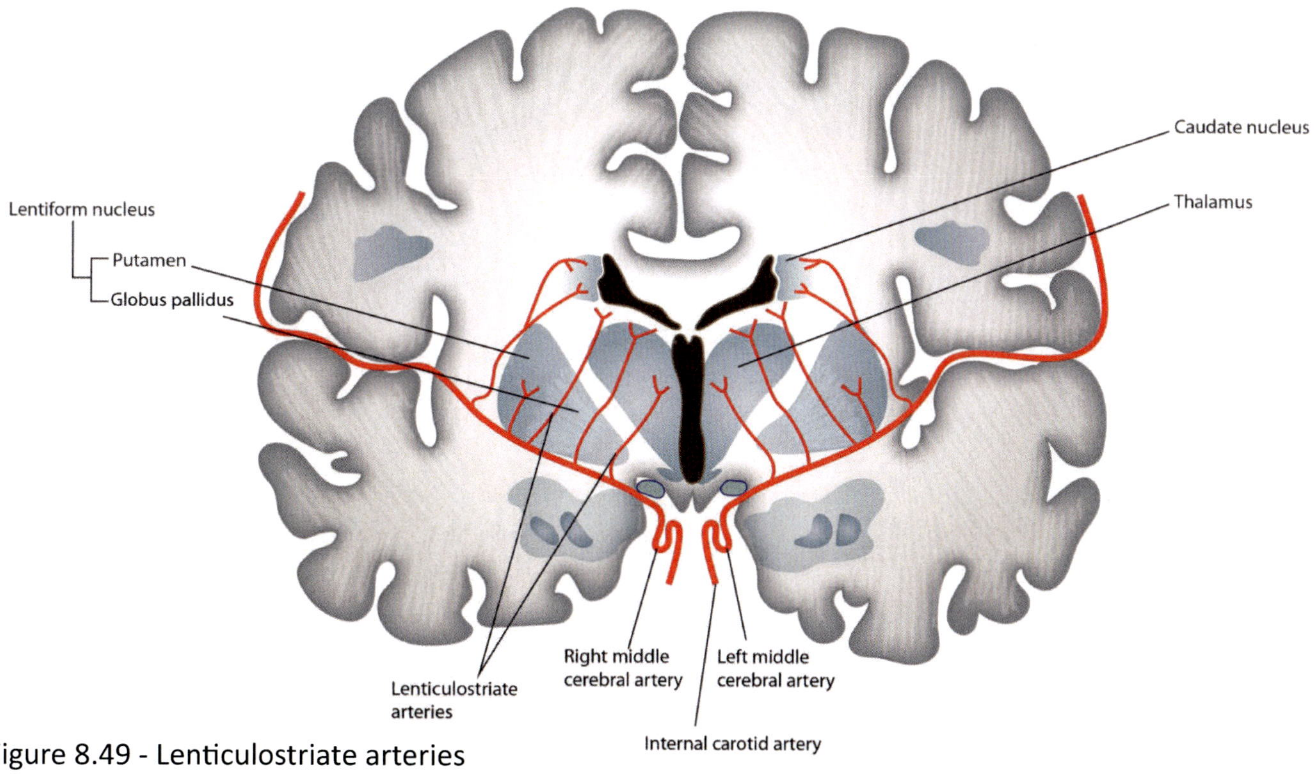

Figure 8.49 - Lenticulostriate arteries

REVIEW QUESTIONS

1. A 68-year-old right-handed woman presents with right sided facial paralysis sparing the forehead and paralysis of the right upper limb. Rupture of an aneurysm likely occurred near what vessel?

   - **Left middle cerebral artery (the MCA supplies blood to the primary motor cortex responsible for facial and upper extremity movement)**

Figure 8.6 - The homunculus

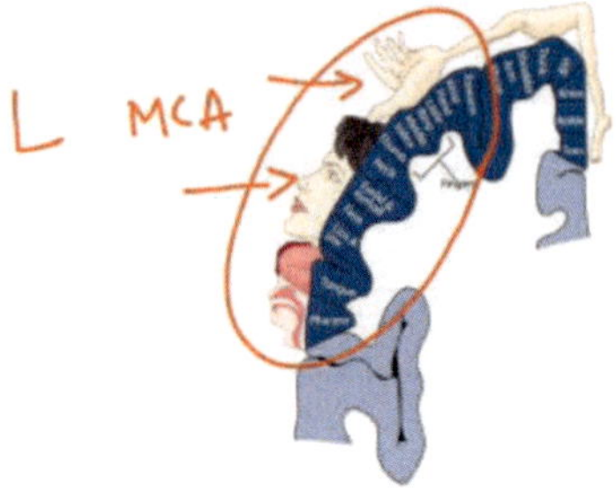

2. A 65-year-old right-handed male with a history of diabetes and a previous MI presents with sudden loss of vision. Fundoscopy shows a cholesterol embolus. From what major branch of the Circle of Willis did the embolus most likely originate?

   - **The internal carotid artery (branches into the ophthalmic artery which supplies blood to the retina)**

Figure 8.46 - Neurovascular anatomy overview

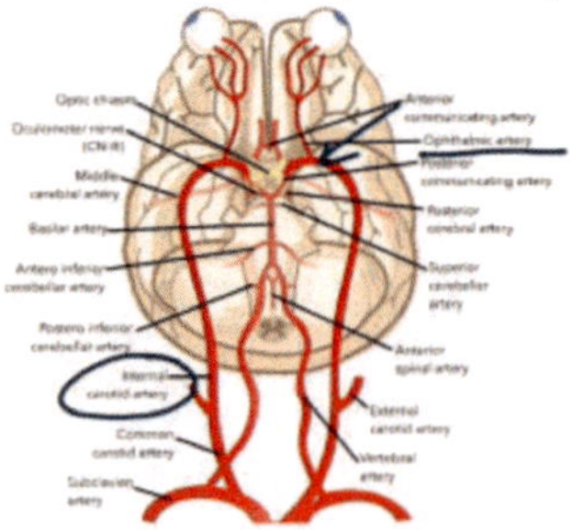

3. A 80-year-old right-handed male presents with paralysis of the right lower extremity. What vessel shown below is most likely occluded?

   - **The anterior cerebral artery (ACA) supplies blood to the lower extremities**
   - **The left ACA is most likely occluded**

Figure 8.6 - The homunculus

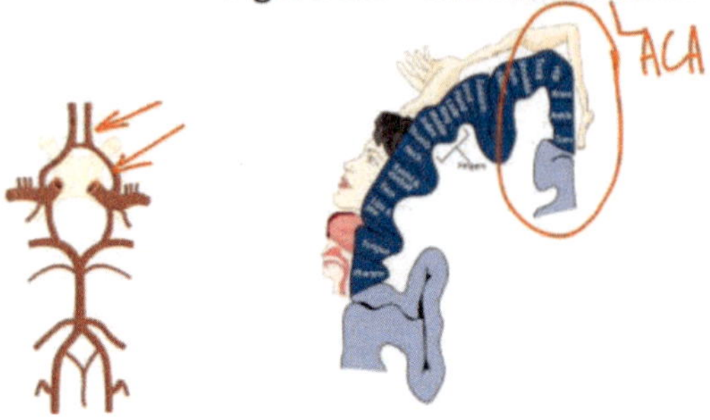

4. A 67-year-old right-handed male presents with a blood pressure of 210/170 and left sided paralysis and sensory loss. Imaging shows hyperintensities near the striatum. What vessel is most likely damaged?

   - **Chronic hypertension commonly results in damage to the lenticulostriate arteries (supplies blood to the basal ganglia)**
   - **The right lenticulostriate arteries are damaged → left-sided paralysis and sensory loss due to damage to the right internal capsule**

Figure 8.49 - Lenticulostriate arteries

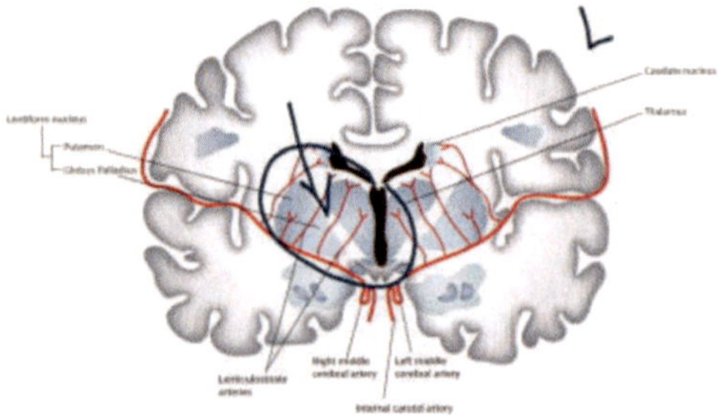

REVIEW QUESTIONS

5. A 77-year-old right-handed male presents with left sided hemiparesis, loss of vibration and proprioception on the left side, and right sided tongue deviation. What vessel is likely occluded?

- **The anterior spinal artery (ASA) supplies blood to the hypoglossal nuclei (responsible for tongue movement), the medial lemniscus (proprioception and vibration), and the corticospinal tract (motor tracts).**
- **The right ASA is most likely most heavily involved**

Figure 8.20 - Transverse section of the medulla

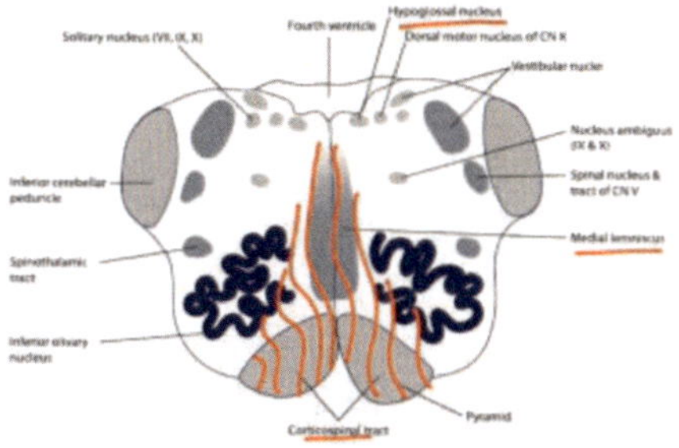

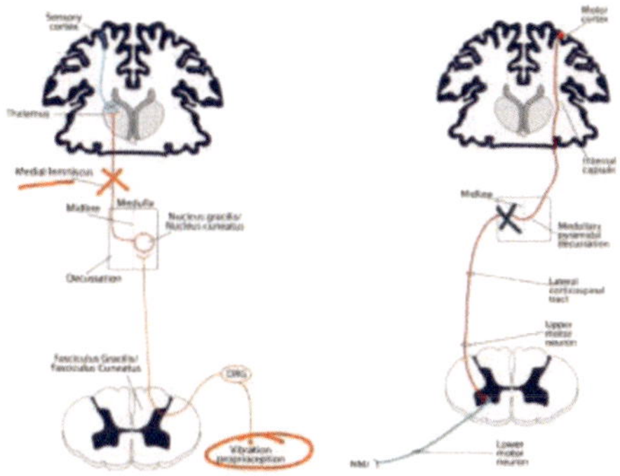

6. A 67-year-old right-handed male with a history of DM and multiple myocardial infarctions presents with a 2 week history of progressive bilateral upper and lower limb paralysis and bilateral loss of pain and temperature. Proprioception and vibration are intact bilaterally. What vascular territory is likely ischemic?

- **Paralysis (corticospinal tract), pain and temperature deficits (spinothalamic tract), and sparing of proprioception and vibration (dorsal columns) → ischemia to the anterior spinal artery (ASA ischemia)**

Figure 8.9 - Spinal Cord Cross Section

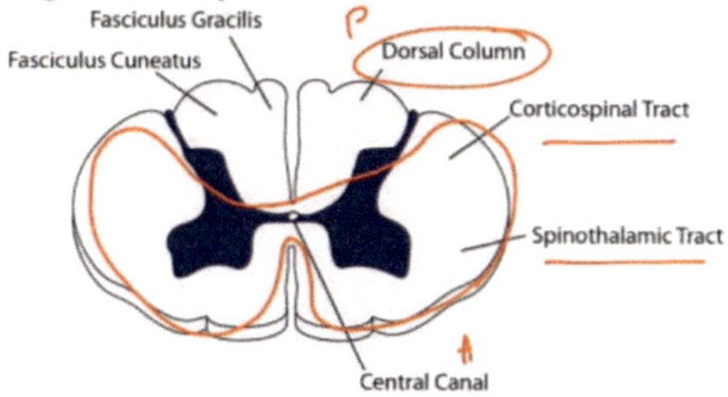

7. A 52-year-old right-handed male with a history of CAD presents with vertigo, ataxia, dysphagia, and difficulty speaking. What vessel is most likely occluded?

- **Dysphagia and dysphonia are unique to lateral medullary syndrome**
- **Lateral medullary syndrome occurs due to occlusion of the PICA or the vertebral artery**

Figure 8.46 - Neurovascular anatomy overview

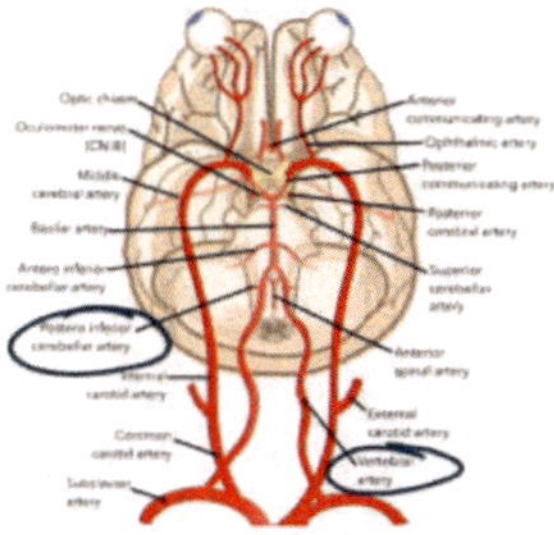

Figure 8.20 - Transverse section of the medulla

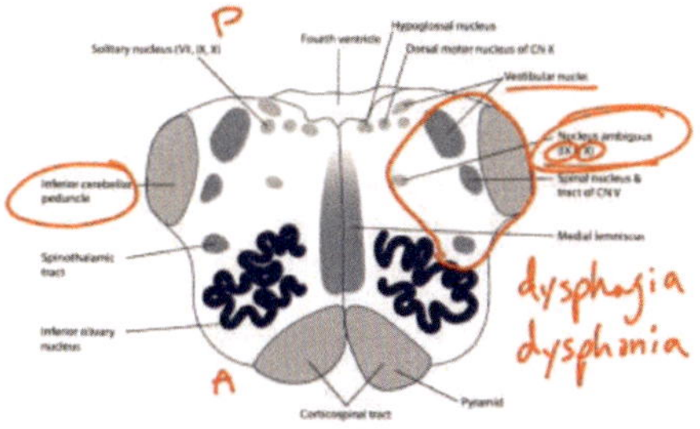

REVIEW QUESTIONS

8. A patient presents with Horner syndrome, nystagmus, right-sided facial paralysis, and taste deficits. What vessel is most likely occluded?

- **Facial paralysis and taste deficits are unique to lateral pontine syndrome**
- **Lateral pontine syndrome occurs due to occlusion of the AICA**

Figure 8.46 - Neurovascular anatomy overview

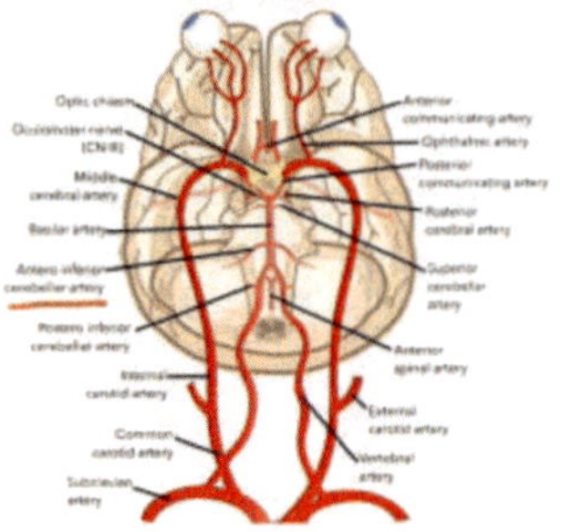

Figure 8.18 - Transverse section of the pons

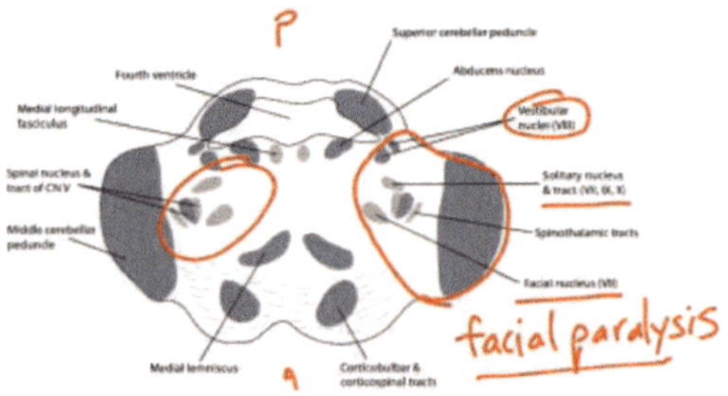

9. An 88-year-old right-handed female presents with quadriplegia and bilateral facial paralysis. An astute medical student notices that the patient has the ability to respond by blinking. What vessel is most likely occluded?

- **Basilar artery → locked-in syndrome**

Figure 8.46 - Neurovascular anatomy overview

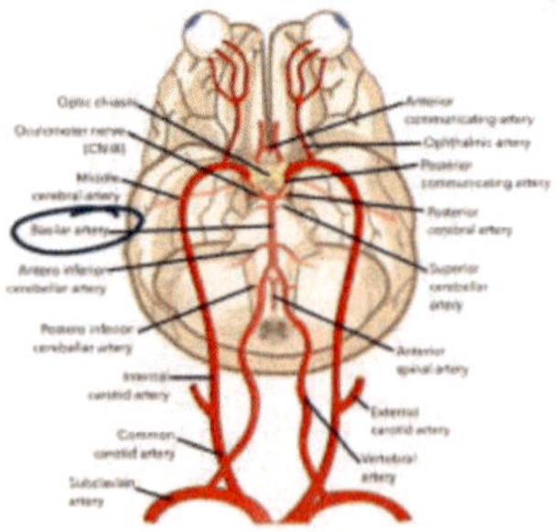

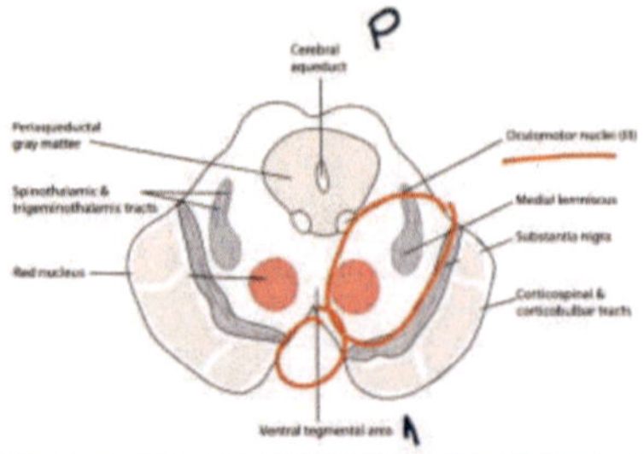

10. A 26-year-old right-handed male presents with abnormalities of the right eye including mydriasis, ptosis, and difficulty adducting the eye. An aneurysm from what vessel is most likely responsible for the patient's symptoms?

- **Mydriasis, ptosis, and difficulty adducting the eye → damage to the oculomotor nerve (CN III)**
- **An aneurysm originating from the posterior communicating artery → compression of CN III**

Figure 8.47 - Circle of Willis

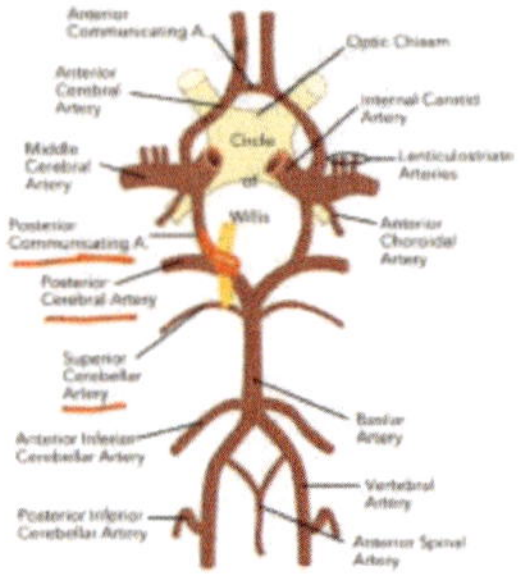

Section X - Ventricular System

I. Sinuses and Ventricular System

A. Ventricular system (Figures 8.50 and 8.51)

1. Lateral ventricles

a) The lateral ventricles empty into the third ventricle via the interventricular foramina of Monro.

2. Third ventricle

a) The third ventricle empties into the fourth ventricle via the cerebral aqueduct.

3. Fourth ventricle

a) The fourth ventricle empties into the subarachnoid space via the foramen of Magendie and the two lateral foramina of Luschka.

b) The area postrema is located near the floor of the fourth ventricle in the medulla. When stimulated, this area causes vomiting.

4. CSF moves from the ventricles → subarachnoid space → arachnoid granulations → superior sagittal sinus.

II. Hydrocephalus

A. Communicating → ↓ CSF absorption due to damage to the arachnoid granulations.

B. Noncommunicating → structural block within the ventricular system.

C. Ex vacuo → enlargement of the ventricular system due to decreased brain tissue, rather than an increase in CSF.

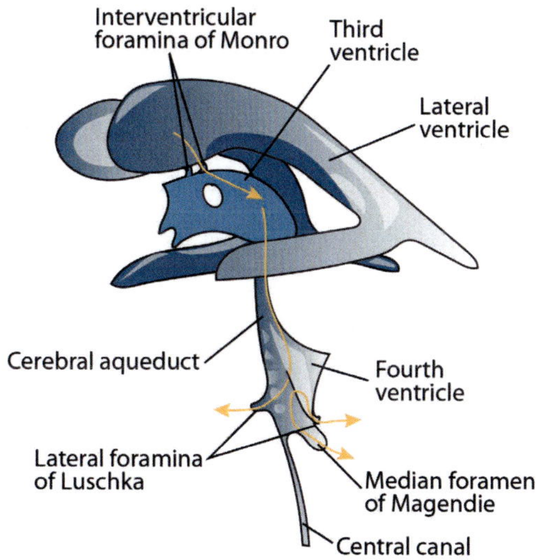

Figure 8.50 - Ventricular system

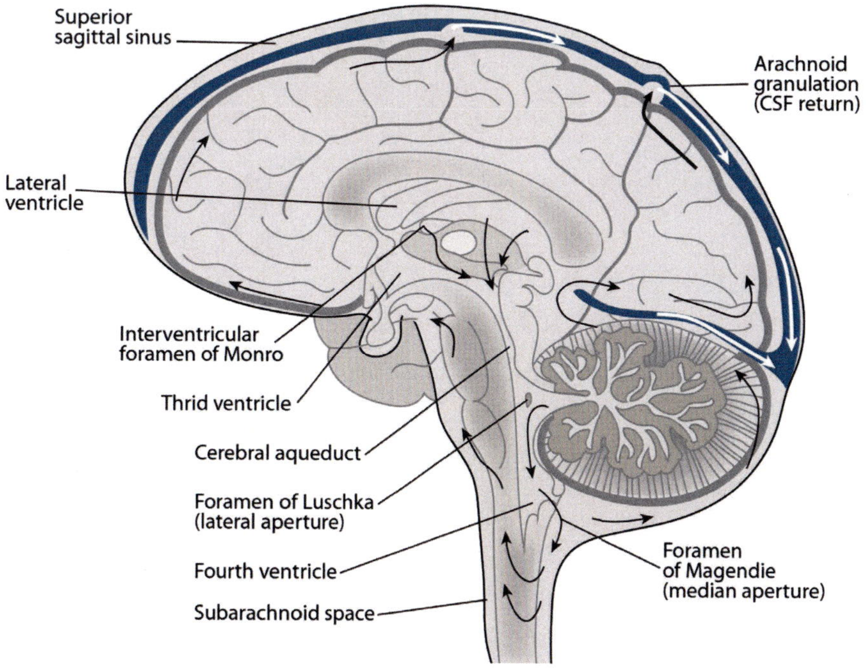

Figure 8.51 - CSF flow overview

III. Dural venous sinuses are formed by spaces within the two layers of dura mater of the meninges (Figures 8.52 and 8.53).

A. The superior sagittal sinus receives blood from the arachnoid granulations.

B. Infections from the eye can spread to the cavernous sinus through the ophthalmic vein.

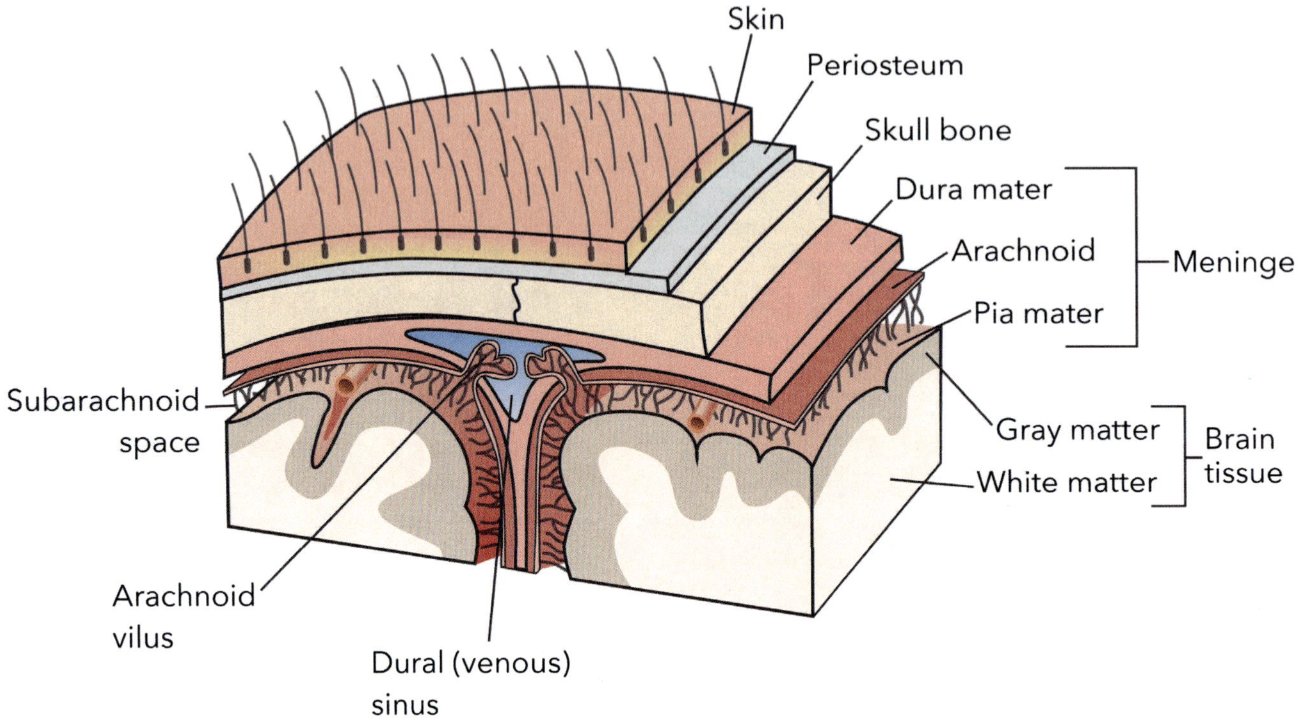

Figure 8.52 - Meninges

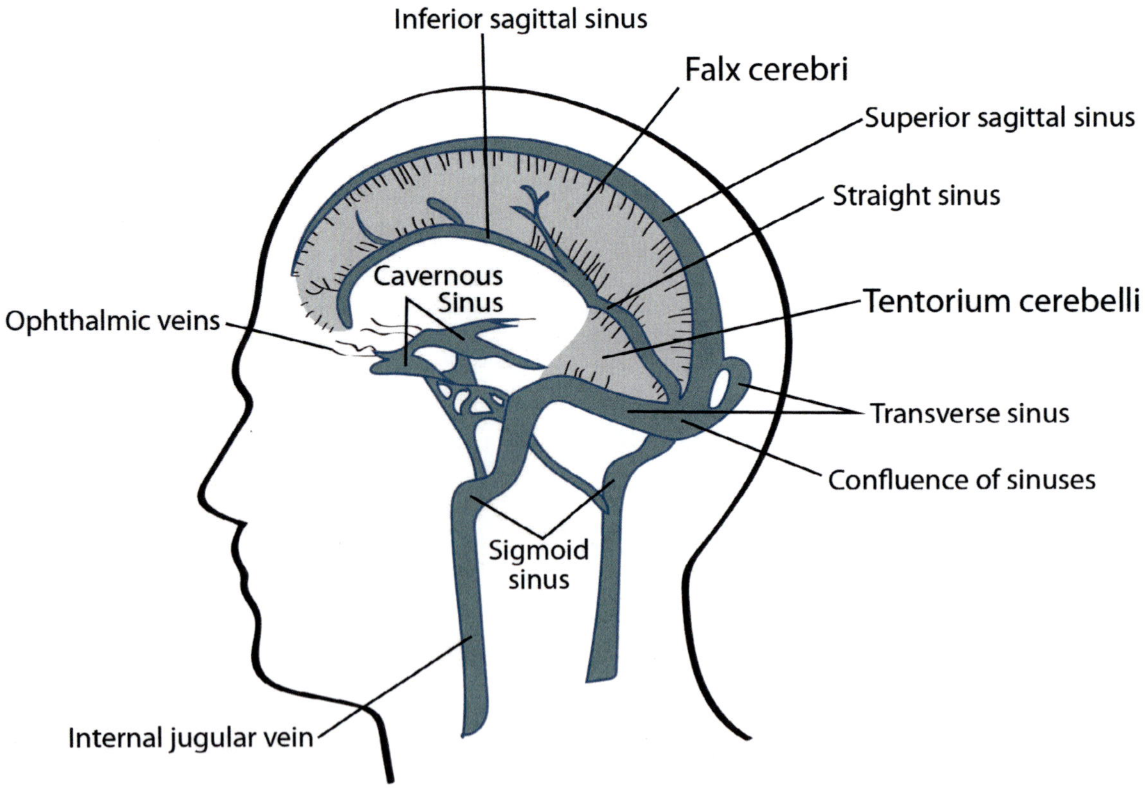

Figure 8.53 - Dural venous sinuses

REVIEW QUESTIONS ?

1. A 2-week-old boy presents with bulging fontanels and papilledema. His history is significant for bacterial meningitis which was promptly treated and appeared to have resolved several days ago. What is the likely cause of the patient's symptoms today?

    - **Meningitis → scarring of the arachnoid granulations → ↓ ability to absorb CSF → ↑ intracranial pressure → papilledema and bulging fontanels**
    - **This patient has communicating hydrocephalus.**

Figure 8.51 - CSF flow overview

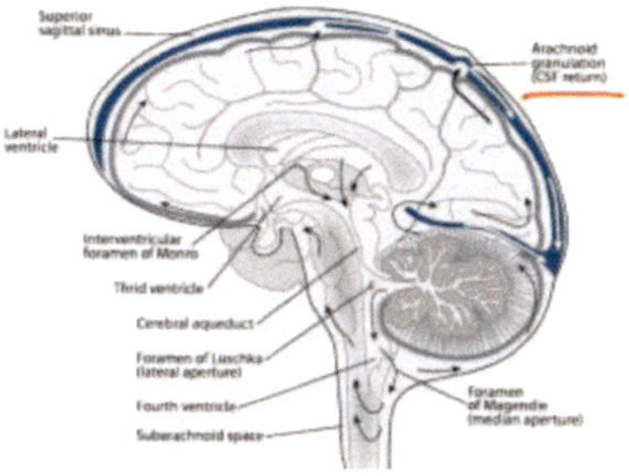

2. An MRI of the brain shows enlarged lateral ventricles and an enlarged third ventricle, but a normal sized fourth ventricle. What structure is obstructed resulting in the MRI findings?

    - **The cerebral aqueduct**

Figure 8.50 - Ventricular system

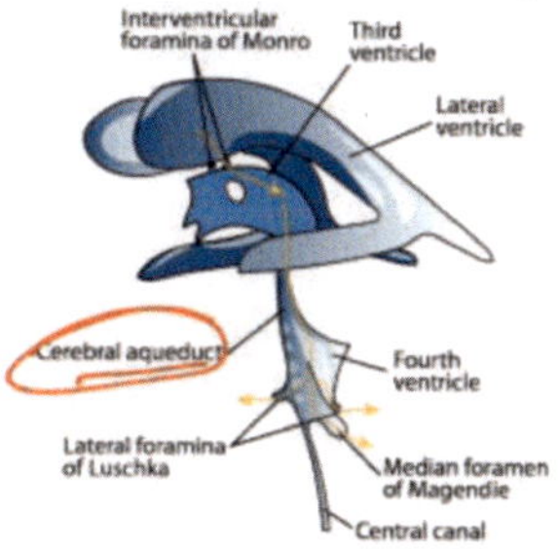

3. A 67-year-old female with Alzheimer's disease received a routine MRI and the radiology technician noticed the patient had extremely large ventricles. What is the most likely cause?

    - **Cerebral atrophy (hydrocephalus ex vacuo)**

4. A 2-year-old boy has an infection of the eye. The physician is concerned that the infection may rapidly spread to the cavernous sinus. Through what structure would this be possible?

    - **The ophthalmic vein (drains directly into the cavernous sinus)**

Figure 8.53 - Dural venous sinuses

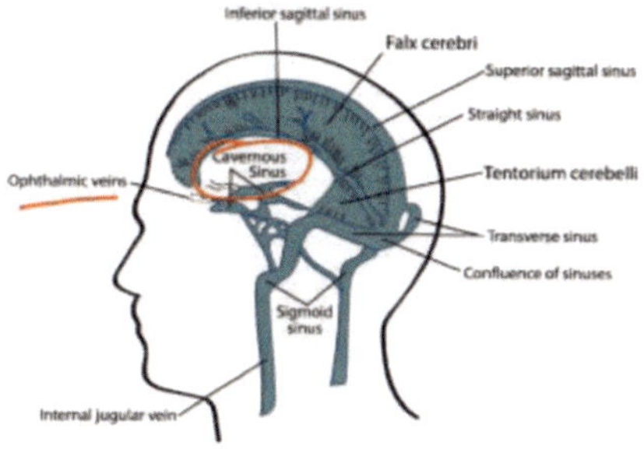

Section XI - Aphasia

I. Aphasia

Table 8.6 - Aphasia

Type	Comprehension	Repetition	Fluidity	Notes
Broca (inferior frontal gyrus)	Intact	Impaired	Impaired	Aware of cognitive deficit. Supplied by the MCA.
Wernicke (superior temporal gyrus)	Impaired	Impaired	Intact	Unaware of cognitive deficit. Supplied by the MCA.
Conduction	Intact	Impaired	Intact	Caused by damage to the arcuate fasciculus.

A. Broca's area is located in the inferior frontal gyrus.

1. Broca aphasia
    a) Able to comprehend verbal and written language
    b) Difficulty with repetition
    c) Unable to speak fluently
    d) Patients frustrated due to their awareness of the cognitive deficit

B. Wernicke's area is located in the superior temporal gyrus.

1. Wernicke aphasia
    a) Cannot comprehend verbal or written language
    b) Difficulty with repetition
    c) Speech is meaningless, but the patient articulates in a melodic and convincing manner (fluidity intact).
    d) Patients unaware of their cognitive deficit

C. Conduction aphasia is caused by damage to the arcuate fasciculus, a fibrous band that relays messages between Broca's area and Wernicke's area.

1. Able to comprehend verbal and written language
2. Difficulty with repetition
3. Fluidity intact

REVIEW QUESTIONS

1. A 67-year-old female with a history of a stroke presents to a neurologist for follow up care. As the history is taken the neurologist notices the woman has difficulty with repetition despite normal comprehension and fluidity. What area of the brain is likely lesioned?

    - **Conduction aphasia (can speak and comprehend but has difficulty with repetition) due to damage to the arcuate fasciculus**

    conduction aphasia
    → arcuate fasciculus

2. A 72-year-old male is brought to the ED by his concerned children. Since admission, the man appears to have asked well articulated questions but they lack meaning. Upon further exam he has difficulty repeating phrases and does not appear to understand the questions being asked. What region of the brain shown below is likely damaged?

    - **Speech lacks fluidity → Wernicke aphasia (superior temporal gyrus)**

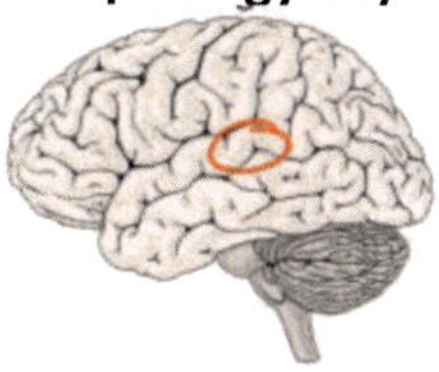

3. An 88-year-old female is brought to the ED due to difficulty speaking. When asked to make a fist she does so. When asked to repeat a simple phrase she becomes highly agitated and shrugs her shoulders in frustration. What area of the brain shown below is likely damaged?

    - **Comprehension intact, difficulty with repetition and speech → Broca aphasia (inferior frontal gyrus)**

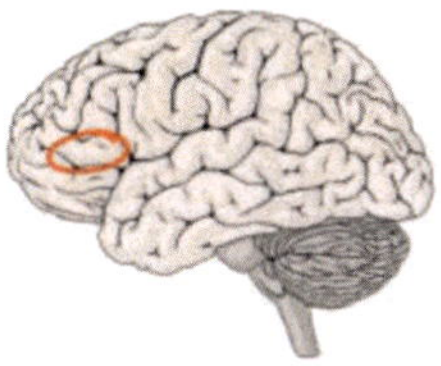

Section XII - Dermatomes, Myotomes, and Clinical Reflexes

I. Dermatomes (Figure 8.54 and Table 8.7)

Table 8.7 - Dermatomes

Spinal Cord Level	Region Innervated
C2	Posterior scalp
C3	Upper neck
C4	Lower neck
C6	1st digit (thumb)
C7	3rd digit (middle finger)
C8	5th digit (little finger)
T4	Nipple line
T7	Xiphoid process
T10	Navel line
L1	Inguinal ligament
L4	Patella and medial malleolus
L5	Dorsum of foot
S1	Lateral malleolus
S2-S4	Perineal region

A. Areas of skin associated with a single spinal nerve

B. Pain in a certain region can implicate a spinal cord level

C. Dermatome sensation includes:

1. Pain and temperature (spinothalamic tract)
2. Proprioception and vibration (dorsal columns)

D. Referred pain

1. Sensation from an *internal* organ enters spinal cord at a given level → pain is felt in the dermatome associated with that spinal cord level
2. Classic examples:
    a) Pancreatitis → diaphragm irritation → sensation sent to C3-C5 spinal nerves → pain within the C3-C5 dermatomes
    b) Appendicitis → sensation sent to T10 spinal nerves → pain at T10 dermatome

E. Radiculopathy

1. Pain resulting from a compression (pinching) of a spinal nerve
2. Can cause paresthesias (tingling sensation)

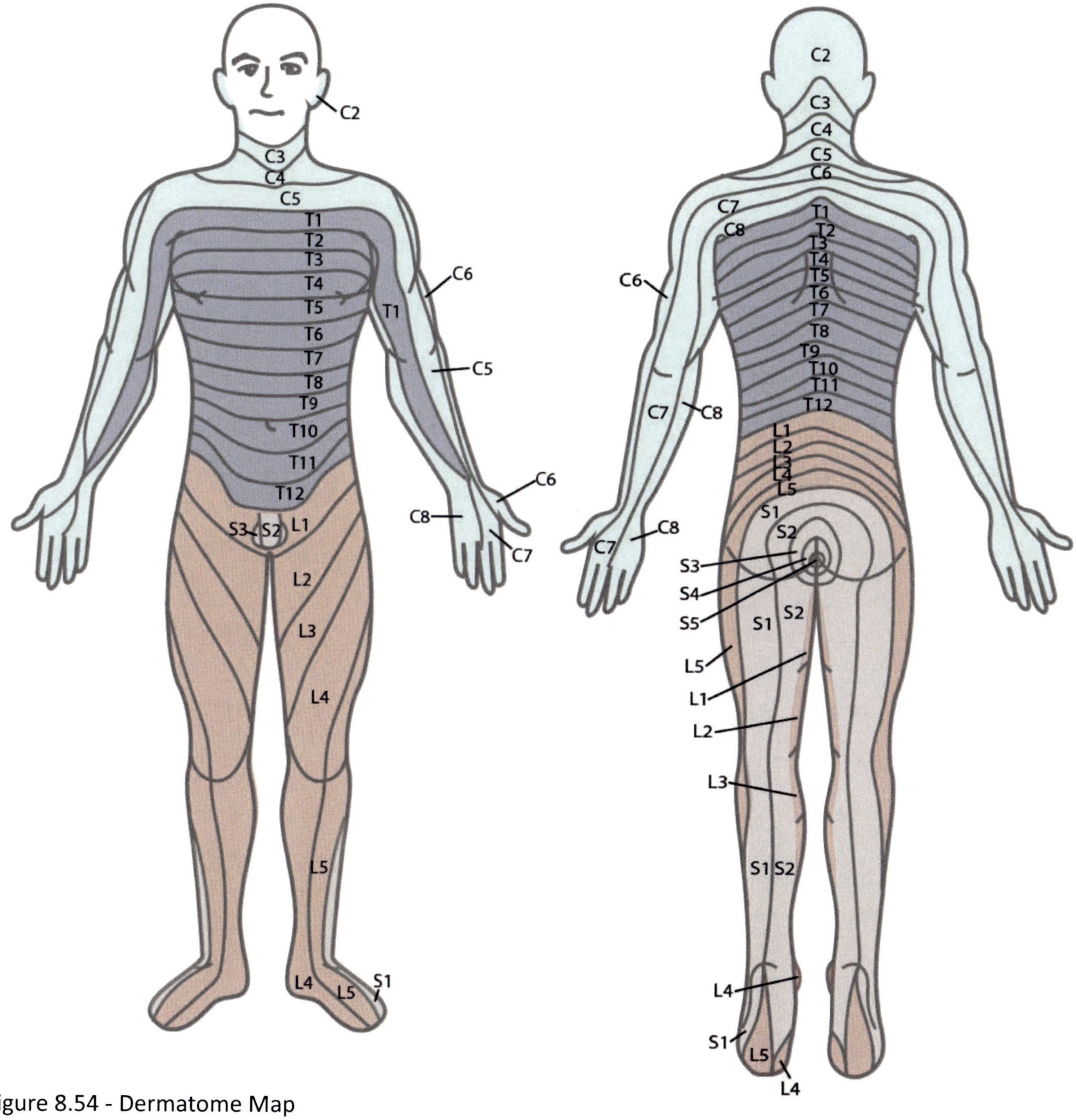

Figure 8.54 - Dermatome Map

II. Myotomes (Table 8.8)

Table 8.8 - Myotomes

Spinal Cord Level	Action
C5	Shoulder abduction
C6	Elbow flexion
C7	Elbow extension
C8	Wrist flexion
T1	Thumb opposition
L2	Hip flexion
L3	Hip adduction
L4	Knee extension
L5	Ankle dorsiflexion
S1	Ankle plantar flexion
S2-S4	Erection and anal sphincter

A. Myotomes are groups associated with a single spinal nerve.

B. Diminished strength in a certain region can implicate a certain spinal cord region.

III. Clinical Reflexes (Table 8.9)

A. Absent clinical reflexes can implicate a specific spinal cord level

Table 8.9 - Clinical reflexes

Spinal Cord Level	Reflex
C5-C6	Biceps reflex
C7-C8	Triceps reflex
L1-L2	Cremaster reflex
L3-L4	Patellar reflex
S1-S2	Achilles reflex
S3-S4	Anal wink reflex

REVIEW QUESTIONS

1. A patient is hospitalized following a car crash. He complains of pain on the surface of the abdomen about 2 inches superior to the inguinal ligament. If a vertebral fracture is the cause of the pain, what vertebral level is likely damaged: cervical, thoracic, lumbar or sacral?

   - **Dermatome along inguinal ligament is innervated by L1. Pain above this level implicates thoracic vertebral damage**

2. A patient is hit in the neck with a baseball bat. Radiograph shows spinal cord damage to the region beneath the C6 vertebrae on the left side. If this trauma has altered sensation on the left side, where would it likely manifest?

   - **C7 spinal nerve exits below C6 vertebra**
   - **C7 is responsible for sensation of third digit**

3. A patient has a known herniated vertebral disc and presents with pain on his lower extremity including the medial ankle. During a neurological exam, where would diminished strength be noticed?

   - **This is radiculopathy of the L4 dermatome**
   - **L4 nerve damage would diminished knee extension**

4. A patient demonstrates hyporeflexia when the triceps tendon is hit with a reflex hammer. The patient also complains of occasional shock-like pain in the hand. Radiograph shows herniation within the cervical spinal cord. What region of the hand is likely experiencing pain?

   - **Triceps reflex is mediated by C7 spinal nerve**
   - **Pain would be seen along C7 dermatome (3rd digit)**

Table 8.9 - Clinical Reflexes

Spinal Cord Level	Reflex
C5-C6	Biceps reflex
C7-C8	Triceps reflex
L1-L2	Cremaster reflex
L3-L4	Patellar reflex
S1-S2	Achilles reflex
S3-S4	Anal wink reflex

5. The anterior root of the L4 spinal nerve is damaged. What reflex would be altered?

   - **L4 spinal nerve is responsible for the patellar reflex**

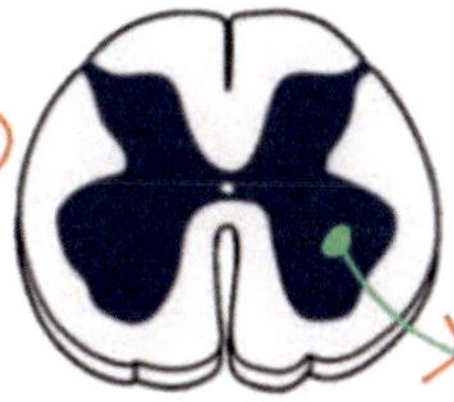

MUSCULOSKELETAL

Section I - Neurotransmission

I. Corticospinal Tract and Alpha Motor Neurons (Figure 9.1)

A. The descending corticospinal tract synapses on alpha motor neurons in the ventral horn of the spinal cord.

B. Descending axons of the corticospinal tract release ACh into the synaptic cleft which binds ACh receptors of an alpha motor neuron.

C. Binding of ACh to the postsynaptic cleft causes Na^+ influx and K^+ efflux resulting in alpha motor neuron depolarization.

D. Depolarization reaches the axon hillock and voltage-sensitive sodium channels open, depolarizing this region of the neuron.

E. Depolarization in the axon hillock causes voltage-sensitive Ca^{2+} channels to open.

F. Ca^{2+} influx allows neurotransmitter vesicles within the alpha motor neuron to fuse to the cell membrane and enter the synaptic cleft.

II. Muscle Stimulation (Figure 9.1)

A. Neurotransmitter vesicles in the presynaptic terminals release acetylcholine (ACh) into the synaptic cleft.

B. Nicotinic ACh receptors of the postsynaptic cleft within skeletal muscle tissue facilitate Na^+ and K^+ exchange.

C. Binding of ACh to the receptors causes Na^+ to enter the cell and K^+ to leave the cell resulting in depolarization.

D. Voltage gated Na^+ channels then open resulting in additional depolarization.

E. The muscle cell membrane (sarcolemma) contains deep invaginations that extend into the muscle fiber which are called T-tubules.

F. T-tubules are an extension of the extracellular space and contain L-type voltage-gated calcium channels that open when intracellular Na^+ concentrations rise resulting in depolarization.

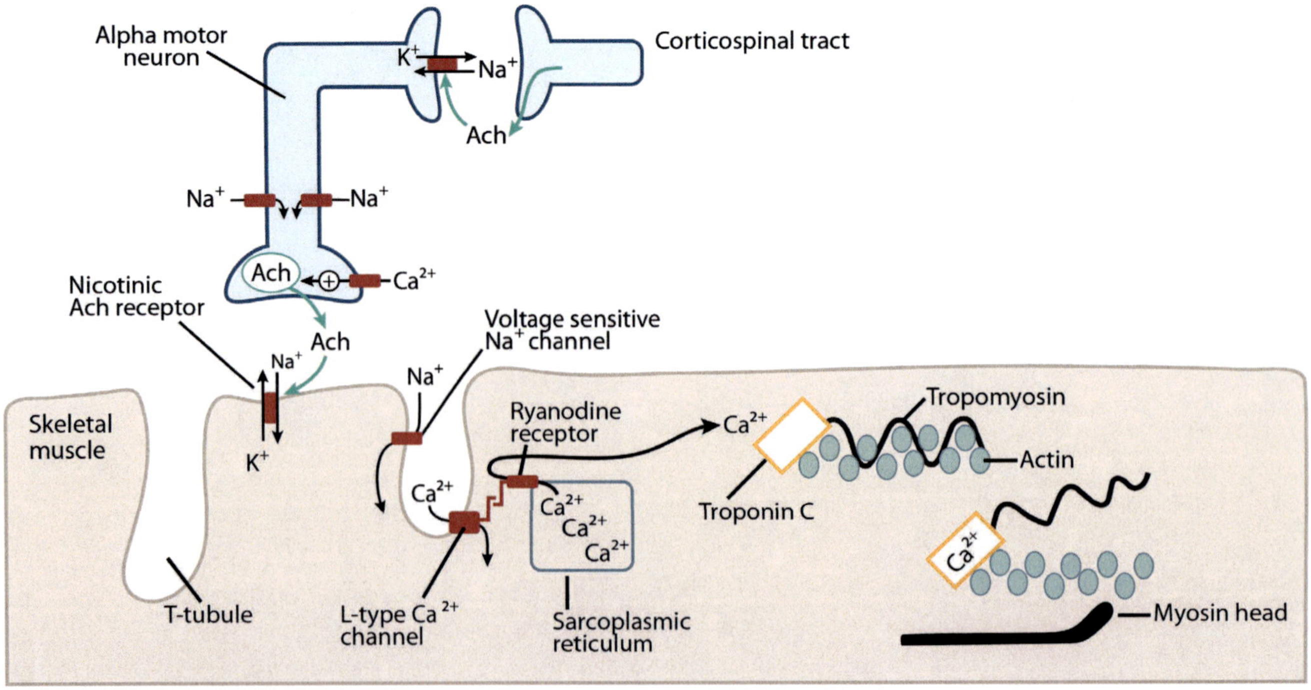

Figure 9.1 - Neurotransmission

G. The expansive distribution of T-tubules allows the entire muscle fiber to contract uniformly because it allows the depolarizing signal to reach all of the myofibrils at the same.

H. Ca^{2+} enters the cell through L-type Ca^{2+} channels, but the release of Ca^{2+} from the sarcoplasmic reticulum (SR) is not directly dependent upon Ca^{2+}. Rather, the L-type Ca^{2+} channel mechanically interacts with the ryanodine receptors resulting in SR release of Ca^{2+}.

I. Ca^{2+} release from the SR results in increased cytosolic Ca^{2+} which binds to troponin C.

J. Troponin C moves tropomyosin from actin allowing myosin to bind actin and cause muscle contraction.

K. After contraction the Ca^{2+}-ATPase pump (SERCA) actively pumps intracellular Ca^{2+} into the SR which allows intracellular Ca^{2+} concentrations to be kept low.

   1. Within the SR is a Ca^{2+}-binding protein called calsequestrin → allowing the SR to store Ca^{2+}

REVIEW QUESTIONS ?

1. A new experimental drug is known to inhibit voltage-sensitive Ca^{2+} channels in the alpha motor neuron. How will this drug likely alter skeletal muscle activity?

   - **The calcium channels described are responsible for inducing acetylcholine release into the synaptic cleft → stimulation of the postsynaptic sodium-potassium channel → muscle contraction**
   - **Blockage of the calcium channels → ↓ skeletal muscle activity**

Figure 9.1 - Neurotransmission

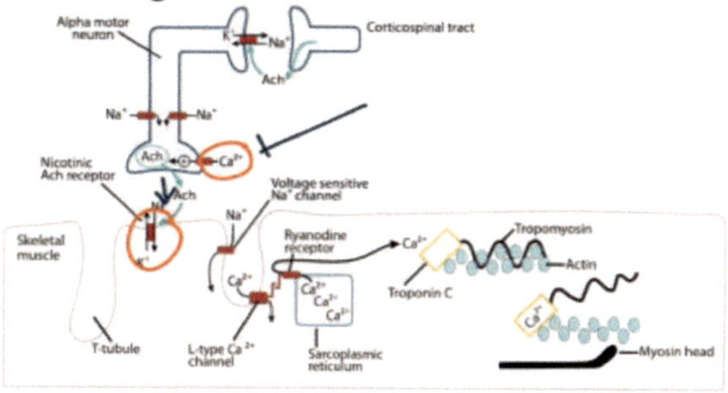

2. A 66-year-old with a 50 pack-year smoking history presents with generalized muscle weakness. He states that it is worse in the morning but gets better throughout the day. What is the underlying explanation for the muscle weakness?

   - **This patient has small cell lung cancer → Lambert-Eaton syndrome (paraneoplastic syndrome that results in antibodies against the presynaptic calcium channels)**

Figure 9.1 - Neurotransmission

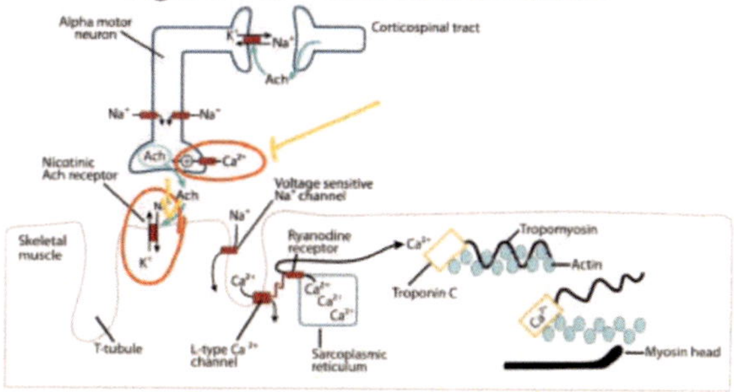

REVIEW QUESTIONS ?

3. Why does myasthenia gravis result in progressive weakening of muscles with repetitive use?

- **Myasthenia gravis → antibodies against the postsynaptic acetylcholine receptors**
- **Dysfunctional receptors → excessive endocytosis**
- **Initially, the acetylcholine binds the few receptors that are available and results in a strong muscle contraction**
- **However, as more acetylcholine is released there are no more available receptors so the muscle becomes progressively weaker**

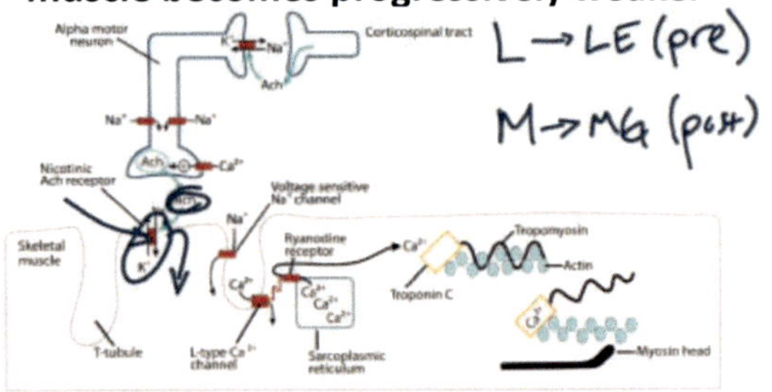

4. A 67-year-old female is being intubated for a hip replacement surgery. The anesthesiologist suddenly notices that she develops hyperkalemia. What drug was likely used to assist with the intubation that resulted in the hyperkalemia?

- **Succinylcholine (activates the nicotinic acetylcholine receptor → sustained efflux of potassium)**

Figure 9.1 - Neurotransmission

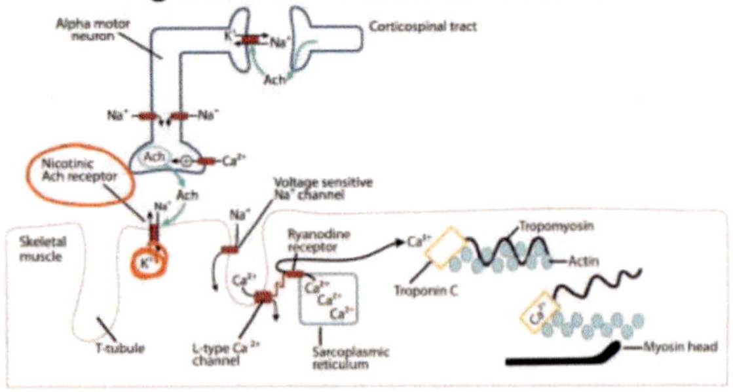

5. The skeletal muscle of a knockout mouse is able to contract despite total depletion of intracellular skeletal muscle calcium concentrations. What protein defect most likely explains the finding?

- **Tropomyosin**
- **This protein normally prevents actin from binding myosin and is released from actin in the presence of calcium**
- **If calcium is not needed for muscle contraction, then tropomyosin must be defective**

Figure 9.1 - Neurotransmission

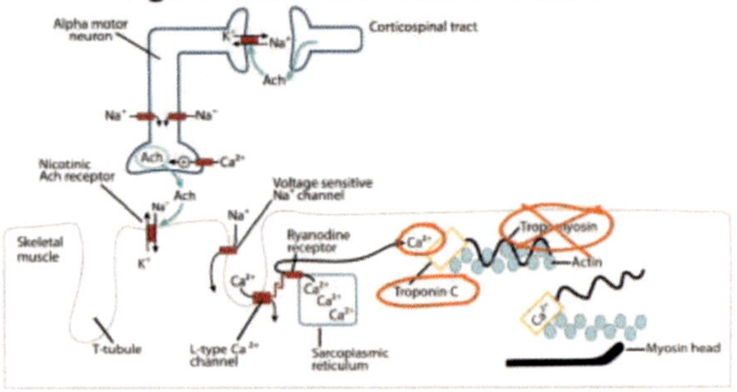

6. A 47-year-old male is administered an inhaled anesthetic and suddenly develops intense muscle contractions. What molecular abnormality explains the sudden change?

- **Inhaled anesthetics can cause malignant hyperthermia (autosomal dominant disorder → mutations in the ryanodine receptor → excessive release of calcium into the cytosol → intense muscle contractions)**

desflurane, isoflurane → malignant hyperthermia

Figure 9.1 - Neurotransmission

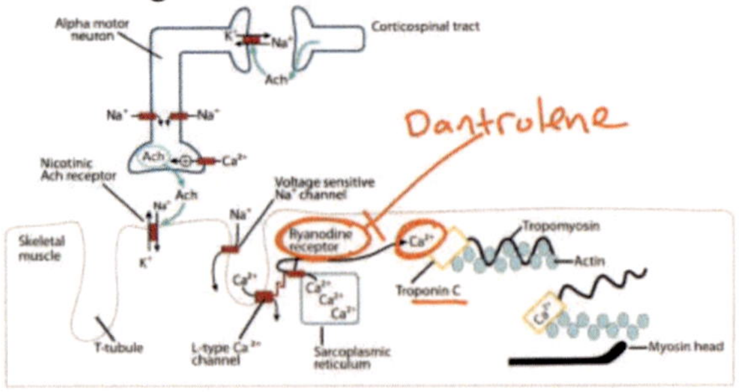

Section II - Muscle Anatomy and Contraction

I. Skeletal Muscle Anatomy

A. Muscle → fascicle → muscle fiber (muscle cell) → myofibril → sarcomere (Figure 9.2)

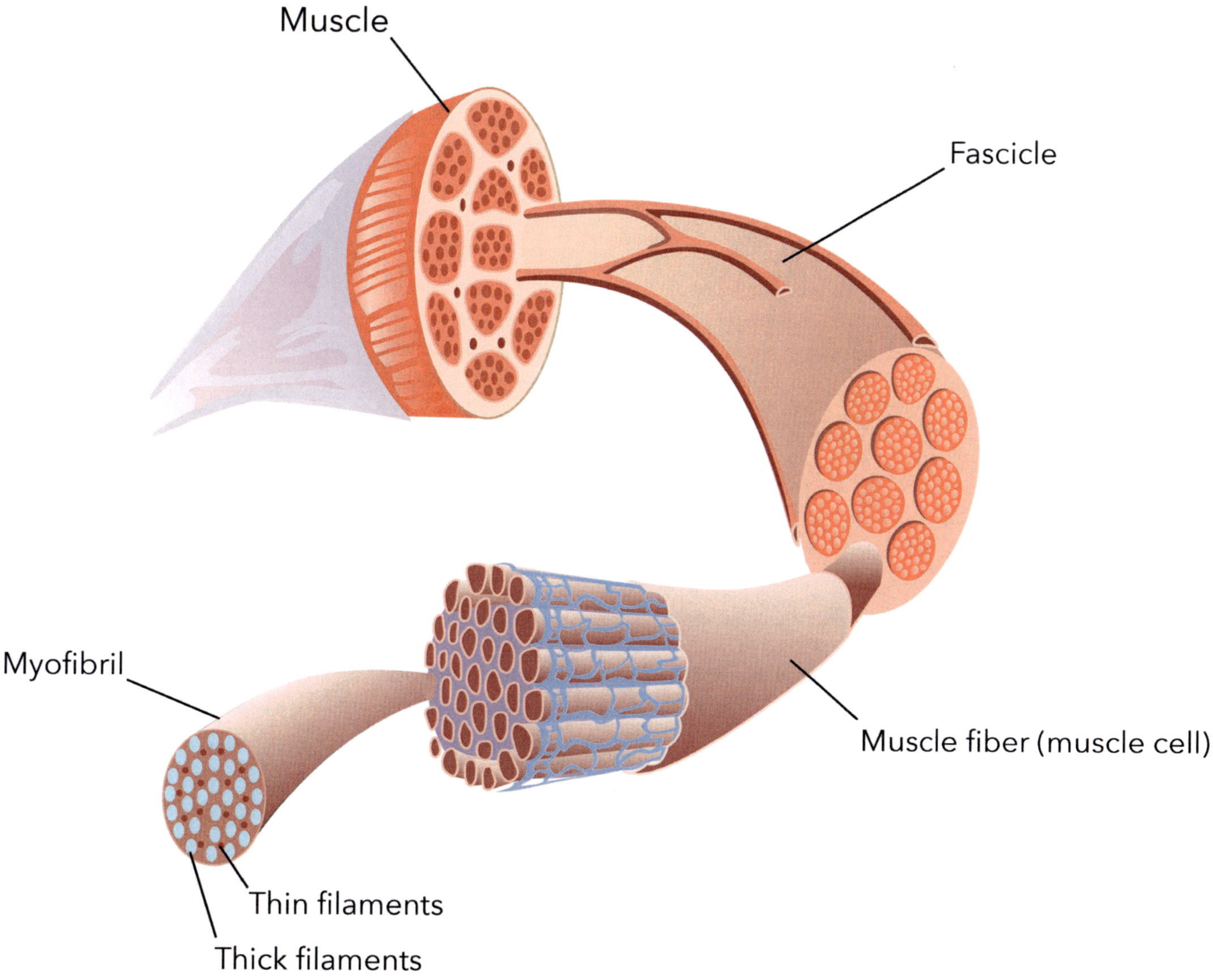

Figure 9.2 - Muscle anatomy

B. A sarcomere is the structural unit of a myofibril (Figure 9.3)

II. Myosin and Actin (Figure 9.4)

A. When ATP binds myosin, the myosin-actin cross bridge is detached (muscle relaxation).

B. ATP is hydrolyzed resulting in "cocking" of the myosin-ADP + P complex.

C. As Ca^{2+} binds troponin C the tropomyosin is removed from the actin, allowing the myosin ADP + P complex to bind actin.

D. Once bound, the ADP + P complex is released from actin resulting in shortening of the sarcomere and ultimately muscle contraction.

III. Golgi tendon organs (GTOs) are an important part of the negative feedback mechanism whereby an excessively stretched muscle can cause forced relaxation (Figure 9.5)

A. are located between the muscle-tendon junction and contain sensory axons.

B. When a muscle contracts, the tension is transmitted to the tendon which causes activation of the GTOs.

C. The afferent sensory axons then send signals to an interneuron within the spinal cord that causes inhibition of the efferent alpha motor neuron of the corresponding muscle.

D. Inhibition of the alpha motor neuron results in muscular relaxation.

IV. Muscle Fibers

A. There are two major types of muscle fibers throughout the body.

1. Slow twitch (type I) muscle fibers contain high levels of mitochondria and myoglobin which facilitate long lasting sustained force.
2. Fast twitch (type II) muscle fibers contain lower levels of mitochondria and myoglobin, but can rapidly metabolize ATP via anaerobic glycogenolysis. These muscle fibers are primarily involved in short forceful movements.

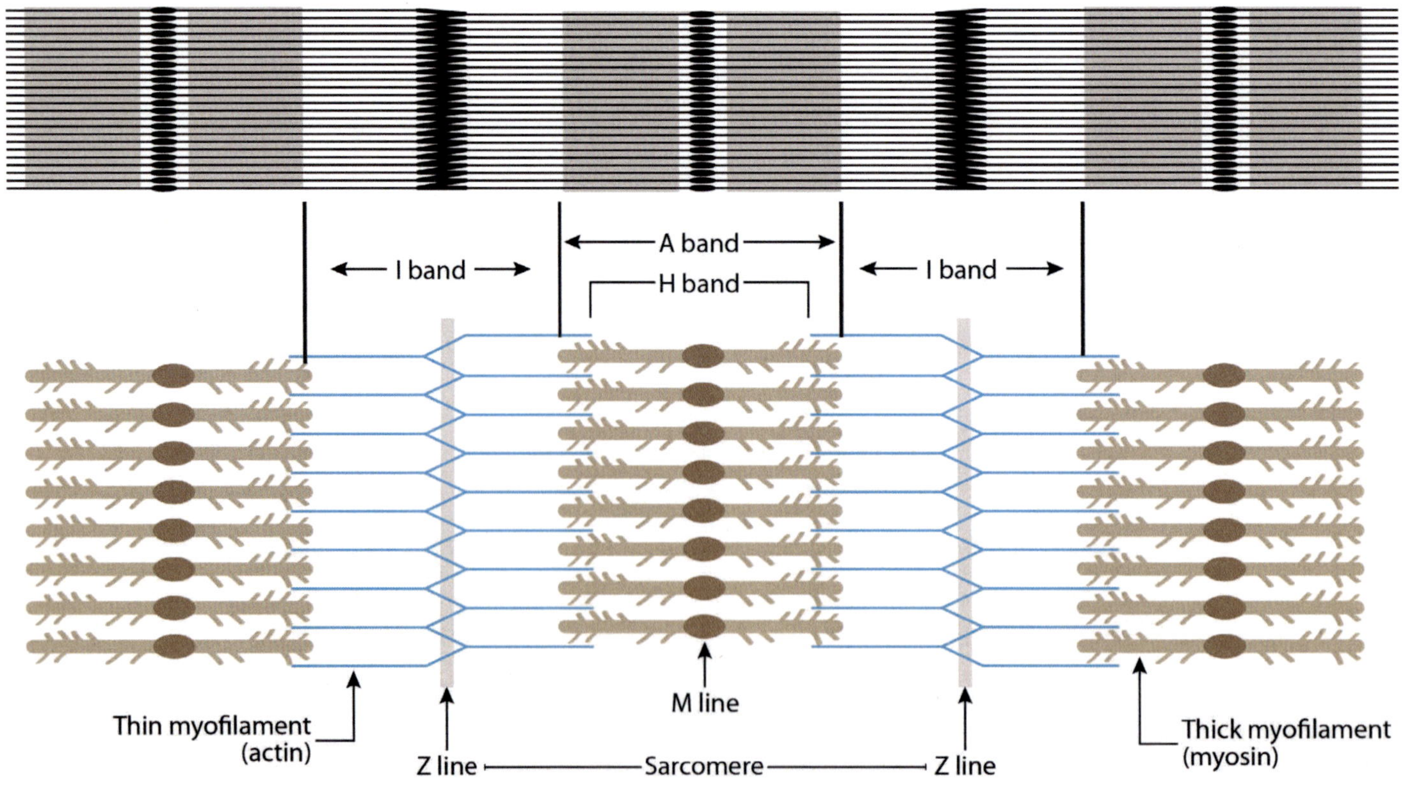

Figure 9.3 - Sarcomere

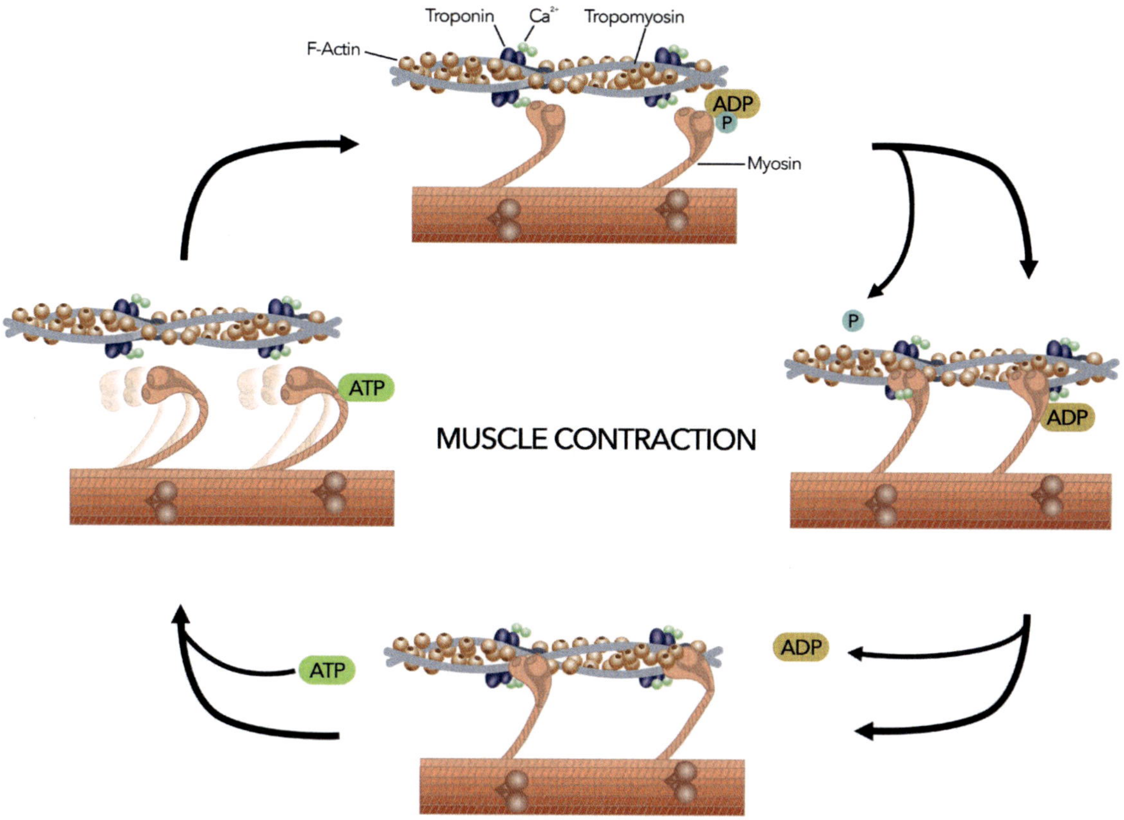

Figure 9.4 - Myosin and actin

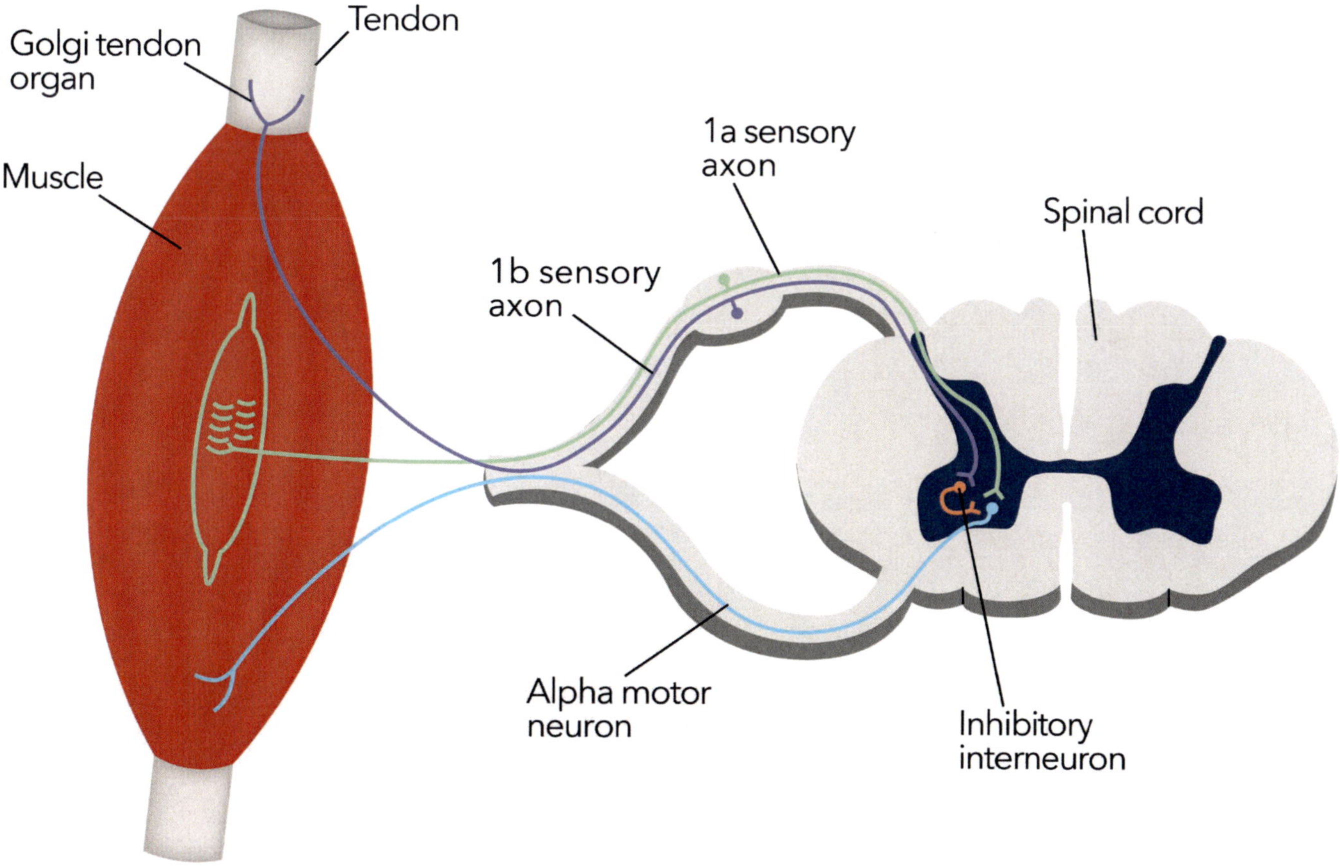

Figure 9.5 - Golgi tendon organs

V. Wave Summation (Figure 9.6)

A. Wave summation - when a muscle fiber is stimulated more frequently the force of contraction increases.

1. When a muscle fiber is stimulated with a single action potential the muscle fiber twitches.
2. When a muscle fiber is stimulated with several action potentials in succession it's referred to as summation of twitches.
3. When a muscle fiber is stimulated by many action potentials for a sustained period of time the muscle fiber produces maximum force, a condition called tetanus.

B. Heavy lifting is made possible through the activation of additional motor units and increased frequency of contraction of muscle fibers.

1. A motor unit is an alpha motor neuron and the muscle fibers it innervates.

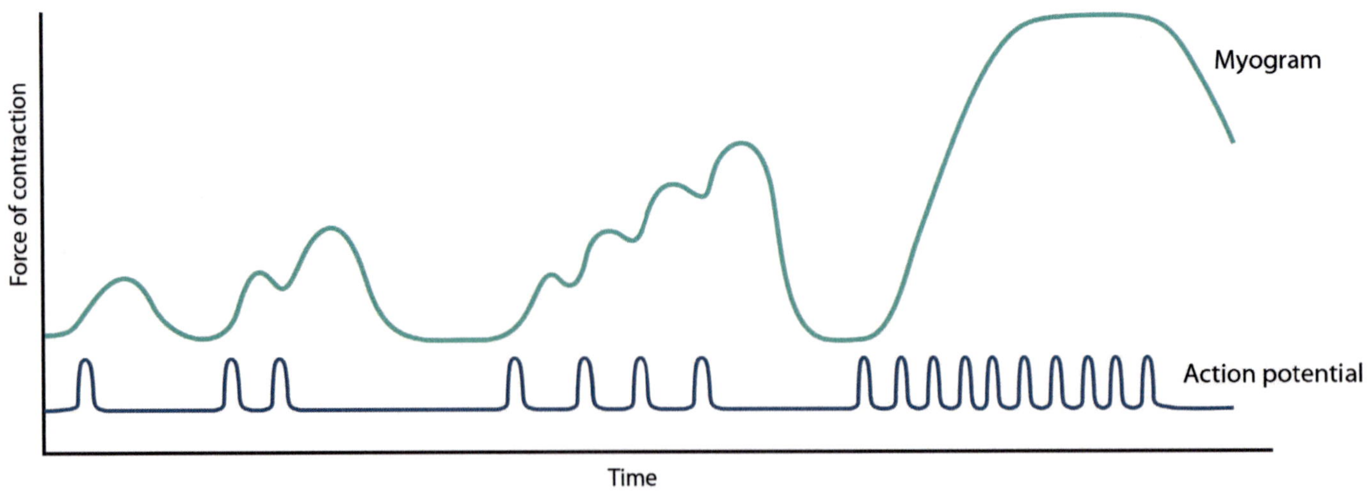

Figure 9.6 - Wave summation

REVIEW QUESTIONS

1. How would the H band and I band change during muscle contraction?

- **I band → shortens**
- **H band → shortens**

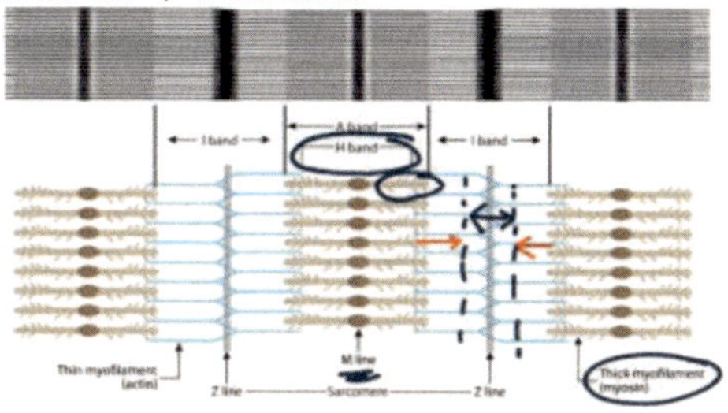

2. What region of the sarcomere only contains thin filaments?

- **The I band**

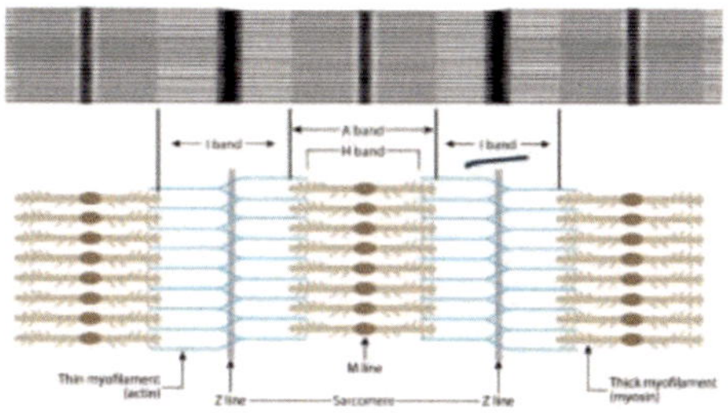

3. What underlying molecular abnormality is responsible for the stiffening of the muscles seen in rigor mortis?

- **A lack of ATP**
- **The binding of ATP to myosin normally allows the myosin heads to be released from actin**
- **A lack of ATP prevents the myosin heads from detaching from actin → sustained muscle contraction**

Figure 9.4 - Myosin and actin

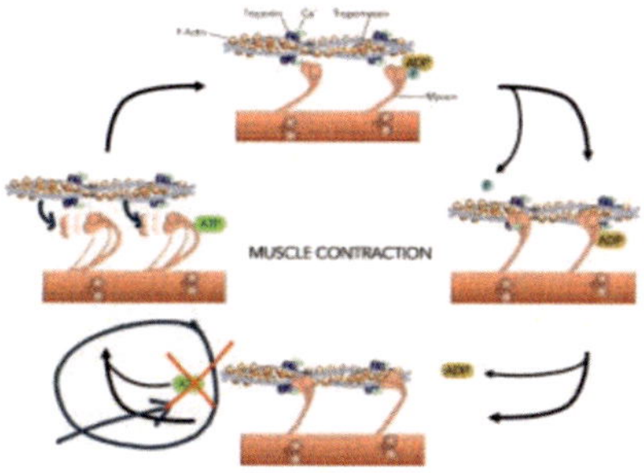

4. A man is involved in an extremely intense arm wrestle when his arm suddenly involves relaxes. Explain the physiologic pathway that caused his arm to suddenly relax.

- **Muscle contraction → activation of the golgi tendon organ → 1b sensory axons stimulate the inhibitory interneuron → inhibition of muscle contraction**

Figure 9.5 - Golgi tendon organs

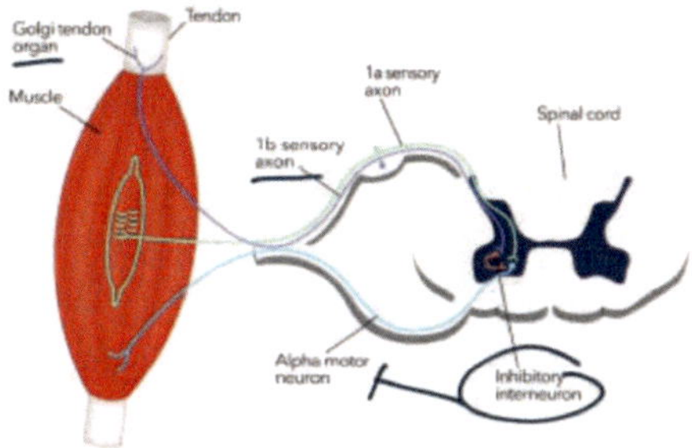

5. Two experimental mice are conditioned on two separate treadmills over a several month period. Mouse A runs at a speed of 2 ft/s for 5 minutes several times throughout the day. Mouse B runs at a speed of 0.5 ft/s for long durations once a day. How will a biopsy of the muscle fibers of mouse A likely compare to that of mouse B?

- **Mouse A: abundance of fast twitch muscle fibers (these are responsible for short forceful movements)**
- **Mouse B: abundance of slow twitch muscle fibers (these are responsible for long sustained movements)**

REVIEW QUESTIONS

6. What two compensatory mechanisms allow the biceps muscle to increase the force of contraction during heavy exercise?

   - **Stimulation of the alpha motor neurons would occur with increased frequency**
   - **Increased recruitment of the motor units**

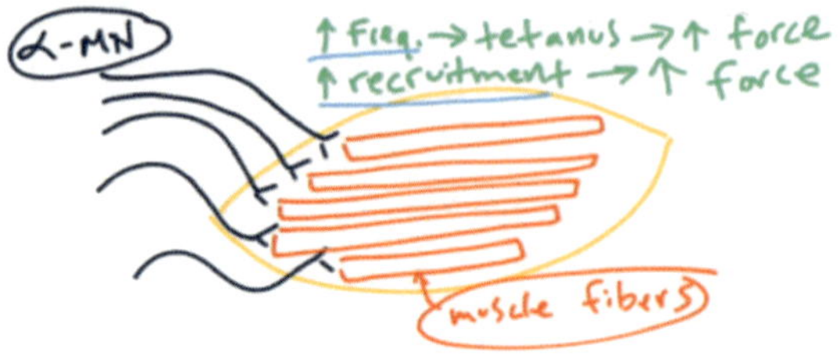

7. How does exercise promote angiogenesis?

   - **During exercise cells are highly active → ↓ oxygen → ↑ release of vascular endothelial growth factor (VEGF) → ↑ angiogenesis.**

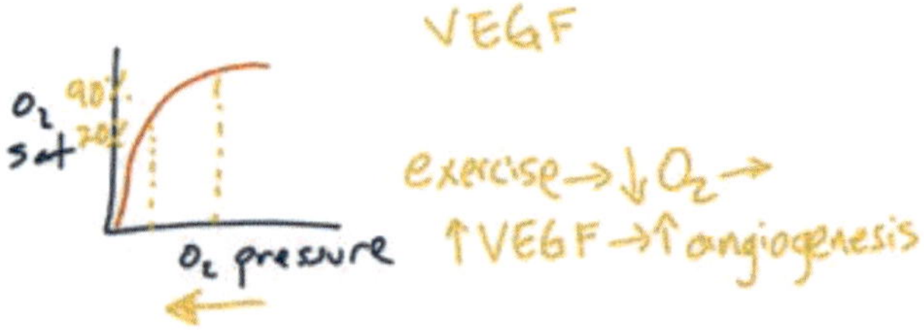

Section III - Osteoblasts and Osteoclasts

I. Osteoblasts

A. Come from mesenchymal stem cells in periosteum (not marrow)

B. Lay down new bone composed of:

1. Hydroxyapatite (calcium and phosphate) → provides hardness
2. Type I collagen → provides flexibility (defect → osteogenesis imperfecta)

C. Express bone-specific alkaline phosphatase (BAP)

1. Functions best in an alkaline environment
2. Can be detected in the serum

D. Upregulated by mechanical stress (weight-bearing exercise)

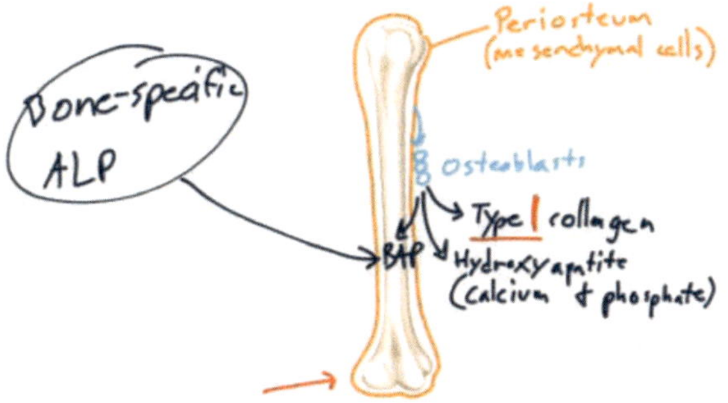

II. Osteoclasts (Figure 9.7)

A. Derived from macrophages/monocyte precursors in bone marrow

B. Resorb bone

C. Stimulated by:

1. M-CSF, RANKL, IL-1, and PTH

D. Inhibited by:

1. OPG and estrogen

E. OPG:RANKL ratio determines activity

III. Factors Contributing to Bone Density

A. Density determined by osteoclast:osteoblast activity

1. Age (bone loss ↑ with age)
2. Gender (woman more prone to bone loss)
3. Ethnicity (African Americans tend to have ↑ bone density)
4. Genetics

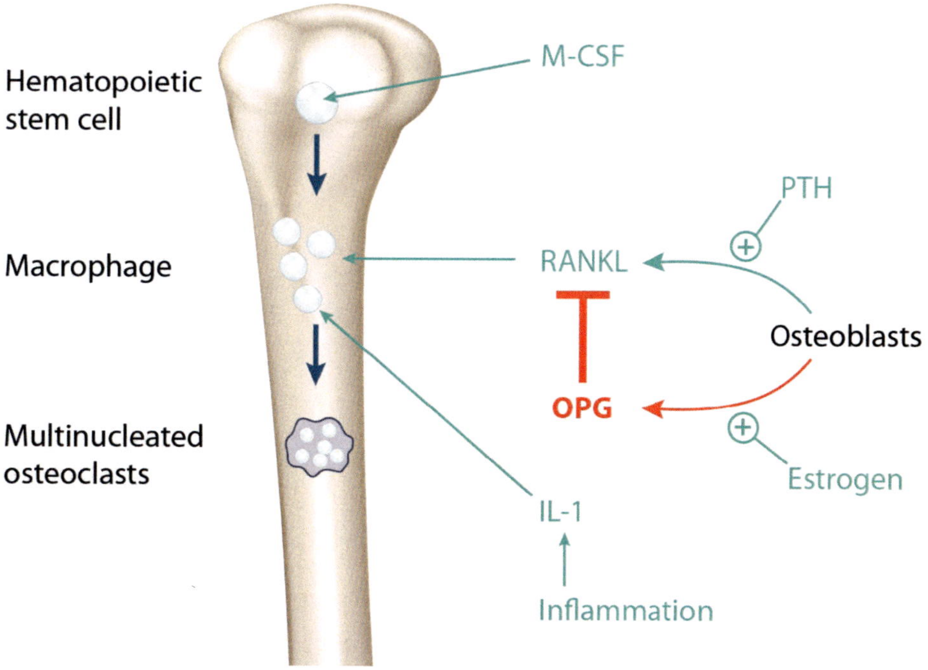

Figure 9.7 - Osteoclast and Osteoblast Physiology

REVIEW QUESTIONS

1. Osteoblasts in an 8-year-old male secrete type I collagen and hydroxyapatite as normal. However, the collagen is defective. What may occur in the bones as a result of the defective type I?

   - **Bones would be hard but brittle**

   Normal mineralization (hydroxyapatite) → Hard bones

   Defective Type I collagen → brittle bones (OI)

2. A patient is unable to produce adequate levels of OPG. What will happen to the bones as a result?

   - **Low OPG leads to higher RANKL and higher osteoclast activity (osteoporosis)**
   - **Note: This occurs in Paget's disease, where osteoblasts will also become overactive and create misshapen bones**

   ↑RANKL → ↑osteoclasts → Osteoporosis (Paget's disease)

   ↓OPG ⊣ RANKL

   ↑osteoblasts → disorganized bone growth → deformed bones

3. A 55-year-old female patient has not had a menstrual period in five years. Her clinician informs her that she has an increased risk for osteoporosis. Why?

   - **Low estrogen results in decreased osteoblast and OPG activity, leading to increased osteoclast activity (osteoporosis)**

   Menopause → ↓ estrogen

   ↓Estrogen → ↓osteoblasts → ↓OPG → ↑osteoclasts → Osteoporosis

4. With decreased OPG levels, what would happen to the level of free RANKL?

   - **Osteoblasts secrete RANKL and OPG.**
   - **OPG normally inhibits RANKL (less OPG means increased RANKL activity)**

   Osteoblasts → ↑RANKL

   Osteoblasts → ↓OPG

Section IV - Endochondral and Intramembranous Ossification

I. Two types of ossification (bone development)

A. Hyaline cartilage → endochondral ossification

1. Long bones (tibia, femur, etc)

B. Fibrous membrane → intramembranous ossification

1. Flat bones (skull, mandible, pelvis, etc)

II. Endochondral Ossification

A. Occurs in long bones (e.g. ribs, tibia, fibula, femur, radius)

B. Begins with hyaline cartilage model surrounded by perichondrium

C. Mesenchymal cells within perichondrium differentiate into osteoblasts → forms bony collar (periosteum) → nutrition to chondrocytes, via diffusion, is blocked → chondrocytes within model release calcium and die → porous holes formed

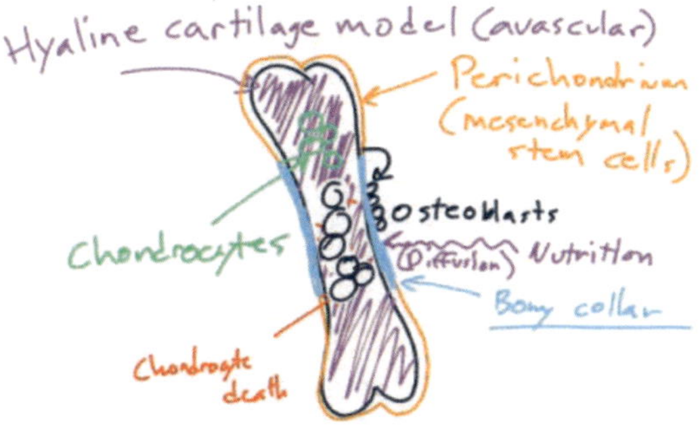

D. Periosteal bud penetrates bone collar providing blood supply to inner portion of cartilage model → osteoblasts travel from periosteum to cartilage model → spongy bone replaces cartilage in diaphysis (primary ossification center)

E. Osteoclasts remove central portion of spongy bone along diaphysis → medullary cavity formed

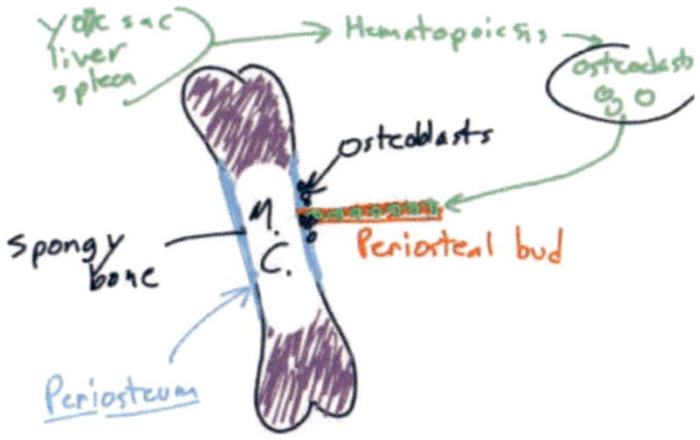

F. Osteoblasts in periosteum continue to lay down bone → compact bone beneath periosteum

G. Secondary ossification centers form after birth at epiphyses → formation of spongy bone filled with hematopoietic stem cells → continued release of osteoclasts, erythrocytes and leukocytes

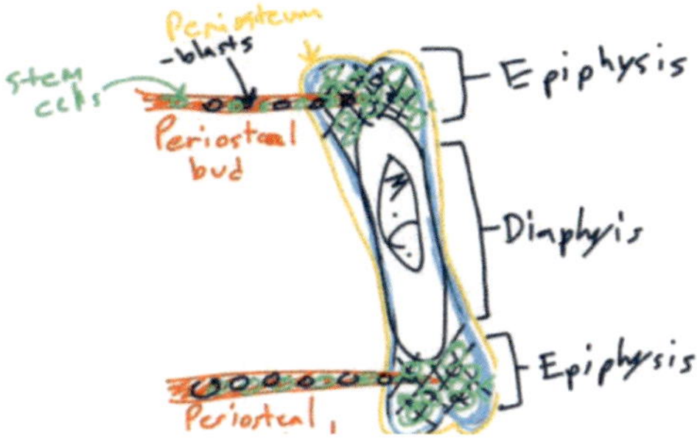

III. Metaphysis

A. Metaphysis = epiphyseal plate

B. Located between epiphysis and diaphysis

C. Hyaline cartilage remains in metaphysis and is the source of new bone growth.

1. Chondrocytes make new cartilage

2. Osteoblasts in diaphysis ossify old cartilage → bone elongation

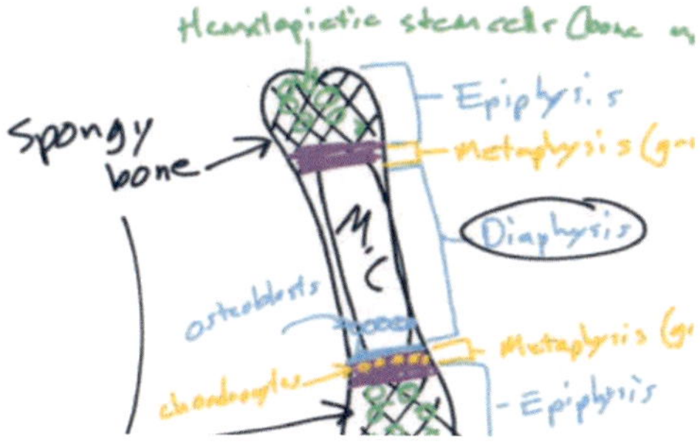

D. Inhibited by FGFR3

1. FGFR3 is hyperactive in achondroplasia → growth plate fails to produce new cartilage

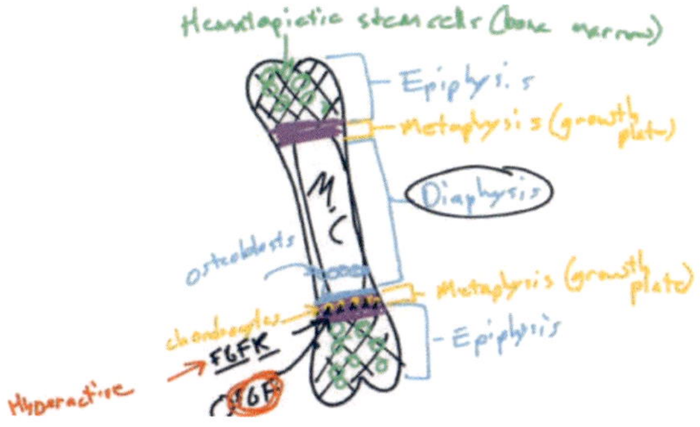

IV. Intramembranous Ossification

A. Occurs in flat bones (e.g. skull and pelvic bones)

B. Dense irregular connective tissue with mesenchymal cells

C. Mesenchymal cells differentiate into osteoblasts which create spongy bone in the center and compact bone on the outside

D. Periosteum surrounds compact bone

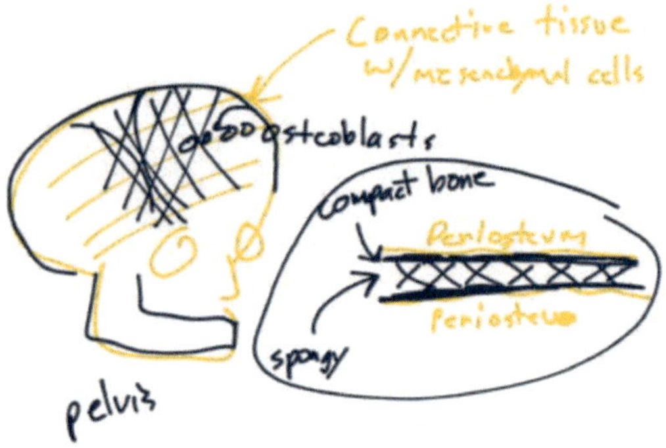

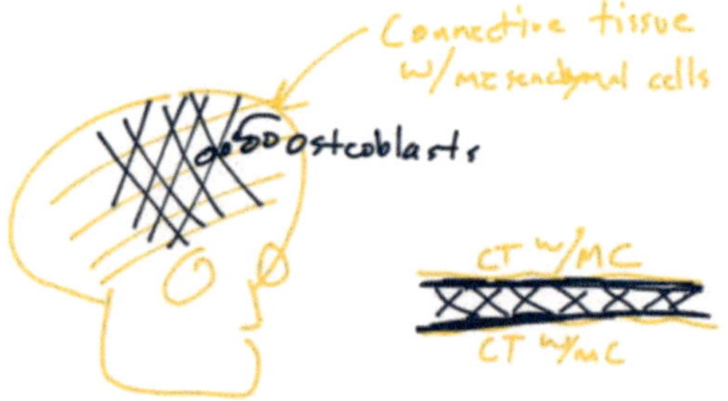

REVIEW QUESTIONS

1. A 10-year-old male patient is hit in the upper left arm with a baseball bat. Radiograph shows a fracture at the metaphysis. If the damage to the metaphysis was irreversible, what would be a long-term consequence of this fracture?

   - **Metaphysis is the growth plate (hyaline cartilage)**
   - **Irreversible damage here would cause decreased bone growth**

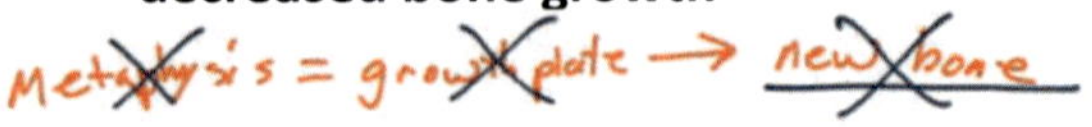

2. Why would an activating mutation in the FGFR3 gene cause short bones?

   - **FGFR3 inhibits chondrocytes, resulting in decreased formation of new hyaline cartilage (short bones)**

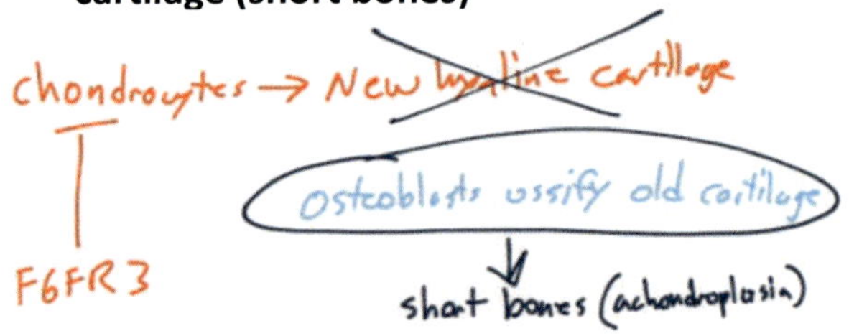

3. Intramembranous ossification is disrupted in a two-year-old boy. Would this disturb normal growth of the phalanges of the fifth digit?

   - **Long bones are formed via endochondral ossification and would not be impacted by disruption to intramembranous ossification**

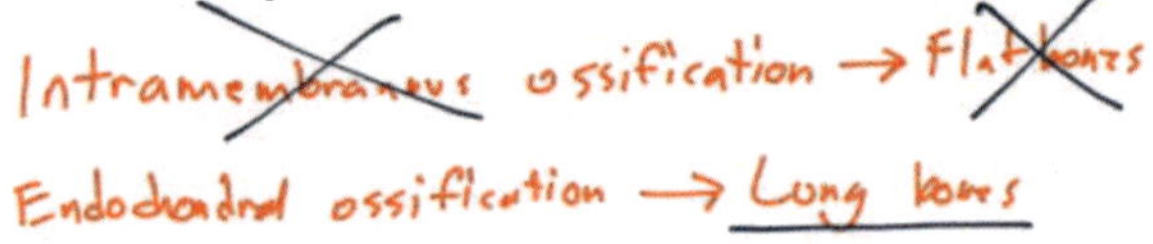

Section V - Skin

I. Skin Layers (Figure 9.8)

A. Epidermis

B. Dermis (fibroblasts)

1. Collagen types I and III
2. Vitamin A upregulates collagen synthesis

C. Hypodermis (adipocytes)

II. Epidermis (Figure 9.8)

A. The epidermis consists of five layers (superficial to deep):

1. Stratum corneum (dead keratinocytes that slough off)
2. Stratum lucidum (dead keratinocytes)
3. Stratum granulosum (keratinocytes)
4. Stratum spinosum (keratinocytes and desmosomes)
5. Stratum basale (melanocytes, stem cells, hemidesmosomes)

III. Melanocytes produce melanin

A. High melanin → darker skin

B. Low melanin → lighter skin

C. Absent melanin → albinism

D. Melanocyte death → vitiligo

IV. Desmosomes (Figure 9.9)

A. Connects adjacent epithelial cells together

B. Connects cells in Stratum Spinosum together and to adjacent layers

C. Contains desmoglein → attacked by IgG → Pemphigus vulgaris

V. Hemidesmosomes (Figure 9.9)

A. Connects basal cell layer of epithelium to basement membrane

B. Connects Stratum Basale (epidermis) to basement membrane (Dermis)

C. Attacked by IgG → Bullous pemphigoid

REVIEW QUESTIONS ?

1. A patient has dysfunctional hemidesmosomes. What will be a visible manifestation of this problem?

- **Hemidesmosomes connect epidermis to dermis**
- **Lack of functional desmosomes results in bullous pemphigoid**

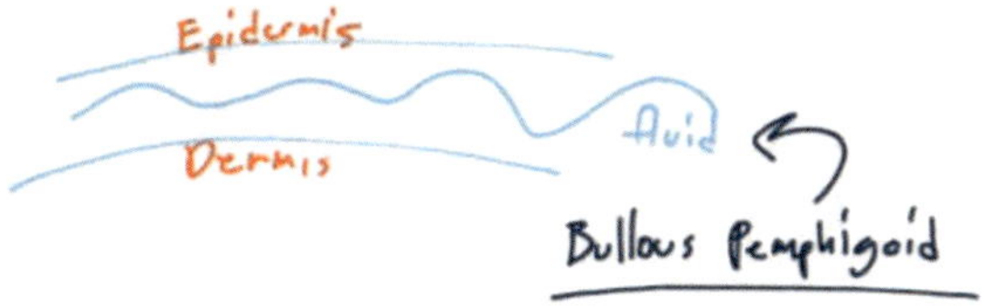

2. The melanocytes in a patient are completely destroyed in portions of her skin. What specific layer within the epidermis is affected?

- **Melanocytes are located in the stratum basale**

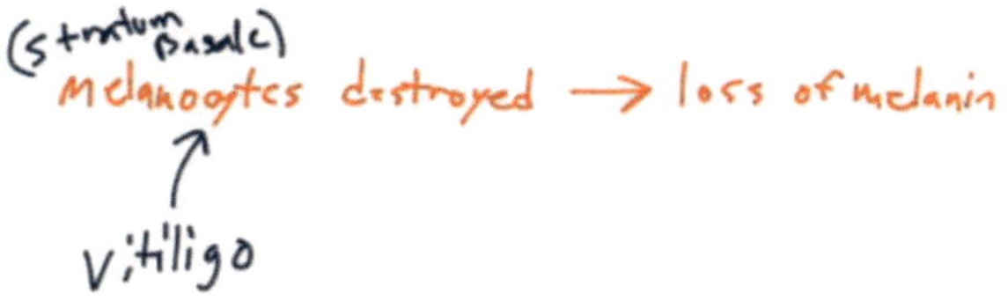

3. A patient is found to have an autoimmune condition in which IgG attacks desmoglein. Would this separate the epidermis from the dermis?

- **IgG against desmoglein indicates pemphigus vulgaris (not bullous pemphigoid), so the dermal-epidermal junction would not be impacted**

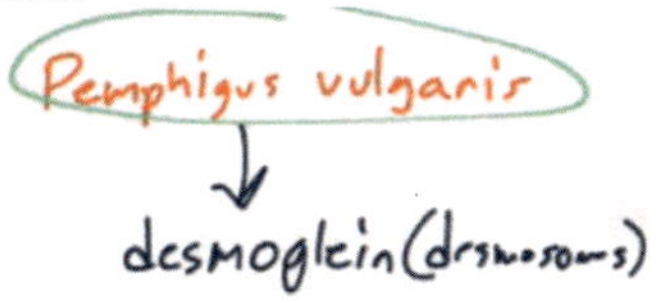

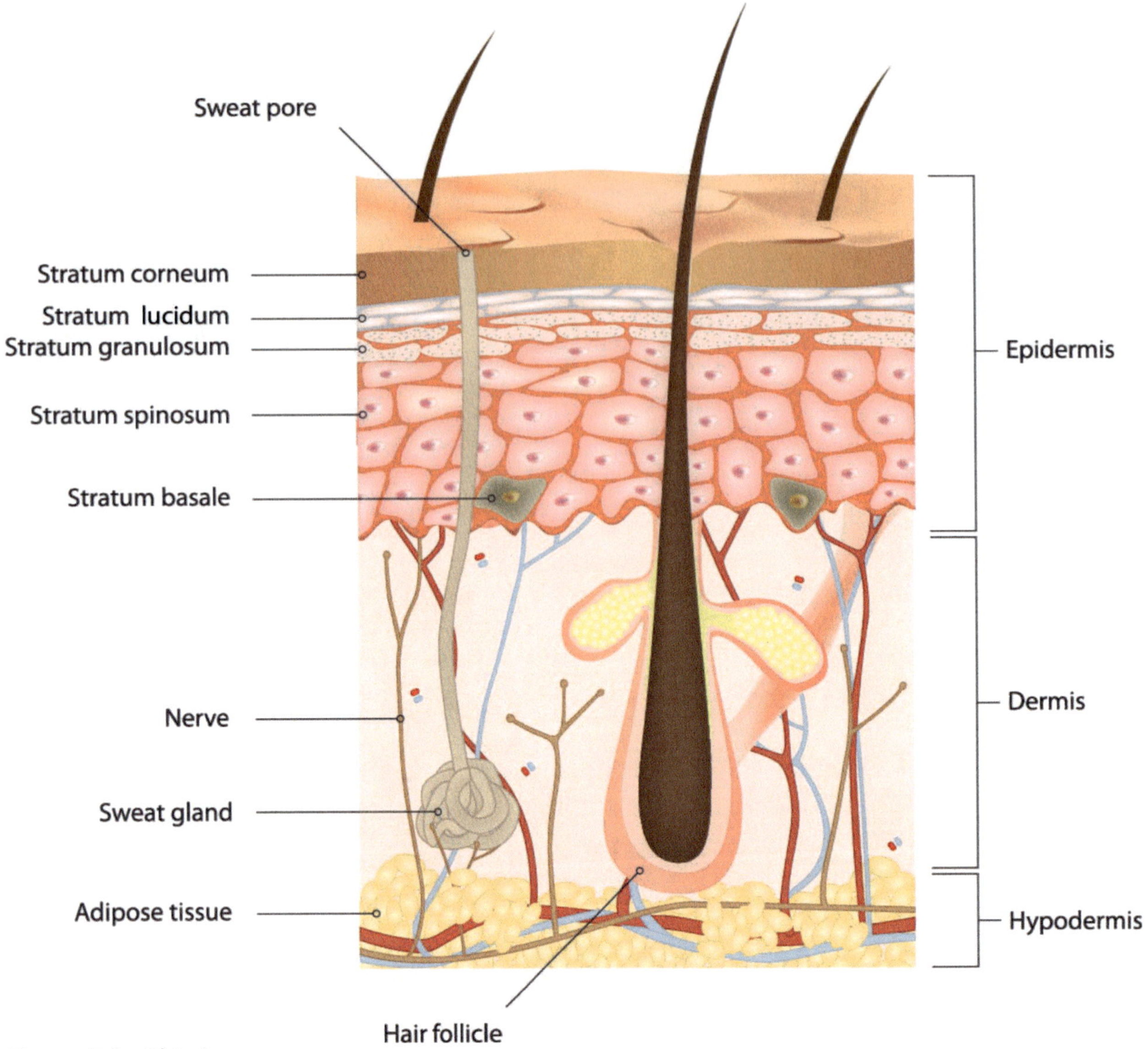

Figure 9.8 - Skin Layers

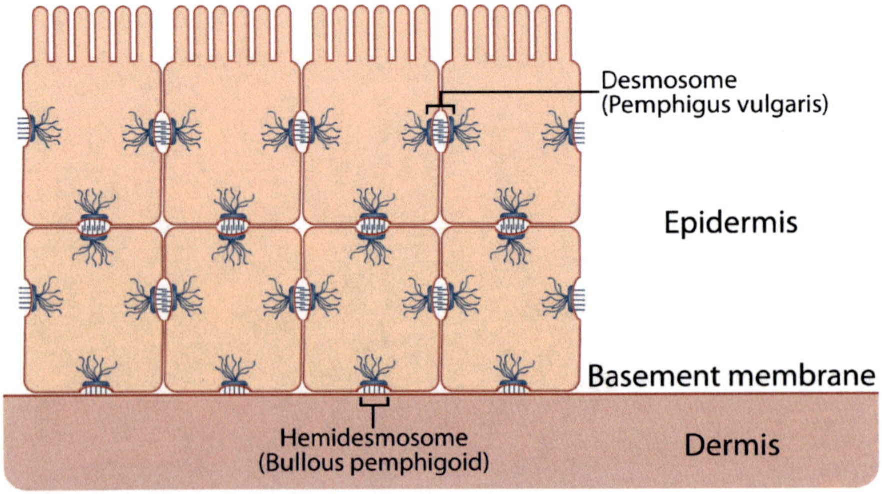

Figure 9.9 - Desmosomes and Hemidesmosomes

TABLES & FIGURES

INDEX

A

B

C

F

G

H

I

O

P

R

Made in United States
Orlando, FL
04 November 2026

90201143R00159